TOUCHING THE RELATIONAL EDGE

TOUCHING THE RELATIONAL EDGE

Body Psychotherapy

Asaf Rolef Ben-Shahar

Routledge
Taylor & Francis Group
LONDON AND NEW YORK

An earlier version of this book was published in Hebrew in 2013 by Pardes, under the name "A Therapeutic Anatomy—Body Psychotherapy" (אנטומיה של טיפול).

First published 2014 by
Karnac Books Ltd.

Published 2019 by Routledge
2 Park Square, Milton Park, Abingdon, Oxon OX14 4RN
52 Vanderbilt Avenue, New York, NY 10017

Routledge is an imprint of the Taylor & Francis Group, an informa business

British Library Cataloguing in Publication Data

A C.I.P. for this book is available from the British Library

ISBN-13: 978-1-78220-094-9 (pbk)

Typeset by V Publishing Solutions Pvt Ltd., Chennai, India

To Cäsar and Theresia, with my love

Telepathy

It gives me a start
whenever you call me
so softly broken the voice
succeeding to install thee
beyond a chance a choice
taking it as a token
beware of the opening line
avoid the sound too consonant
a poem neither yours nor mine
claims to be learned by heart

distance drives us to grow
reaching far and further out
timeless quick spaceful slow
premonitions oh so trying
make us double
second sighted
visions born in love
borne in dying
in the breeding souls
when I trust my part

make my life
off course—of course
ever so lighted

—*Theresia Mestmäcker*

CONTENTS

ACKNOWLEDGEMENTS

I wish to thank Steven Knoblauch for his willingness to engage with the material and write a preface for this book. It is my hope that this book will be accessible for psychotherapists and psychoanalysts from different modalities and deeply value Steve's openness and curiosity. Thank you to Jacqueline Carleton for her support, encouragement, and for writing her preface. To Silke Ziehl, my dear teacher and inspiration—thank you for your ongoing love to me as a person and as a therapist, and for your preface.

Thank you to David Boadella and Stanley Keleman; both of you were professional inspirations—thank you for your recommendations. Thank you to Sharon Ziv-Beiman for her open and generous recommendations. Thanks to Stephen Gilligan for inspiration and generative horizons.

Thank you to Shoshi Asheri for your kind and loving reading of my book and for your support, and to Nick Totton for your inspiration and willingness to enter into dialogue (and for a recommendation which made me blush). Thank you Theresia for your encouragement!

Thank you to Ruth Ben-Asher and Liora Bar-Natan for their contribution to Chapter Eight. Thank you to Ronen Levy and Guy Timor for personal and professional friendship, for critical and supportive reading, the feedback and the comments, and for accompanying me throughout the process of writing and beyond it. Thank you for contributing to Chapter Eight.

To Elad Hadad and Shai Epstein, my dear friends, colleagues, and partners in the *Relational Body Psychotherapy* programme at the Israeli Centre for Body–Mind Medicine; thank you for your friendship, your criticism, your personal and professional brotherhood, and for writing the vignettes for Chapter Eight.

To Carmella Keet, thank you for your support and for the image in Chapter Seven. Thank you to Lika Filtser for your beautiful cover image: you have depicted a precious, sacred moment.

Special thanks to Efrat Even-Tzur who edited the Hebrew version of this book, for her meticulous work and for her friendship. Special thanks to dance and movement therapist Sharon Zack for your dialogue and reading of the English version, for helping me look at my prejudiced assumptions and make this extended version more gender-minded; I really enjoyed our connection.

Thank you to Oliver Rathbone, Constance Govindin, Kate Pearce, and Rod Tweedy at Karnac for taking the risk and supporting the publication of this book. Thank you to James Darley for his keen eye and careful editing of the book.

To my wife Tom, my first reader, thank you my love for your support, for giving me time and space to write, for encouraging me and putting your faith in me, for your friendship, your love, and the home you give me. To Zohar and Shuy Grace, my beautiful daughters, thank you for the wider mind and the internal hope.

Last, a very special thanks to clients who allowed me to use material from our work together, thus giving this book depth and colour. To my teaching assistants, students, supervisees, and clients: thank you for teaching me how to love and be afraid, how to want and need, how to dare to relate. This book was written thanks to you, and it is yours.

ABOUT THE AUTHOR

Dr Asaf Rolef Ben-Shahar is an Israeli-born psychotherapist living in the UK. Asaf is one of the leading clinicians and writers in the field of relational body psychotherapy. He is the training director of the Relational Body Psychotherapy Programme at the Israeli Centre for Body–Mind Medicine, and runs a parallel programme in London called Touching the Relational Edge with the Entelia Institute. Additionally, Asaf teaches and lectures in clinical and academic settings in Israel and Europe. Asaf's doctoral dissertation, *Surrender to Flow*, examined the juxtapositions of relational psychoanalysis, body psychotherapy, and hypnotherapy.

Asaf has published numerous papers in professional journals and a number of book chapters; he is on the international editorial board of Body Psychotherapy Publications, and a member of the *International Body Psychotherapy Journal* editorial team. He is an associate editor for *Body, Movement and Dance in Psychotherapy* and *Self & Society*. This is his first book in English, an extended version of *An Anatomy of Therapy*, which was published in Hebrew in 2013.

Asaf is married to Tom and is a father to two daughters—Zohar and Shuy Grace. He is vegan, loves animals and birds, music, and dancing, and is obsessed with getting new tattoos.

PREFACE

I offer these brief reflections as a psychoanalytically trained practitioner having gained a window into the worlds, past and present, of body psychotherapy through this informative text—and having enjoyed this book immensely. First, what is most significant here, is the historical and contemporaneous tracking of an ongoing relationship, sometimes distant, sometimes almost *touching*, between the development and practice of body psychotherapies and the development and practice of psychoanalytic psychotherapies. From Freud to Ferenczi and especially in the seminal contributions of Reich, we are introduced to the continuous, and seemingly obvious, impact of the body as catalytic to subjective experience and thus to the disorders with which both fields of therapy are concerned. Asaf Rolef Ben-Shahar traces the developing diaspora of therapeutic approaches that subsequently have emerged from these seminal psychoanalytic thinkers, particularly Reich. It is fascinating to see the range of theory and method developed over the last century in North America and Europe that has expanded the initial contributions of Reich concerning the value of attention to the body in therapeutic treatment.

But, what is most significant and unique to this text for me is Rolef Ben-Shahar's focus on contemporary developments emerging from the influence of post-Freudian-Ferenczian-Reichian work, particularly the contributions of seminal thinkers from the relational perspective emerging in North America and now spreading across all schools and regions where psychoanalysis is practised. As a participant in and contributor to this development, I find *Touching The Relational Edge* capturing a critical area of attention expanding both body psychotherapies and relational psychoanalyses, and that area concerns the body of the practitioner and the emergent embodied experiences intersubjectively produced in any therapeutic interaction. I and several others including Orbach in the UK, the Nebbiosis in Italy, Sletvold in Norway, Anderson, Aron, Dimen, Harris, LaBarre, Petrucelli, Sonntag, Wrye, and Katie Gentile among others in the United States, have been offering theoretical visions and clinical narratives harvesting the therapeutic impact of attention to the analyst's as well as the patient's body and their rhythms of interaction in psychoanalytic treatment. Now with so many illustrative clinical narratives and exercises as central to this text, the importance of embodied registrations interactively generated on intersubjective dimensions of the clinical exchange is given the critical importance it deserves in body psychotherapy. This contribution makes clear that future developing expansions and refinements of treatments for emotional dys-regulation in patients will necessarily include this widened focus. Such a development is particularly significant as we grapple with the emerging emotional impact of electronically produced disembodied dimensions of interactive experience on persons and their relationships. Here, we have an invaluable contribution towards this growing field of awareness for practice, first, for body therapists, but ultimately, for all practitioners.

Steven H. Knoblauch, Ph.D.
New York, USA

PREFACE

The trajectory along which psyche and soma have travelled over the past century has not been without its perils. Over the almost half century during which I have been professionally involved with it, body psychotherapy has evolved from a little known and/or much denigrated form of psychotherapy to an object of acute interest to mainstream psychotherapeutic circles as well as the lay public (see Greene & Goodrich-Dunn, 2013; Heller, 2012; Young, 2011a, 2011b).

The Cartesian dualism that dominated much of Western thought over the last couple of centuries formed the backdrop against which psychotherapy, beginning with Freud himself, had to labour. Fearing for the future of the new paradigm he was proposing, Freud in his later years neglected and/or rejected ideas which he had formed earlier on, but which he judged dangerously radical. Among those formulations were the ideas of the importance of the body and sexuality in both the cause and cure of what were then termed "neuroses".

His brilliant pupil, Wilhelm Reich, refused to abandon those concepts and was thus himself ejected from psychoanalytic circles, first in Vienna, then in other parts of Europe, until he landed upon the ultimately no less inhospitable American shores. And, twenty years after Reich's death, in the process of dissertation research in the US, I found that many of his followers were still afraid to acknowledge their prior connections with him or admit that they even still owned journals and books published while he was alive. In celebrating this introduction to body psychotherapy originally written in Hebrew and first published in Israel, I cannot help but note that at least one if not more of Reich's followers fled to Israel after his unfortunate incarceration and death in the US in 1957.

Although the relationship between psyche and soma had been frequently explored previously, most notably by Pierre Janet, Reich is generally considered the progenitor of body psychotherapy today. That does not mean that most or even many of the modalities of body psychotherapy, to which you will be introduced in this volume, followed or incorporated his ideas. You will meet many which developed independently of or in reaction to Reich's ideas.

Especially since the explosion of neuroscientific research in the 1990s, psychoanalysis and body psychotherapy have begun to approach each other, even if still somewhat warily. Psychoanalysts reading interpersonal neurobiology began to realise that the body held information inaccessible by words alone. In the meantime, body psychotherapists, tired of their own small world, had begun to explore and incorporate ideas and techniques from psychoanalysis, especially and most fruitfully, relational psychoanalysis. Particularly in institutes such as the Chiron Centre in London, this marriage was being fruitfully consummated.

Somehow, over the course of his training, private practice, and considerable teaching experience, Dr Rolef Ben-Shahar has managed to incorporate many of the most cogent and profound concepts and methods from these two worlds and many more. Readers can look forward to encountering his thoughtful distillation of these worlds, but in an unusually evocative, relational, and embodied form. Clinical vignettes and exercises are included in each chapter, thus drawing us into the embodied relational world its author is conveying. As he suggests, "Somatic processes become a focal point for the clinician's curiosity [until] … the body ceases being seen as an object and becomes a pulsating dialogue between bodies-in-relation, revealing themselves to one another." A one-person psychology has evolved into a dialogical process. "At best, body psychotherapy is not a set of therapeutic tools but instead a living, pulsating dance of presence and shared becoming—materialising the intersubjective field and embodying it together."

This book will introduce body psychotherapy to psychologists, psychotherapists, and interested others through an attachment based, object relations, and primarily psychoanalytic and relational framework. The material is approached in three Parts through historical, theoretical and clinical perspectives. In this textbook conceived in the spirit of relational writing, questions are posed and dialogues encouraged. Biological and neuroscientific concepts are offered as metaphors, allowing us to think more deeply about the bodymind, allowing different angles of understanding, none of which is Truth. It is hoped that this will be one of many bridges between psychodynamic thinking and body psychotherapy.

Jacqueline A. Carleton, Ph.D.
New York City

FOREWORD

For those who want to know more about body psychotherapy, this book is a rich gift. For Asaf Rolef Ben-Shahar manages to bring the *whole* body back into body psychotherapy, and to talk lucidly, with passion and commitment, about the dynamic, complex, and ever-changing reality of the body that is the primary basis from which our sense of self develops, and the ground and matrix and outcome of our being in relationship.

This is innovative territory—to give the somatic, the nonverbal as well as the verbal, the unconscious as well as the conscious full honour of place and to treat the body as part of the most deeply meaningful and influential aspects of being human and of being and becoming in relationships.

For in the context of a culture which deeply holds a perspective that divides the body from the mind, from the soul, and from the matrix of relationships, a culture which loves the word and the mind and abhors bodily processes and bodily fluids, it is easy to get hooked into such a worldview.

Most writing which focuses on how the body influences the mind, or the mind influences the body, is stuck in that cultural perspective. So is writing which looks at techniques for "contacting" the mind, or changing the mind or the body, through working with the body—for it somehow misses the wonderful complex reality that exists beyond those concepts. Our language itself makes it difficult to switch out of that old perspective—for the way in which our language carves up reality goes with that implicit worldview.

Asaf Rolef Ben-Shahar in this book on body psychotherapy suggests that we need to make an end to some very old divisions that are still very powerful:

- the division between psychoanalysis and body psychotherapy
- the division between conscious and unconscious processes
- the division between the individual and the other

... so that we can "make a beginning".

The beginning which this book proposes and explores is to bring the whirling world of continuous becoming, of intersubjective processes, of resonance and shared realities and communications, of shared responsibility, into mainstream body psychotherapeutic enquiry. That is an exciting enterprise!

There are practitioners who work at this developing paradigm. There are writers who offer holistic and integrated theoretical thinking. There are few who do both with such enthusiasm, commitment, clarity, and creativity as Asaf Rolef Ben-Shahar does.

This book presents a body psychotherapy which is rooted in a much richer and more complex understanding of what it means to be a "body" than the Cartesian worldview so prevalent in Western thought has made us believe—a worldview where the body is seen as quite separate from the mind, and from the soul.

The body as it is portrayed in the pages of this book is a very different kind of body. This body is not only physical and biological, it is also a body with feelings, with a mind (a "bodymind"), with intentions, with spirit. Moreover, this body is always a body in relationship, arising out of relationship, formed by relationships, and forming relationships. No body lives and exists alone. This body is multi-faceted, multi-layered, meaningful and feelingful and soulful.

This is a body which talks (to itself and to other bodies) with words, with gestures and movements, with waves of energy, with changes in temperature, in colour, in smell, in heartbeat, in breathing, in the willingness or unwillingness to open, with thoughts and intentions and feelings. All these often nonverbal and often unconscious processes go on continuously in the body, and between bodies in relationship.

For example, thinking something makes energetic waves and changes reality, not only inside the person's bodymind, but inside the body of the other person in the relationship. By changing one's thinking, without noticeably changing one's doing, one changes irrevocably what the other can or cannot perceive, and even what the other can or cannot do.

Here the concept of body reaches from the most visibly physical aspect to the most "invisible" but clearly perceived and shared, interconnected, and intersubjective space. Its domain reaches, for example, from the physical sensation of a hand on the hip to the very real yet immaterial—though jointly acknowledged and jointly created—transformation of the therapeutic endeavour.

This is the art and science of a body psychotherapy which proposes that the body is as much involved in transference and countertransference as the mind is—or rather, that *bodymind* is the proper level at which to explore these phenomena, as there is no such thing as a mind without body, nor a body without mind. There is only bodymind. Or bodymindsoul—for, as William Blake said, *"Man has no Body distinct from his Soul; for that called Body is a portion of Soul discerned by the five Senses."*

This book poignantly highlights how deeply we miss the real encounter with another when we work with that person's body as if that body were nothing but a physical object. For in working *on* a body, we make the other into a "thing", an object—and we simultaneously invite the other to treat themselves, and others, as an object too. When we do that, something vital leaves the scene. It becomes like a wood without the song of life, without the birds and insects and the wind rustling in the leaves, all singing the song of life. When this quality of aliveness, of life, is not there, we miss it. When it is there, it is like rain on a parched earth, deeply satisfying.

When we are willing to engage fully, as one human being with another, in the context of the therapeutic relationship, when we dare to open ourselves to this encounter and the other dares too, both to the best of our abilities and as deeply and fully as is possible and desirable for both at that moment—then magic can happen, and healing. Then too, both will be moved, and be changed.

This book, therefore, describes a body psychotherapy which is a joint enterprise for therapist and client, an enterprise that neither can enter without risking change. To be challenged by the encounter to redefine oneself, to re-envision oneself, to be willing to get to know oneself anew, again and again, that is the invitation to both client and therapist. Only if I enter with this willingness to engage can I truly meet the other, can I be part of the "I–thou" relationship that Martin Buber defines as the only truly human relationship.

Asaf Rolef Ben-Shahar makes a powerful argument for this vision and brings together an extensive oeuvre of academic writing to support this vision of the body, of bodies in relationship, and of body psychotherapy.

He also brings clinical vignettes to clarify and to ground his theoretical writings. These vignettes show his willingness to fully engage in the encounter with another, to trust himself and the other in the joint exploration, to let go of old certainties and an old role, to "glide on the strings that connect": such a willingness to go to the edge is what makes his work so very alive, so very exciting, and also so very scary at times. It is "riding by the seat of one's pants", trusting that we will be able to do something useful together, even as we may not yet know where we are going and what is at stake. But that joint space will open up possibilities of choice again and again, and to trust our ability to choose wisely, and to deal with any situation that arises.

This book offers a path to a deeper way of connecting with your clients, a more challenging and more transparent way to relate. This book, if you will let it, will change the way you think about and practise body psychotherapy, and it will inspire you to bring more of yourself into your work and into your relationships!

Silke Ziehl, London

INTRODUCTION

Without anatomy, emotions do not exist. Feelings have somatic architecture.

—*Stanley Keleman* (1985, p. xii)

A churned up stomach

Peter is sitting with me in the clinic. His shoulders are inwardly collapsed; his breathing—short and quick. He shares with me a happy moment with his wife and son; a picnic in the park. James, his son, is lying between him and his wife and they are tickling one another. Upon hearing Peter, I find myself contracted and uneasy. My stomach is churning and my neck hurts really badly. I am busy with self-deprecating internal dialogues ("What kind of therapist am I? Where is my empathy?"). My experienced incoherence is amplified as we speak; my body is inexplicably shaken by Peter's story. "You seem to be suffering," Peter tells me. Embarrassed, I confess: "My stomach churns up as I am listening to you, Peter, I am sorry." Peter smiles, "Mine too. There was such an intolerable gap between what was happening and the way I responded to it. James was tickling me and I noticed that every time he touched me I contracted—as if I was preparing to be hit. I was lying down there, with Dianne and James; it was the most secure and loved place I could have in this entire world, yet I kept feeling as if someone is going to hit me." I can breathe more comfortably now, my stomach relaxes. Peter is smiling too. Our anatomies can finally loosen and we resume our attempt to at reclaiming inner security.[1]

This short vignette from my clinical work with Peter demonstrates working with resonance, or somatic countertransference. Resonance occurs in many affect-laden relationships and is not limited to psychotherapy, as it is a manifestation of our bodily responses to the environment and the relationships therein. At the same time, it is also a skill that can be honed and practised, and is one of the central skills used in body psychotherapy in general, and particularly in relational body psychotherapy. It expands the psychoanalytic concept of transference (the way in which the therapeutic relationship acquires characteristics of the client's previous relationships) into somatic spheres. Resonance is a complex therapeutic skill requiring understanding and exploration of therapist-client psychodynamics, and is presented here from my own therapeutic orientation—of relational body psychotherapy. According to relational body psychotherapy, in encountering another person (or anything around us with which we have an affective connection) we affect one another mentally, emotionally, cognitively, and bodily. The other moves through us, and we move through the other. Therefore, my churned up stomach becomes a relevant and important object of discussion in our therapeutic dialogue.

Therapeutic encounters are naturally saturated with both dread and potential. On one level, the therapeutic relationship can be deep and intimate, revealing and loving. On another level, the rigid therapeutic boundaries create a distance—safeguarding (at times) the therapeutic dyad, thus allowing a limited yet liberated exploration. Therapy takes place on these two levels and in the tension therewith.

And what happens when a churned up stomach enters therapy? What happens when the intensity of our somatic sensations, our bodily needs and bodily expressions receive focused attention in psychotherapy? The immediate and unmediated nature of body-to-body meeting could be very powerful, and for those who encounter relational body psychotherapy here for the first time, it might at times feel overwhelming or confusing.

I wrote this book in order to provide historical, theoretical, and clinical background to the work of the relational body psychotherapist. The book is divided into three Parts, each presenting a different angle of exploration; each providing the reader with opportunities to dive in and engage both professionally, personally, and bodily with the material. In choosing this structure I was inspired by Nick Totton's excellent *Body Psychotherapy: An Introduction* (2003).

Part I—*Historical*—begins by examining the relationship between psychoanalysis and body psychotherapy. This historical Part explores the juxtaposition between psychoanalytic perspectives and trancework, and hints towards some of the ways in which body psychotherapy can utilise altered states of consciousness. Next, the roots of body psychotherapy are presented. Part I tracks the early history of body psychotherapy primarily through the work of Sándor Ferenczi and Wilhelm Reich. Concluding Part I, the third chapter presents a roadmap for the main types of body psychotherapy practised today.

Part II—*Theoretical*—outlines some of the main concepts in body psychotherapy. First, I present my theory of bodymind (psychosomatic) organisation, describing three levels of organisation: somatic, cognitive, and relational. The mutual relationship between these elements is explored too, laying the foundation for the body psychotherapeutic theory of mind. The theory of mind is illustrated through the transition of *mind* to *bodymind* (or psychosoma). Bodymind is explained and developed using both monistic philosophies (wherein body and mind are one inseparable whole) and dualistic philosophies (viewing the body and mind as two separate identities), as well as via the phenomena of embodiment, intersubjectivity, and emergence. Chapter Six briefly reviews the bodymind character-structure organisation in body psychotherapy. The last chapter of this Part reviews some of the basic concepts and principles in the body psychotherapeutic terminology and practice. This entire theoretical Part is dedicated to cultivating a dialogue between body psychotherapy and contemporary psychoanalysis.

Part III—*Clinical*—allows the reader a window to the clinical setting through case vignettes and their analysis. Part III aims at allowing the reader to deepen the integration between context, theory, and clinical practice, all the while paying particular attention to the complexities that accompany working with the body and the ways body psychotherapy confronts such complexities. Further in this Part, body psychotherapeutic skills are exemplified and demonstrated. Attention is given to ethical and practical questions that may arise in psychotherapists from other modalities, for whom the breathwork, movement, and touch might feel foreign, as well as in body psychotherapists. Part III is sealed with two chapters expanding on two therapeutic skills that are particularly close to my heart: touch and resonance. These chapters also illuminate the conflicts and challenges that psychotherapists face when working with the body in the clinical setting.

The primary body of knowledge

Both my daughters were born in water, nearly four years apart. They both grew and developed in internal water, protected and shielded from the full impact of gravity, allowing them both to explore movement, connection, and growth in an environment which was relatively gentle—with few stimulations and friction. During their respective births, Zohar (in the UK) and Shuy Grace (in Israel) both transitioned into the bathwater a moment before their lungs were asked to take a first breath, marking the beginning of life outside the womb: a life where separation and connection were continuous movements and pulsation.

When the umbilical cord is not immediately severed, the newborn baby can take its time to breathe through the lungs: for a few precious moments, while the placenta still pulsates blood and oxygen, the newborn baby can choose to embody its breath at its own pace. Zohar emerged into the world full of wonder; her big eyes were wide open with curiosity. Shuy Grace, too, was born without crying; softly clinging to her mother's skin, as both mother and daughter breathed together. In this transitional stage of neither inside nor outside, the breath was not in Zohar's body or in Shuy's body; instead, the body that breathed was this intersubjective body, of mother–daughter: the placenta which was still alive and connecting the oneness who will soon become two. The journey from inner world to outer world was gradual, and the respective breaths of both Zohar and Shuy Grace were chosen rather than forced: they chose to live—and to separate.

My daughters were both born in water and those two labours were connecting and moving spaces for me—opportunities to relate to my wife, Tom, as well as to foster the connection with my daughters. I was not merely a spectator during these births, but a partner—and this partnership was as bodily as it was emotional. We emerge into the world and our being is primarily bodily and sensory. Within moments, both respiratory and digestive systems kick in autonomously; within moments we activate our surroundings (our parents …) which usually hasten to provide us with an environment that is as close as possible to the womb we have just left: warm, enveloping, nourishing, protecting, and loving. Intrauterine development could be and often is, of course, complex and includes unpleasant and disturbing experiences. The good enough womb experience depends on many factors, including the mother, her relationships, and the environment, and is—like life—never perfect, and frequently traumatic to an extent. All our human experiences, beginning with the first breath we inhale and concluding with our last breath, contain bodily, real, and concrete dimensions which often allow us to connect to places inside us that words alone cannot reach.

The term body psychotherapy covers a spectrum of psychological modalities in which the body and bodily processes are a central axis for the curiosity of therapist and client alike. The field includes varied theoretical and clinical methodologies, as well as different styles of therapeutic interventions and toolkits, ranging from body language analysis and breathing techniques, to accompanying somatic processes, and a variety of touch techniques. As a distinctive therapeutic field, body psychotherapy endeavours to present a systematic approach to connecting narrative content, therapeutic relationship, and anatomy and movement, and includes a model of mind (or, to be precise, of bodymind), developmental theory, specific perspectives on psychopathology, and varied skills for therapeutic intervention. The two main global organisations of body psychotherapy, the European Association of Body Psychotherapy (EABP) and the United States Association for Body Psychotherapy (USABP) both use the same formal definition to present the field (C. Young, 2011b):

> Body Psychotherapy is a distinct branch of psychotherapy, well within the main body of psychotherapy, which has a long history and a large body of literature and knowledge based upon a sound theoretical position. It is an ethical and scientific method of professional practice for relieving emotional and mental distress and for human growth.
>
> It involves a different and explicit theory of mind-body functioning, which takes into account the complexity of the intersections and interactions between the body and the mind. The common underlying assumption is that the body is the whole person and there is a functional unity between mind and body. The body does not merely mean the "soma" and that this is separate from the mind, the "psyche". Many other approaches in Psychotherapy touch on this area. Body Psychotherapy considers this fundamental. Body Psychotherapy recognises the continuity and the deep connections in which all psycho-corporal processes contribute, in equal fashion, to the organisation of the person. There is not a hierarchical relationship between mind and body, between psyche and soma. They are both functioning and interactive aspects of the whole human being.
>
> Body Psychotherapy involves a developmental model, a theory of personality, hypotheses as to the origins of disturbances and alterations, as well as a rich variety of diagnostic and therapeutic techniques used within the framework of the therapeutic relationship. There are many different and sometimes quite separate approaches within Body Psychotherapy, as indeed there are in the other branches of Psychotherapy.
>
> It is also a science, having developed over the last seventy years from the results of research in biology, anthropology, proxemics, ethology, neurophysiology, neuro-psychology, developmental psychology, neonathology, perinatal studies, and many more disciplines.
>
> Body Psychotherapy exists as a specific therapeutic approach with a rich scientific basis on an explicit theory. There are also a wide variety of techniques used within Body Psychotherapy and some of these are techniques used on the body involving touch, movement and

> breathing. There is therefore a link with some body therapies, somatic techniques, and some complementary medical disciplines, but whilst these may also involve touch and movement, they are very distinct from Body Psychotherapy.
>
> Body Psychotherapy, as a mainstream branch of psychotherapy, has been "scientifically validated" by the European Association for Psychotherapy (EAP) and several modalities within Body Psychotherapy have also been scientifically validated by the EAP. (Young, 2011b, pp. 25–26)

Body psychotherapists use somatic-attunement skills to deepen their awareness of themselves and their clients as bodies. A basic presumption in body psychotherapy is that in the very act of attending to ourselves as bodies we create a connecting movement: between body and mind, between feelings, sensations, and thoughts, and in the interface between us and the world. Developing a felt-sense allows us to experience ourselves as bodyminds, and the more we are able to embody our experience in our somatic reality, the greater the chance we stand to liberate ourselves from both somatic and psychological rigidities, since we acquire more than one language with which to encourage change and movement (the somatic alongside the cognitive-affective language). Thus, the main skill in body psychotherapy is not about a specific therapeutic technique of one kind or another, but instead it is a therapeutic position, characterised by alive and active curiosity towards somatic processes, which take place in the client, the therapist, and the dyadic space that opens within and between the two.

Psychoanalyst Donald Winnicott (1949) believed, not unlike Freud, that the body was the home of our psyche. He perceived the body–mind relationship as a matrix of psychosomatic influences. Winnicott claimed that mind was not a separate entity but instead: "Mind is then no more than a special case of the functioning of the psyche-soma … One can look at the developing body or at the developing psyche. I suppose the word psyche here means the imaginative elaboration of somatic parts, feelings, and functions, that is, of physical aliveness" (p. 244).

However, despite the fact that the somatic aspects of our psyche have been thoroughly discussed in psychoanalytic literature since the days of Freud, and even though body psychotherapy has presented a distinct field of practice since the first decades of the twentieth century, psychoanalysis adopted the hierarchy of the thinking self over the sensing self, as Chapter One will demonstrate. Bodily expressions in therapy are still frequently interpreted by psychoanalysts in psychological terminology alone, thus—as identified by psychoanalyst Susie Orbach (2004c)—important aspects of the client's experience may be neglected. Furthermore, seminal psychoanalytic writers who did choose to directly relate to the body—and meticulously so—such as Didier Anzieu (1989), Joyce McDougall (1989), and Wilma Bucci (1994), have done so while giving minimal acknowledgement to or, more often than not, completely ignoring the significant body of work and research accumulated in body psychotherapy.

Many types of bodywork and somatic therapies maintain a holistic approach, aiming at integrating body–mind processes with their clients. However, as argued by the EABP and USABP definition, there is a principle that is different between those methods and body psychotherapy: the techniques used may differ too, but more—so, the therapeutic positioning and the understanding of the therapeutic relationship differentiate the two ways of working with people. Many types of bodywork, like massage, physiotherapy, and others, aim at improving the client's bodily state. While the psychological benefits of these methods cannot be denied, they are neither necessarily a central axis of the work, nor are they part of the contracted relationship, as they are in the clinical practice of the body psychotherapist. Other somatic therapies invite the client to attain higher somatic awareness, yet body psychotherapy differs from these too, as it holds a double focus: the body psychotherapist relates to the client's subjective experience as it manifests in various dimensions (body, feelings, thoughts)—yet this reality is examined and understood in view of the therapeutic relationship. Hence, the body psychotherapist is not an expert of her client's body (or mind), and the therapeutic interventions are not done *to the client* or *on the client*; instead, the body psychotherapeutic interventions form part of a complex matrix of subject-to-subject relationship, of two people who are willing to allow for a shared exploration (asymmetrical, but still shared) and transformation. Therefore, unlike bodywork methods, the understanding of transference and countertransference, the intricate complexity accompanying the therapeutic relationship and the use of interventions, is central to the clinical work of the body psychotherapist.

During the last two decades, theoreticians and clinicians began to directly relate to body psychotherapy as a distinct field of psychotherapy and a respectable body of knowledge. In her characteristically bold (and sometimes blunt) style, Susie Orbach (2004a) mused: "Sometimes psychoanalysis comes to the ordinary sense embarrassingly late. To tell someone not in the field that touch is crucial to human psychological and physical development and you'll get a contemptuous 'daa' and yet we within the non-body, and particularly within the psychoanalytic wing, get singularly jittery and uneasy when touch comes to therapy" (p. 37).

Who is this book for?

This book was written with psychotherapists in mind, out of my desire to offer a textbook that could connect two fields I love and appreciate—relational psychoanalysis and body psychotherapy. I wanted to explore relational body psychotherapy in its wider developmental, historical, theoretical, and clinical context. Therefore, although the book covers many modalities of body psychotherapy, it is not a neutral text, nor is the work representative of other modalities of body psychotherapy. Different body psychotherapeutic modalities, theoretical concepts and their clinical applications are all delivered through my own subjective orientation of relational body psychotherapy. In writing this book, I had four types of readers in mind:

First, body psychotherapy students, experienced body psychotherapists, or those who are interested in acquiring such training. I hope that you will enjoy a theoretical and conceptual framework that will help organise the knowledge you have gathered or will have gathered by the end of your training. Additionally, it is my hope that this book will form a bridge between body-psychotherapeutic language and the psychodynamic one, easing the dialogue between the two fields. Very little has been written about relational body psychotherapy and in writing this book I wish to contribute to the literature in this field.

Second, psychotherapists from other modalities, psychologists, and psychoanalysts. I hope that you can deepen your understanding of body psychotherapy and integrate the historical, theoretical, and clinical knowledge, hopefully getting a taste from the clinical experience of relational body psychotherapy. The book was written with a deep appreciation of and respect for psychoanalytic and psychodynamic thinking and with my desire to engage in dialogue with these perspectives. I attempted to write about body psychotherapy in a manner accessible to dynamic and relational professionals, hopefully igniting in you curiosity and interest in the potential that lies within relational body psychotherapy.

Third, for bodyworkers and those who work with the body from a non-psychotherapeutic perspective. It is my hope that this book will support the richness, integrity, and understanding of your work and invite you to notice the shared fields of interest and work between your work and body psychotherapy. Many bodyworkers discover the depth of psychological complexity soon after they begin their practice, and perhaps this book can organise some thoughts and answer some questions regarding these issues.

Fourth and last, this book was also written for the curious non-professionals. Among these are probably clients of body psychotherapy, who are interested in psychology and psychotherapy. I hope that you will find the field of body psychotherapy promising and inviting, and that by the end of the book you will have more questions than answers, wanting to find out more. Therapy is such a deeply moving experience, and understanding the guiding principles behind it and the rationale behind the application of interventions may deepen the therapeutic experience, organise it and sometimes soothe some fears or balance therapeutic expectations.

Internalising a body of knowledge is not unlike digestion. Here, please take a bite of this apple. Once you allow the apple inside, you already begin to process it and digest it: enzymes are secreted in your saliva, for the coarse disintegrating of food as you chew the apple. Swallowing sends the apple to your stomach where it is further disintegrated and dissected, a process which continues throughout the gastrointestinal tract. You may adopt some chosen parts of the apple; you dismantle the apple until it loses its original form and becomes a part of you. No longer is it an apple, instead it is a part of you—or of me. Other parts of what used to be an apple find their way out. In experiential learning, something of the "appleness" of the apple stays inside me: I not only transformed the apple, I was changed by the apple too.

To assist in the digestive process, at the end of each chapter I added a bodily exercise, which offers an experiential way of connecting with the theoretical and clinical content of that chapter, bringing some movement and sensation to the words of this book. You can practise some of these exercises on your own, and most of them could be used in training or therapy. I thank you for choosing this apple and invite you to take a bite, allowing the apple to nourish you while throwing away the parts you do not wish to make yours. Bon appétit!

Note

1. All the vignettes in this book are taken from my own clinical work. Names and identifying details have been changed. Permission to use material has been given. In other cases, vignettes are amalgamations of case material which was composed for the sake of exemplifying theoretical and clinical material.

PART I

HISTORICAL

You said: One day follows another; each night followed by night.
The days are upon us, you spoke in your heart.
And you shall see eves and morns attending your sight
And declare: there is no news under the sun.

Here you are, having aged, a grey elderly man
And your days are but few, and their number is dear,
You shall now know that each day is the very last
You shall now know that each day is new under the sun.

—Poems at the End of the Road, *Lea Goldberg* (1973, p. 152).*

---

* All translations from Hebrew are the author's.

CHAPTER ONE

Blanche Wittman's breasts[†]: tracking the historical split between body psychotherapy and psychoanalysis

> The traditions of all the dead generations weigh like a nightmare on the brain of the living.
>
> —*Karl Marx* (1852, p. 15)

> Nine souls
> I am all but shadow
> In your shadow I can rest
> I am all death
> In your death I might live
>
> Eternally tied amongst your shadows, between my deaths
> Stopping for a brief moment at your feet
> Then I shall know comfort, in your need for me to relieve your loneliness
> With your blessing
>
> —Asaf Rolef Ben-Shahar

The birth of a split

We were not always as apprehensive of touch and body as we are today. While attention to the body and somatic processes and practices of breathwork and touch were immanent in many

[†]An earlier and amended version of this chapter was published in *Psychotherapy and Politics International* (Rolef Ben-Shahar, 2010a).

Eastern and non-dualistic religions and philosophies, serving as an integral part of personal growth and spiritual development, in orthodox Judaeo-Christian monotheistic traditions the body played a marginal, indirect, and almost insignificant role in personal and spiritual development (Mindell, 1982).

The seventeenth-century philosopher René Descartes, considered by many the father of modern philosophy, struggled to integrate our animalistic bodily-existence with our mental-spiritual aspects. The conclusion of his deductive philosophy, the famous *cogito ergo sum* (I think, therefore I am), identified the self with the cognitive, thinking self (Descartes, 1636). According to Descartes, the body was a corporeal machine and the appropriate platform to explore it was science, while the psyche belonged to the spiritual dimensions and was therefore the property of the church. While this dualistic perception created a split between body and mind, it had at the same time "liberated" the body from the trapping claws of the church in general, and the Inquisition in particular (Rolef Ben-Shahar, 2012b; Withers, 2008), allowing for real and unthreatened scientific enquiry. Additionally, the body–mind split has also gendered roots and origins, as women were considered "body", "nature", while men were "spiritual", "transcendent", superior by nature (a split that was justified by religious institutions defiling women as "body") (Balsam, 2012; Beauvoir & Parshley, 1949).

Following our adoption of Cartesian philosophy and Newtonian physics, it had taken us Westerners centuries to catch up with the non-dualistic notion of body–mind (and self-other) unity. Medical and paramedical treatments of the body have reached inspiring sophistication and technological brilliance and, at the same time, psychological sciences and spiritual philosophies have independently reached seminal contributions and understanding regarding our psyche and spirit. However, such explorations tended to be separated from our embodied organismic experience (Capra, 1975); we still kept the divide marked by Descartes, and therefore such contributions remained limited.

Indeed, some Western philosophers and clinicians have spoken about the human being as a bodymind organism, vouching for bodymind unity, but the clinical applications of these holistic perceptions was still greatly underdeveloped. Philosopher Ludwig Wittgenstein (1953), for example, suggested that language attained meaning only in the act of speaking ideas, thus arguing that the body (and relationship) was a necessary context for language. This was the grounds for his rejecting the Cartesian subjectivist picture, which isolated "thought from action, private thought from public speech, mind from body, one mind from other minds" (Cavell, 2006, p. 64). The phenomenologist Maurice Merleau-Ponty (1962), whose writing was central to the development of body psychotherapy, made an even more radical claim, arguing that the body was our medium for having a world—the means with which we experienced the world, therefore the means through which we had a world. Moreover, these philosophers primarily related to the male body–mind, bodies who were actively operating in the world; however, the female body–mind was still largely denied of its integration and remained objectified (Butler, 1988; Irigaray, 1993; I. Young, 2005).

Despite these refreshing voices, the understanding that bodymind was (also) a single unity frequently got lost in the clinical settings. In the traditional psychoanalytic and psychodynamic therapy, the bodies of both client and therapist tended to be absent. In this chapter I will suggest that the resistance to including the body in psychotherapeutic practice largely resulted from

Freud's (necessary) political and strategical choice to disavow the body en route to establishing psychoanalysis as a valid scientific field. Pre-psychoanalytic psychiatry was largely an attempt to alter the mind through physical interventions and laying on of hands (Kertay & Reviere, 1993). Yet it was Freud who legitimised the psychotherapeutic use of touch. His unequivocal capacity for cohesive and methodical theory, the breadth of his thinking, his clinical practice—and no less important, his charismatic personality—all these opened a door for embodied practices and touch within psychotherapy, as a methodical and organised science.

Sigmund Freud perceived himself first and foremost as a medical practitioner and a scientist. While medical practitioners could not ignore the body, as a serious scientist operating under the Cartesian–Newtonian paradigm, the knowledge that Freud acquired—and his relation to such information—was mechanistic and physiological. Accordingly, Freudian theory and practice were highly informed by bodily process. "The greatest thing that ever happened in psychiatry" wrote Wilhelm Reich (1967) about Freud, "was the discovery that the core of the neurosis was somatic" (p. 70). In *The Ego and the Id*, Freud (1923b) stated that the ego was "first and foremost body-ego" (p. 16). Freud further expanded on the matter: "The ego is ultimately derived from body sensations, chiefly from those springing from the surface of the body. It may thus be regarded as a mental projection of the surface of the body" (ibid.).

Many years earlier, in 1885, when he was but a young man of twenty-nine, Freud won a travelling scholarship to Paris where he studied the effects of hysteria under the supervision of the greatest neurological star of his time, Professor Jean-Martin Charcot at the Salpêtrière in Paris. Freud was in awe of the magic that was revealed to him during his research with Charcot. Freud's involvement with these maverick and innovative techniques marked the beginning of psychoanalysis and arguably the birth of Western psychotherapy.

The emergence of the forbidden body

The Parisian scene that Freud joined was full of vibrancy, charisma, and power trips. In many ways, Charcot's hypnosis resembled traditional shamanic work more than scientific medical procedures (yet it lacked the traditional belief system that supported shamanic rituals, and gave them meaning). Freud was exposed to highly dramatised, overly technical, and very simplistic form of hypnosis. Charcot, Hippolyte Bernheim, and Josef Breuer were practising hypnosis that involved methodical passing strokes and physical pressure points, and giving suggestions in an authoritarian style. These practices were direct derivatives of the work of Franz Anton Mesmer, the father of medical hypnosis. They also heavily relied on the therapist's charisma: the hypnotist's authority and control over his clients were considered preconditions for therapeutic success.

The rituals and practices which were used in the hypnotic treatment of the time (and the beautiful women who were the subjects of these experimental treatments) sparked the interest and curiosity of the global medical and scientific community, but also attracted artists and celebrities who swarmed to Salpêtrière from all over the world, to witness Professor Jean-Martin Charcot delivering his therapeutic hypnotic show. Among Charcot's students are found some of the most influential scientists and pioneers of the time, including Joseph Babinski, Pierre Janet (who was, for a while, Charcot's laboratory head), William James, Alfred Binet (who created the first widely used intelligence test), George Gilles la Tourette (Tourette syndrome is called after his name), Paul Broca, and, of course, Sigmund Freud.

These (chauvinistic and objectifying) demonstrations of hypnosis and touch, as portrayed in Brouillet's famous 1887 painting *A Clinical Lesson with Doctor Charcot at the Salpêtrière* (Figure 1) fell nothing short of a spectacular circus show. The painting, a lithograph of which was hung in Freud's consulting room, presented the part-woman part-guineapig Blanche Marie Wittman. The histrionic pressure points required (how curious) a certain intimate exposure, thus the white and beautiful body of Wittman was publicly exposed to the doctors: a beautiful and wild hysterical woman, hypnotically collapsing into the strong arms of the kind doctor's assistant. All the while the crowd, consisting of serious-looking male doctors, all in black, watched mesmerised. We may be left wondering whether these good doctors actually focused on the stage performance and the cutting-edge scientific discovery, or perhaps used the opportunity to stare at the wild woman's perfect breasts (Bonduelle & Gelfand, 1999; Pérez-Álvarez & García-Montes, 2007).

Brouillet's painting is a disturbing document reflecting the scientific, chauvinistic, and socio-political zeitgeist. It reveals the time's attitudes towards women and regarding the body as much as it tells us about hypnosis and Charcot. At a time when touch and sexuality were forbidden, doctors were given the liberty to hypnotise their patients, undress them and caress them (for medical purposes, of course). What an inflation of excitement and fear! How hard it was to sustain a grounded ethical standing (both internal and external) faced with such drives and forces!

As a side note, it is interesting to learn that patients at the Salpêtrière were known to occasionally disappear with a swelling belly and return to the hospital after an unspoken period (Bonduelle & Gelfand, 1999). This detail may shed some new light on the case of Anna O, whose

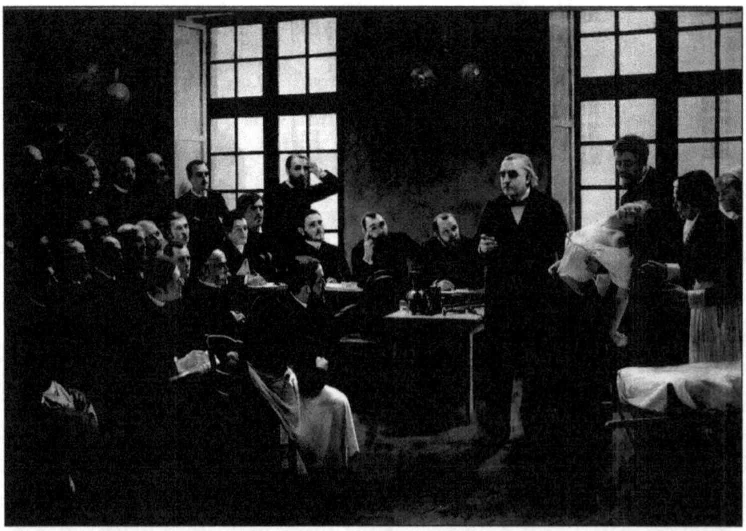

Figure 1. *A Clinical Lesson with Doctor Charcot at the Salpêtrière* (Brouillet, 1887).

treatment was described by Freud and Breuer in *Studies on Hysteria* (1895d). Her treatment was terminated when erotic feelings developed between Anna O and her doctor, Breuer, climaxing in her declaring that she was pregnant with Breuer's child. Could Breuer and Freud have become so terrified of the erotic transference also because of Salpêtrière's abominable history?

Examining his performance more than 120 years on, we can easily identify that the forces at play in Charcot's demonstrations at the Salpêtrière were far greater than hypnotic suggestions. Political and gender leverage, authoritative transference dynamics, peer pressure, narcissistic saving fantasies, and erotic transference were just as influential and meaningful in creating the impact of the work as the hypnotic suggestions administered so charismatically and assuredly by Charcot. I would dare suggest that his hypnotic suggestions were actually far less influential than the other factors mentioned here.

Charcot's hypnotic performances provided a rare legitimised peep-show, an official opportunity for voyeuristic drives and power trips, ethically approved by an authoritative figure, in a sexually oppressive and oppressed society. Imagine a room full of sexually excited men, hungry for action, in a Victorian setting. Doctors who were trained and forced to be "talking heads" alone were "forced" to witness this wild and liberated (and half-naked) woman who "willingly" submitted herself to the mercy of the powerful doctor. This painting depicted a drama that offered the spectators a particularly intimate show; in many aspects, as close as you could get to watching coitus. It is easy to see why both trance and touch were thereafter considered dangerous: the charge was too high to contain, the participants were playing with fire.

Influenced by Charcot, Freud's early clinical work involved extensive use of hypnosis as well as some therapeutic touch. In fact, his passing and stroking techniques incorporated both touch and trance (1890, 1891). These two techniques were old-fashioned hypnotic induction techniques, involving slow passing movements over the body of the subject in a downward direction while giving suggestions to sleep, or applying touch on hypnotic pressure points. The following is a fascinating description from a letter Freud had written to his friend, otolaryngologist Wilhelm Fliess (Masson, 1985): "Yesterday Mrs K again sent for me because of cramplike pains in her chest … In her case I have invented a strange therapy of my own: I search for sensitive areas, press on them, and thus provoke fits of shaking that free her" (p. 120).

But Freud felt ambivalent about hypnosis; he became increasingly uncomfortable with its suggestive nature and the impact-laden relationship that was created between hypnotist and subject, as well as the potentially manipulative nature of such a relationship. Watching a particularly authoritative demonstration by Hippolyte Bernheim, who yelled hypnotic suggestions at his patients, Freud (1921c) reported feeling astonishment and hostility: "I said to myself that this was an evident injustice and an act of violence" (p. 89). Freud's sensitivity to the person's autonomy and to the therapeutic relationship was already apparent then, and indeed these touch techniques (and hypnosis techniques) were inconsistent with the therapy Freud wished to establish. Furthermore, the type of hypnosis and touch he was exposed to was procedural and mechanistic. When human touch, so rich in potential for deepening human contact, is applied mechanistically and procedurally, it can easily seem a futile, dissociating, and possibly dangerous methodology, certainly irrelevant to the psychoanalytic process.

Our theoretical and clinical positions and decisions are saturated with our biographical strengths and challenges, and indeed it seems that Freud's primary reason for abandoning hypnosis and touch was more complex than the professional account presented above. In *An Autobiographical Study*, Freud (1925d) narrated the following incident:

> And one day I had an experience which showed me in the crudest light what I had long suspected. It related to one of my most acquiescent patients, with whom hypnotism had enabled me to bring about the most marvellous results, and whom I was engaged in relieving of her suffering by tracing back her attacks of pain to their origin. As she woke up on one occasion, she threw her arms round my neck. The unexpected entrance of a servant *relieved us from painful discussions* but from that time onwards there was a tacit understanding between us that the hypnotic treatment should be discontinued. (p. 27, my italics)

Note that this reported event was so unsettling for both parties that Freud deemed it to remain unspoken! This incident, which led Freud to abandon hypnosis around 1896, was an excellent example of the power of transference (and countertransference), which may arise in psychotherapy. Realising the complexity of the therapeutic relationship, Freud no longer thought that real trauma was always at the base of neurosis and concluded that many of his patients unconsciously fabricated their abuse stories in order to satisfy the desire of the hypnotist. He therefore found the hypnotic work potentially masking and confusing the analytic process.

Melvin Gravitz (2004) suggested that it was Freud's discomfort with the degree of transference, particularly erotic transference that pushed him to abandon hypnosis. Thus, the very phenomenon that was to later become the central axis of psychoanalytic work—transference dynamics—was at first rejected by Freud, considered as an obstacle to the therapeutic process, and moreover deemed taboo.

After he ceased using hypnosis, Freud continued for a short while to work with the pressure technique, which was based on the hypnotic protocol. He believed that the pressure technique assisted the patient to reach an energetic discharge (catharsis) quicker, thus freeing pent-up emotional and bodily energy (Hinshelwood, 2002). However, within a short while Freud deserted cathartic work altogether, forbidding the psychoanalytic use of touch and hypnosis thereafter.

Psychoanalytic technique was at first affective and abreactive, incorporating techniques that actively sought to encourage cathartic expression for emotional and bodily experiences. In order to establish and deepen the psychoanalytic relationship, Freud shifted the focus of the psychoanalytic practice from the affective and abreactive to the interpretive. He chose to turn to gentler and more subtle therapeutic tools, of free associations and transference interpretation. Not unlike Blanche Wittman, the woman on whom Charcot demonstrated his work to his fellow doctors, hypnosis and touch were both considered wild; too wild to be therapeutically tamed; too unstable to allow for conscious psychotherapeutic use. Choosing to incorporate hypnosis and touch, tools that were associated with Charcot and Bernheim, but also with charlatanism and danger, would not have been a wise choice for a man who desperately sought for his ideas to be adopted by the scientific and medical community.

Autonomy, emancipation, and the biological science of the psyche

Freud fought boldly and wisely to establish psychoanalysis as a science, all the while proudly leaning against the medical-physical model of Descartes and Newton for support. The influential psychoanalyst Hans Loewald (1977) claimed that Freud, who was deeply prejudiced against any type of religious position, was diligently engaged in "the disenchantment of the world" (p. 518), and was strongly committed to the demystification of the unconscious. Freud aspired to create psychoanalysis in the image of natural sciences, and was hoping that one day all psychological processes could be understood and explained by biology.

The hope that biological processes would one day suffice to describe psychological processes is still commonly held, both by professionals and the public. Psychiatrist, neurologist, and Nobel laureate Eric Kandel, for example, summarised his current biological thinking about mind-brain relationship, stating that: "All mental processes, even the most complex psychological processes, derive from operations of the brain" (1998, p. 39). Kandel's causal logic and belief that biology could one day provide the biological foundations of our psychological and mental life, represents a similar yearning that Freud expressed in his theory: a human desire for absolute form (although some may argue that this—as science in itself, is a gendered desire—man's desire (Sharon Zack, personal communication, 2013)).

To achieve such an enormous task, Freud aspired to create a value-free psychotherapy, as clean as possible from the therapist's influence. Seen through this endeavour, hypnosis and touch were now highly criticised and were seen as saturated with suggestive and authoritarian influences. Like Blanche Wittman, the hypnotised and touched person was perceived as a passive object, awaiting the hypnotist's forceful commands. To use a gestalt terminology, hypnosis and touch became the background against which psychoanalysis defined itself. Freud wanted to demonstrate that, unlike hypnosis, the effectiveness of the psychoanalytic treatment was independent of the psychoanalyst's suggestive influence. Stephen Mitchell (2005), one of the most important contributors to and creators of relational psychoanalysis, suggested that Freud wished to differentiate psychoanalysis from hypnosis precisely because psychoanalysis emerged out of hypnotic work. Therefore, wrote Mitchell: "It was crucial for psychoanalysis to differentiate itself from its ancestor, hypnotism, and its reliance on the personal power and influence of the therapist" (p. 8). The hypnotic techniques Freud was exposed to were similar to the type shown in Charcot's demonstration: powerful cathartic dynamics, which heavily relied on the charismatic influence of the therapist, laden with indecent touch and energetically charged seizures. Freud wanted to emancipate psychoanalysis from such influence. Mitchell continued: "Where hypnotism added influence, psychoanalysis removed historical influences; where hypnotism directed and shaped, psychoanalysis liberated and released" (ibid.).

Freud's efforts to minimise the analyst's impact (if not to eliminate it altogether), resulted from his aspiration to establish an objective scientific model whereby understanding brought cure. Even though the objectivist aspect of his theory and practice was refuted as dogmatic over the years, the mere attempt to minimise the therapist's influence significantly contributed to the acceptance of psychoanalysis by the scientific community. However, the psychoanalytic emancipation from hypnosis and touch brought with it an almost hermetic rejection of hypnosis from the psychoanalytic field, and alongside it, touch techniques too were rejected as inappropriate for the treatment of the mind. The body was left behind.

From its inception, psychoanalysis has always placed the greatest importance on the patient's autonomy and self-direction. Nevertheless, today it is widely accepted that influence, not least therapeutic influence, is unavoidable. Relational psychoanalyst Irwin Hoffman (1996) acknowledged that "Whatever the analyst does is invariably saturated with suggestion" (p. 106). Systemic psychotherapist Bradford Keeney (1983) reiterated a similar position: "Therapists affect the systems they are treating whether they intend to or not. On the other side of the relationship, the systems treated always affect the therapist" (p. 129).

The wish to find an absolute truth, and the accompanying fantasy for an absolute and static science, characterised the history of human thought, and highlighted one of the most fundamental psychological (culturally enhanced and carrying strong gender bias) human needs: for certainty, consistency, and external authority. One of the most prominent and influential scientists of our time, the late palaeontologist and evolution theorist Stephen Jay Gould, worked vigorously against the objectivist perception of science, claiming that the belief that science could (or should) be objective is merely a fantasy: "I criticize the myth that science itself is an objective enterprise, done properly only when scientists can shun the constraints of their culture and view the world as it really is" (1996, p. 53).

One of the reasons for the current blossoming of body psychotherapy within the general field of psychotherapy concerns the conceptual and clinical openness brought by the relational turn in psychoanalysis. Relational psychoanalysis shattered the sterile fantasy which typified the first decades of psychological treatment. Mitchell (2000) wrote:

> The analytic relationship is no longer usefully understood as the sterile operation theatre Freud believed it could be. The analytic relationship is not as different from other human relationships as Freud wanted it to be. In fact, the intersubjective engagement between patient and analyst has become increasingly understood as the very fulcrum of and vehicle for the deep characterological change psychoanalysis facilitates. (p. 125)

No less influential in challenging psychoanalytic drive theory was the feminist critique of psychoanalysis, from De Beauvoir, Juliet Mitchell, through to Kristeva, Irigaray, and Cixous. They all demonstrated how "neutral" was illusive, and how gender played a central role not only in the therapy room but also in theoretical formulations and conceptualisations (Cixous & Clement, 1986; Kristeva, 2001; J. Mitchell, 1974).

Following the splits

The splits between psychoanalysis, hypnosis, and touch rippled on, creating alongside those splits many prejudices among and between these three professional fields. The body has almost disappeared from the classic psychoanalytic practice. Although some psychoanalysts who were close (at some point) to Freud's inner circle (primarily Georg Groddeck, Sándor Ferenczi, and Wilhelm Reich) continued to emphasise the importance of the body and used touch in their work, the development of psychoanalytic thinking and its clinical models by and large marginalised the body (and with it, Reich's and Ferenczi's contributions).

Ferenczi (1929), for example, suggested that non-erotic touch (including hugging and holding) was invaluable in repairing early developmental injuries. Freud (who was Ferenczi's analyst) first supported Ferenczi, but once he recognised the potential for erotic interpretation to the touch (and considering the fact that Ferenczi had an affair with one of his patients and later married her mother), he withdrew his support.

Abstaining from touch in psychoanalysis became one of the main rules of conduct, and developed into a central taboo in psychoanalysis and psychodynamic psychotherapy. The renowned psychiatrist Karl Menninger (1958), for instance, wrote: "Transgression of the rule against physical contact constitutes evidence of the incompetence or criminal ruthlessness of the analyst" (p. 40). Touch, which is widely recognised today as a crucial aspect of our early development, imperative for our regulatory capacities in childhood and adulthood, became a dangerous therapeutic prohibition. Hypnotic work, too, once announced as suggestive by Freud, almost completely disappeared from the clinical psychoanalytic practice (excluding research), and was often presented as manipulative, dangerous, impermanent, or otherwise inappropriate.

In his later writing, Freud related to hypnosis as one of the forces that could prevent or obstruct organic analytic process. "Hypnosis" he wrote, "had screened from view an interplay of forces which now came in sight and the understanding of which gave a solid foundation to my theory" (Freud, 1925d, p. 29).

The same fabric that weaved psychoanalysis, touch, and hypnosis together also set them apart. To better understand the long-lasting and far-reaching effects of Freud's rejection of touch and hypnosis, let us turn to physicist, historian, and philosopher of science Thomas Kuhn (1962), whose book *The Structure of Scientific Revolutions* was one of the classic texts in the history and philosophy of science. A new paradigm shift, as Kuhn showed, required a societal turn, a cultural reorganisation of major perceptions, beliefs, and sociocultural schemas; a true surrender to the flux of change. Therefore, societal changes required similar stable structures to those of personal changes (and vice versa). Just as a baby required both internal and external stable organisations and a safe space in order to move and explore, so did social structures. Flexing in one place was usually accompanied by the tightening of another. We could not change everything in one go, and Freud had brought about an important, yet highly uncomfortable, societal paradigm shift; and it came with a pricetag.

Four major paradigm shifts challenged humanity's firm hold on certainty and the human narcissism. Copernicus disenchanted the sacredness of skies by challenging the geocentric astral organisation and demonstrating that Earth was merely a planet revolving around the sun, and that Earth was not the centre of the universe, as it was previously believed. Darwin similarly disenchanted the primacy of human biology by showing that we were a product of an ever-unfolding evolutionary development and furthermore that evolution will not stop with us, that we were not the final and most astute product of divine creation. Einstein, too, challenged the illusion of objectivity by demonstrating that even time and space were relative in nature, dependent on the observing subject; and that in the very act of observation we created a systemic change. Flow (uncertainty) hence became an essential characteristic of the universe—we lived in an ever changing, relating, and pulsating world. Freud was the fourth iconoclast, by disenchanting our fantasy of liberty and freedom. Freud (1917a) himself saw psychoanalysis as "the third blow" to our anthropocentrism, seeing the world as the centre of the universe, following Copernicus and Darwin. According to Freud, humans were primarily acting unconsciously, unaware of the drives, anxieties, and desires that motivated them. For me, this was one of Freud's greatest achievements: a call for humility, resulting from perceiving the human journey as a process of growth. Thus, self-awareness was not a given but had to be worked at and gained: we were required to pursue self-knowledge, with diligence and integrity, in order to fully assume the human potential inherent in us all.

The same characterological traits, which enabled Freud to embark on and follow through such a humongous societal paradigm shift, also involved exclusiveness. In discussing Freud's personality, Reich (1967) described—with genuine fondness and love for his teacher—a very lonely man. Freud was highly intolerant of differentness, and throughout the years many of his closest students were rejected by him when they expressed opinions or theories different to his own. Alfred Adler, Sándor Ferenczi, Carl Jung, and Wilhelm Reich, for example, have all been close to Freud before being expelled—implicitly or explicitly, from the inner circles of psychoanalysis. This rigidity, which was probably necessary when establishing psychoanalysis as a discipline, still deeply influences the professional milieu today, as hypnotic clinicians, professional bodyworkers, medical practitioners, and psychotherapists receive limited and partial theoretical and clinical education in the huge knowledge gathered by each of the other disciplines (D. Johnson, 1998).

The juxtaposition of therapeutic touch and therapeutic hypnosis was not merely found in their crucial meeting within the psychoanalytic field and their subsequent exile from psychoanalysis, but was moreover marked by the great potential these two practices offered for unmediated work with unconscious processes. For example, in his revolutionary psychoanalytic work, Ferenczi (1925) recognised the connection between muscular relaxation and the quality of free association, and consequently made use of relaxation techniques as part of his psychoanalytic work. In the last few years, I have published a number of papers exploring and illustrating the theoretical and clinical resemblance of these two fields (Rolef Ben-Shahar, 2001a, 2001b, 2002a, 2002b, 2008a, 2008c, 2009, 2010c).

Reich's excellent biographer Myron Sharaf (1984) drew similar parallels between the psychoanalytic free association technique and the different patterns of breathing identified and differentiated by Reich. Both systems aimed at encouraging flow and flexing structural rigidities, thus allowing the patient to soften and restructure fixated body–mind organisations.

The pounding heart

> The pounding heart, the sweaty palms, the tight stomach, the tensed muscles are the emotions.
>
> —Deane Juhan (1998, p. 368)

Another unfortunate consequence of exiling hypnosis and touch from the psychoanalytic mainstream was the impact on the relationship between these two exiled fields. Despite their affective similarity, cross-fertilisation between these practices has been minimal. Psychotherapeutic touch and hypnotherapy have as a result thereafter developed in two separate and parallel routes, with scarcely any meeting points.

On the one hand, we can find clinical yet non-psychotherapeutic applications of both bodywork and hypnosis, mostly drawing from traditional philosophies (such as Eastern disciplines). Traditional Chinese medicine, Shiatsu, Tai Chi, and Yoga (among others) have extensively flourished in the West in the last few decades. These practices, however, seldom engaged in dialogue with the Western body of psychological knowledge, as they relied on alternative philosophies. Similarly, psychodynamic psychotherapy scarcely dialogued with these types of therapies. Parallel dynamics were found in hypnosis too, and many types of trancework, such as meditation, yoga, ecstatic dance, shamanic practices, and various systems of healing regularly utilised non-ordinary states of consciousness outside the field of psychotherapy.

Many practitioners of hypnosis (whether we call their practice hypnosis or give it other names, such as NLP and guided visualisation) and bodyworkers could fit this category, as they used these tools therapeutically, yet not within a psychotherapeutic relationship. Psychotherapeutic conduct required, among other things, appropriate therapeutic training, sufficient theoretical grounding, and awareness of the complexity of therapeutic relationship and transference dynamics. While these therapies often proved highly effective and useful, their practitioners rarely engaged in fertile and reciprocal dialogue with the psychotherapeutic and psychoanalytic body of knowledge.

On the other hand, the last few decades saw the development of relational and integrative ways of working—both in body psychotherapy and in trancework, informed and influenced by both traditional (non-dualistic) and modern psychotherapeutic perspectives.

When the therapeutic focus on embodied processes is carried out alongside the understanding of the complexity of the therapeutic relationship, it poses significant challenges to the psychotherapist: as therapists we are being seen by as well as seeing the other, being examined and analysed as well as examining and analysing our clients. In fact, we lend ourselves to the scrutinising gaze of our clients in the hope of remodelling a less defensive surrender, thus permitting the internal and external pressure to change and flex to touch us, so that we may soften our rigidities and flow. Neither Freud nor the culture he was operating in were ready for such a radical shift, as demonstrated in Freud's (1913c) writing:

> I hold to the plan of getting the patient to lie on a sofa while I sit behind him out of his sight. This arrangement has a historical basis; it is the remnant of the hypnotic method out of which psycho-analysis was evolved. But it deserves to be maintained for many reasons. The first is a personal motive, but one which others may share with me. I cannot put up with being stared at by other people for eight hours a day (or more). Since, while I am listening to the patient, I, too, give myself over to the current of my unconscious thoughts, I do not wish my expressions of face to give the patient material for interpretations or to influence him in what he tells me. (pp. 133–134)

As a product of his time and culture, Freud was terrified of his clinical visibility and this inevitable bodily presence must have been highly challenging for him. It is not too speculative to assume that Freud was not particularly aware of his own body or his somatic countertransference: these two aspects were perceived as irrelevant to the clinical enquiry and were beyond the scope of contemporary cultural dialogue. However, when body psychotherapy was practised from a psychodynamic or relational stance, the clinician was positioned against concrete and sometimes destabilising expressions of transference and countertransference: we may experience real emotional and physical discomfort and pain, excitement, fears, and hopes. Transference dynamics between psychotherapist and client no longer remained the convenient and interesting conceptual framework: just like any other real and non-therapeutic relationship, the relational therapy provided a space within which we could actually matter to one another—as well as get hurt (Asheri, 2004; Soth, 2005).

Living and practising in Victorian times, although Freud recognised the relative transparency of his unconscious processes, he refused to allow these (and himself as a subject) to be fully expressed in the therapeutic relationship. He resisted the development of attachment to his patients and perceived it as unprofessional; only their attachment to the analyst was permitted, and even encouraged by the analyst. The split from hypnosis and from the body was arguably a necessary step for creating a clinical and applicable science of the mind. Perhaps, not unlike Descartes, Freud's dissociative tendencies might have been facilitative for the early stages of psychoanalytic research and clinical growth. However, these splits and dissociation also bore a grave price. Psychoanalyst (and Buddhist) Harriet Kimble Wrye (1998) illustrated:

> Freud discovered psychoanalysis, the "talking cure", and freed his fledgling science from hypnotic touch. At the same time, in his effort to make his scientific project within the Victorian culture of, and with his own perchance for, Cartesian dualism, he fostered an inadvertent splitting off of the body. (p. 114)

Given Freud's personal and cultural background and his unequivocal contribution to the fields of psychology and psychotherapy, it is most likely that Freud could not have worked differently without risking the establishment of psychoanalysis. Relational psychotherapy, whose roots began to sprout over fifty years later, required maturation that was yet impossible for Freud to attain, a maturation that demanded a period of post-Freudian brewing and fermentation—which has characterised the last two decades, out of which relational body psychotherapy was born.

Reclaiming touch in psychotherapy

> Your body is your subconscious mind, and you can't heal it by talk alone.
>
> —Candace Pert (1997, p. 30)

An increasing number of clinicians recognise today that the transformative experience in therapy is taking place in the tension between the spoken (the narrative) and the resonant. More than anywhere, healing and growth occur in the undercurrent and nonverbal communication spheres—currents which manifest the wider minds co-created by client and therapist, within the body and between the bodies.

Attending to the body of the client, and of the therapist, and the ongoing attention to internal organisation, the deconstruction of these and reorganisation (not merely in the client but also in the therapist and the therapeutic dyad) are taxing and terrifying processes. Such work forces us to walk on the edge of safety and never cease from exploring our boundaries. We are called to stretch our own person in a continuously dialectic organisation between our enmeshment with the client's material—to sufficient differentiation of ourselves; between our own personal processes and those of our clients. By doing so, we genuinely risk having our own lives changed in the process of doing therapy.

For the last few decades, thanks to three main factors, body psychotherapy has been making its way back into mainstream psychotherapy and psychoanalytic thinking. The first concerns the huge advances made in neuroscience, particularly in the field of mirror neurons and trauma research. The second factor involves the maturation of body psychotherapy and the development of psychodynamic and relational body psychotherapy, as a field committed to continuous dialogue with psychoanalytic theory and practice. The third agent relates to the fact that relational psychoanalysis and psychotherapy brought a fresh wind to the analytic and therapeutic field, together with a more inclusive and curious attitude towards external influences in general, and becoming open to somatic influences in particular (Rolef Ben-Shahar, 2008a).

Neuroscience

Over the last twenty years, research in brain sciences began to point to the inextricable bond between psychological development and somatic organisations. Of particular interest were the research projects of Allan Schore (1994, 2003), who examined the connection between attachment, affect regulation, and the development of both body and mind. The extensive research in mirror neurons (for example, Gallese, Ferrari, & Umiltà, 2002; Rizzolatti, Fadiga, Fogassi, & Gallese, 1996) also contributed to strengthening the growing interest in body–mind connection. Furthermore, therapeutic research has shown that bodily interventions were highly effective in traumawork (Levine & Frederick, 1997; P. Ogden, Minton, & Pain, 2006; Rothschild, 2000; F. Shapiro, 1989).

These studies provided body psychotherapists with acknowledgment, validation, and appreciation from both the scientific and the psychotherapeutic fields; as well they attracted serious and learned practitioners to body psychotherapy (Chapter Three will expand the discussion on body psychotherapy and trauma. Mirror neurons will be discussed in Chapters Five and Eleven).

Relational body psychotherapy

Relational body psychotherapy (which will be expanded on in Chapters Four and Five) is a relatively new development in body psychotherapy that maintains a close dialogue with psychoanalytic developments, particularly relational psychoanalysis. This cross-fertilisation within contemporary body psychotherapy created a new generation of therapists who are able to use psychodynamic terminology, and therefore could engage and discuss with psychotherapists from other disciplines, influence them, and be influenced by them.

Relational psychoanalysis

The term *relationality* (within psychoanalysis) was coined by Jay Greenberg and Stephen Mitchell in 1983 in their book *Object Relations in Psychoanalytic Theory*, which celebrated one of the most important developments in contemporary psychoanalysis. The flexibility shown by the pioneers of relational psychoanalysis, who challenged some of the unquestionable taboos of classic psychoanalysis, opened a door to external influence of therapeutic methods, which were not seriously considered before within psychoanalysis, including body psychotherapy (for example, see Evelyn Rappoport's (2012) paper on integrating *Somatic Experiencing* within psychoanalytic work). In the last few years, relational psychoanalytic journals have further been publishing papers by body-oriented psychotherapists (King, 2011; Krantz, 2012; Rolef Ben-Shahar & MacDonald, 2011; Sletvold, 2012). Relational psychoanalysis presented a "softer" clinical position than traditional psychoanalysis, which allowed body psychotherapists to identify with this professional field without feeling patronised or ostracised, renewing the organic connection with their roots, which was sadly severed towards the end of the nineteenth century. Relational psychoanalysis is currently allowing itself to directly engage with theoretical and some clinical applications of body-centred psychotherapy.

Relational psychoanalysis and the disciplines from which it emerged—attachment theory, object relations, and self-psychology—receive extensive referencing throughout this volume. In the Appendix, I present a short review of relational psychoanalysis, while focusing on aspects which are relevant for body psychotherapy.

Severing the connections between body psychotherapy, psychoanalytic psychotherapy, and hypnosis had adverse effects on all three disciplines. Many contemporary practitioners of hypnosis were unaware of research, understanding, and advances in system theory, attachment theory, and relational research—or in body psychotherapy. Many hypnotherapists perceived themselves as positioned outside the system, doing things to the client—maintaining a similar illusion held by Freud decades beforehand, and disregarded the interactive and mutual nature of the therapeutic relationship. Traditional and authoritarian hypnosis incorporated a fantasy of bypassing the clients' consciousness, reorganising unconscious habitual patterns for them, and bringing them back into the world (S. Gilligan, 1987). The fantasy that such reorganisation could be a singular process which did not impact the therapist and was disconnected from the therapeutic relationship created a great deal of fear, scepticism, and eventually led to avoiding hypnosis in psychoanalysis altogether. Many body psychotherapists too maintained a prejudicial opinion regarding psychoanalysis on the one hand and hypnosis on the other, despite the resemblance between those practices.

The relational-embodied paradigm is neither convenient nor pleasant. It presents a world of relations that is far more opaque and less knowable than we might have wanted. The shift from understanding the world as flat to seeing it as round, confronted humanity with many illusions. In a similar way, the relational paradigm challenges us to acknowledge the (at least partial) illusion of our separate individual self. Such a paradigm shift requires a societal maturation, with greater capacity for tolerating not-knowing and flow. Embodiment disenchants the Cartesian hope that our mind and soul could be separated from the body; hope for attaining a level of objectivity independent of the world we observe. Influential physicist Fritjof Capra (2002) argues that embodiment demonstrates how "the very structure of reason arises from body and brains" (p. 53).

British psychoanalyst Susie Orbach, who is a crucial ambassador for reclaiming the body in psychoanalysis, challenges the Freudian notion of the body as a dustbin for what the psyche cannot tolerate. Instead, argues Orbach (2004a, 2004b), all our actions are inevitably dependent on bodies in relations: our bodies, and ourselves, are only made in relationships, assuming meaning through connection. We become bodies when we relate, and we relate thanks to our somatic reality.

As the distant great-grandchildren of Freud, we are currently occupying a unique position: we can be grateful for his canonical contributions, and at the same time let go of some of the presuppositions he was forced to adopt, either due to personal limitations or because of political and cultural limitations or stigmas. We can now return and be bodies in relations; we can now surrender to flow, we can allow ourselves to touch and be touched—impact and be impacted—in life, and in psychotherapy.

Exercise: embodying somatic identity

(Best done in pairs—an explorer and a guide)

The chapter has dealt with the historical split between body and mind. The following exercise offers a possible means to reintegrate the two. It assists in deepening our identification with the somatic, sensory, and motoric self, thus expanding our resources beyond thoughts and feelings. This exercise can also help down-regulating emotional flooding. Coming back to the senses may help ground us and soothe highly charged affective processes.

1. The explorer lies down comfortably and for a few moments is simply allowed to slow down, while paying attention to his breathing cycles. If closing the eyes is possible and safe, then this is encouraged.
2. Internal scan: the guide helps the explorer to direct his attention inwardly, developing a felt sense, by asking the following specific questions. To maintain the exercise's effectiveness, I strongly suggest that the ritualistic structure and simplicity of questions are maintained (you can read them aloud). During this stage, interpretations or verbal discussions should be avoided.

GUIDE: how are your feet feeling?
EXPLORER: my feet are ____ (for example: warm)
GUIDE: how are your calves feeling?
EXPLORER: my calves are ____ (for example: hurting)
GUIDE: how are you knees feeling?
EXPLORER: my knees are ____ (for example: weak)

Continue with: thighs, pelvis, lower back, stomach, upper back, chest, shoulders, arms, forearms, hands, neck and head (and feel free to be more specific than suggested).

3. So who are you, really? The guide now repeats the same questions, but this time the explorer answers by identifying with the body part, in the first person—as if he is the body part that speaks.

GUIDE: how are your feet feeling?
EXPLORER: I feel/am ____ (for example: warm)
GUIDE: how are your calves feeling?
EXPLORER: I feel/am ____ (for example: hurting)
GUIDE: how are you knees feeling?
EXPLORER: I feel/am ____ (for example: weak)

Continue with: thighs, pelvis, lower back, stomach, upper back, chest, shoulders, arms, forearms, hands, neck and head (and feel free to be more specific than suggested). Notice differences in sensations and thoughts. Are there parts with which it is easier to identify? Are there body parts that feel foreign?

4. You may choose to swap roles and share with your partner. The exercise could be done alone, by doing two internal body scans.

CHAPTER TWO

The melting pot of body psychotherapy

Come into my hand
By your mild power; descending down the Nerves of my right arm
From out the Portals of my Brain, where by your ministry
The Eternal Great Humanity Divine planted his Paradise

—*William Blake,* Milton, 2: 5–7

Cosmic magnetism and Mozart's piano concerto no. 18

Attempting to accurately portray the history of body psychotherapy is a complex task. First, some modalities of body psychotherapy developed independently of the main historical roots of body psychotherapy. Georg Groddeck, Arnold Mindell, and Stanislav Grof, for example, created their therapeutic practices without directly relating to the developmental route presented in this chapter, namely, of Freud and Reich. Second, as a field that integrated theoretical and clinical perceptions stemming from psychology with bodywork and somatic methodologies, body psychotherapy was not only influenced by and developed from psychotherapeutic models but also from bodywork disciplines. Wilhelm Reich, for instance, was deeply influenced by German bodywork and breathwork traditions (D. Johnson, 1995). Gerda Boyesen was influenced by psychiatric physiotherapy in Norway; Jack Painter—from Ida Rolf's structural integration ("Rolfing") and more.

In this review of the early history of body psychotherapy I have chosen to focus on the mainstream of body psychotherapy, which clearly and distinctly identifies itself as body psychotherapy and has developed alongside (and been saturated with influences from) psychoanalysis. I shall begin my review with the pre-Freudian sources of somatic therapeutic intervention and then focus on the theoretical and clinical stances of Sándor Ferenczi and Wilhelm Reich. For readers who are interested in learning more comprehensively about the history of body psychotherapy, Courtenay Young's (2011d) edited book, *The Historical Basis of Body Psychotherapy*, offers an excellent collection of historical review papers on the subject.

As Chapter One illustrated, the history of psychotherapy was weaved with those of body psychotherapy and hypnosis. Neurologist and hypnotist Hippolyte Bernheim was probably the first person to use the term *psychotherapy*, in his discussions on ideodynamism, the curious phenomenon whereby a thought or idea was translated into a bodily event: a movement, a feeling, or a sensation (Bernheim, 1887). Ideodynamism is an everyday phenomenon, marking a deep connection between body and mind. Suffice it to think about and imagine biting a lemon, for example, to begin salivating. Upon hearing a compliment (or an insult), many of us blush. Usually, ideodynamism correlates to an autonomic nervous system response, that is, an unconscious somatic reaction. For example, when after a sleepless night I asked Zohar, my daughter, why she couldn't sleep all night, she answered: "The thoughts confused my body, daddy."

The body–mind connection, which is axiomatic in many traditional non-Western cultures and healing methodologies, became unravelled and severed in the West following our adoption of Cartesian philosophy and Newtonian physics. One of the first attempts to reintegrate the body–mind connection in modern science was led by the Viennese doctor Franz Anton Mesmer (1734–1815), considered the father of modern hypnosis and one of the pioneers of energetic healing in the West, who argued for inseparable connections between body and mind. In his uniquely unconventional ways, Mesmer wished to retrieve psychological healing from the hands of priests and magicians and reclaim their relevance to science and medicine. Mesmer believed that there was a magnetic energy (animal magnetism) that flowed throughout the universe and that it was possible to use and utilise it. Mesmer speculated that a fine and invisible magnetic fluid moved through all things in the cosmos and connected us all. This fluid was also flowing in our own bodies, and contributed to our regulation and maintenance of our wellbeing (Mesmer, 1766). As we shall later see (both in this chapter and in Part II (Theoretical)), this idea strongly resembles Reich's understanding of the "orgone energy".

Mesmer's efforts to harness this cosmic magnetic energy to healing involved dramatic rituals, saturated with pathos. The rituals incorporated touch, ecstatic drumming, playing atmospheric music, and delivering hypnotic suggestions. All these were designed to create bodily and affective charge. In order to utilise this cosmic magnetic energy, believed Mesmer, an affective triggered state was necessary: an actively charged bodymind state (Gezundhajt, 2007). The belief that affective charge was necessary for healing has been central in body psychotherapy since its inception, and has regained popularity in the last few decades, as well as supported by neuroscience research (particularly mirror neurons, about which you can read in Chapter Five).

Mesmer's therapeutic reputation and success, his charismatic character, and the great popularity his methods gained, attracted both positive and negative attention: particularly envy attacks and unforgiving criticism by both scientific and medical circles. In 1777, following a highly publicised scandal, Mesmer left Vienna and moved to Paris. The scandal involved an unfortunate therapeutic failure with the talented young musician Maria Theresia von Paradis, for whom Mozart (allegedly) composed his piano concerto no. 18. The young pianist suffered from—how relevant to our discussion—hysterical blindness. Using his touch and hypnotic rituals, Mesmer managed to cure von Paradis, and his star immediately shone, gaining him greater reputation than ever and attracting more interest. However, the cure quickly turned out to be temporary, von Paradis's blindness returned and Mesmer's standing dropped as quickly as it climbed, reaching pit bottom almost in an instant. Doctors and scientists descended on Mesmer like hungry scavenging vultures, and the criticism and persecution followed Mesmer to Paris too. A few years later, King Louis XI of France summoned a commission of inquiry, headed by the US Ambassador to France, Benjamin Franklin. The commission declared Mesmer's work fraudulent and scientifically unsubstantiated (Franklin, 1785). He was subsequently shunned as a charlatan and lost his licence to practise medicine.

Mesmer was possibly the first body–mind celebrity to be crowned and then be publicly dismissed and shamed, but he was certainly not the last one. Almost 200 years later, in August 1956, in an unusual political exercise of censorship and information control, the US Food and Drug Administration (FDA) burned a few tons of Wilhelm Reich's books and published papers, while Reich was rotting in jail under similar accusations to Mesmer's.

Although Mesmer's research methods and their clinical applications were extreme, it was his professional insistence that emotional and bodily symptoms were interlinked that set the ground for the studies in hysteria by Freud and Breuer more than a century later. Mesmer offered the first scientific validation for conversion phenomenon—an emotional disturbance which manifested as a bodily symptom. In fact, it was not only his theoretical concepts that were central in the studies of hysteria, but also Mesmer's unique methods of practice, made subtle perhaps, but still utilising a systematic building up of bodily charge and emotional affect. In reality, Jean Martin Charcot's dramatic rituals were not that different from Mesmer's rituals of animal magnetism. However, Charcot was a seasoned and astute politician, and a much cleverer strategist than Mesmer. Perhaps, too, the times they were a changin' … Charcot's practice and theory did not result in expulsion or dismissal, but instead positioned him as one of the most famous and appreciated neurologists in the world, a position that attracted the best scientists and clinicians to Salpêtrière and liberated those around him to explore and experiment in methodologies that were considered, until Charcot normalised them, too extreme to practise.

As described in Chapter One, Charcot established his neurological laboratory at Salpêtrière hospital in Paris in the mid-1880s. I enjoy imagining this hospital as the (politically and gender deviant, but nonetheless) delivery room of psychoanalysis, modern hypnosis, and body psychotherapy. The pioneering French psychologist Pierre Janet, for example, who was the head of Charcot's laboratory, used deep tissue massage to prevent muscular atrophy and taught movement exercises as part of the therapy he offered hysterical patients (Boadella, 1976). Janet furthered the work of Bernheim and William James, researching ideomotor (an idea that became a movement) and ideodynamic phenomena. Janet presented his findings in 1885, at the first French conference on psychology and physiology. Ideodynamism is still researched today within studies of hypnosis (Rossi & Cheek, 1988).

This electrifying and exciting atmosphere (circus-like, for sure) where studies in hypnosis were conducted alongside experiments in therapeutic touch and deep scientific exploration of body–mind connectedness, was the environment into which the young Freud was introduced upon his arrival in Paris. In Freud's early work, hypnosis and touch were not only theoretically validating the inseparable connection of body and mind, but also formed a central route for his clinical practice. Similarly to Mesmer, and certainly influenced by his work, Freud identified that treatment that encouraged energetic response from his hysterical patients (emotional-bodily expression such as crying, shaking etc.) facilitated a quicker recovery. The idea of emotional discharge (catharsis) has since disappeared from mainstream psychoanalysis, but is still preserved and has been practised in many body psychotherapy modalities.

Chapter One traced the historical split between those three fields, all "born" during the end of the nineteenth century at the Salpêtrière: psychoanalysis, modern hypnosis, and body psychotherapy. Freud's discovery of transference phenomena and his subsequent conclusion that not all his patients suffered sexual abuse, led Freud to exercise greater therapeutic caution and withdraw from using touch and hypnotic techniques. Another factor impacting his avoidance of those potentially explosive techniques was his understanding of the importance of, and centrality of sexual development in our lives. The coarse touch techniques of the time, and the Victorian zeitgeist of sexual repression, turned these unskilled touch techniques to a flammable gas of erotic transferences. Freud's verbal interpretation and the free association techniques were safer means of working with such emotional charge, and so the *talking cure* was clearly established as a distinctive therapeutic methodology (Fenichel, 1945).

In spite of Freud's stern resistance to using hypnosis and touch in psychoanalysis, a few notable clinicians continued to work directly with the body and with touch; two of them will be discussed here. The first was Hungarian analyst Sándor Ferenczi. The second was that man who was usually considered the father of body psychotherapy: the psychiatrist and psychoanalyst Wilhelm Reich. Both men were profoundly influenced by the work of Georg Groddeck (1931), an analyst who used deep tissue work to facilitate his patients' emotional and bodily expressions.

Sándor Ferenczi (1873–1933)

The Jewish Hungarian psychoanalyst Sándor Ferenczi was at certain stages a close member of the prestigious Viennese inner circle, intimately sponsored and endorsed by Freud (who was also his psychoanalyst), and was particularly known for his work with difficult patients. Over the years, Ferenczi was extremely critical of the therapeutic passivity which was commonplace in traditional psychoanalysis. He blamed psychoanalysis for sacrificing clinical performance (i.e., the patient's best interests) for the sake of research and theoretical advancement (Tosone, 1997). A solely intellectual stance, claimed Ferenczi (Ferenczi & Rank, 1925), might indeed foster self-awareness but at the same time it strengthened intellectual defence mechanisms against emotional expressions.

Together with Otto Rank (whose research on birth trauma provided important theoretical and experimental background to the development of body psychotherapy), Ferenczi developed his *Active Technique*, which made an important impact on many therapeutic fields, among them Carl Rogers's client-centred therapy, the psychoanalytic object relations theory, and also relational psychoanalysis. His work influenced studies in trauma, dissociation, and hypnosis (Bányai, 1998), the formation and establishment of short-term psychotherapy (Malan, 1963), and—of course—was a pivotal (if sometimes indirectly so) influence on body psychotherapy. Ferenczi and Rank (1925) recommended that the therapist was active and encouraged amplification and intensification of the client's emotional expression, since an insight without experience was insufficient for healing; what goes around comes around, so it seems ...

In addition to emphasising the therapist's activity, Ferenczi's active technique positioned the analyst and the processes taking place within the psychoanalyst at the centre of the analytic process. Thus, he perceived countertransference as a central process in psychoanalysis—an approach that was radical and far reaching at the time. Ferenczi's positions, influential and significant as they might have been for so many therapeutic fields, gradually distanced him from the central melting pot of analytic discourse, as well as attracting violent and piercing criticism towards him. Freud's renowned biographer Ernest Jones (who happened to be Ferenczi's patient), went as far as claiming that Ferenczi was mentally ill.

In a similar vein to British psychiatrist Ian Suttie (1935), Ferenczi believed that the analyst's love was necessary for the patient's development and healing, and he frequently used non-sexual touch, including holding his patients and hugging them, as ways of expressing this love. Ferenczi suggested that many of the patients, who Freud considered inappropriate for analysis on account of their being too narcissistically wounded, actually suffered the real trauma of love deficiency. For him, in these conditions therapy demanded that the analyst provide some of these needs by expressing tender love towards her patients. Ferenczi was one of the first psychoanalysts who recognised the importance of affective expression in the therapeutic process and of creating the facilitative environment for reparative regression. He held (Ferenczi, 1932) that an important therapeutic role was allowing the patient to experience regressive processes without shame, thus being attentive (and attuned) to provision for these patients' early developmental needs—serving, for a temporary period, as the good enough parents until the object was internalised as part of the patient's self-regulatory processes.

To attain such therapeutic goals, Ferenczi's *Active Technique* (1930) incorporated relaxation exercises and guided visualisation together with somatic interventions, including touch. As mentioned before, the physical contact Ferenczi offered was primarily in his work with regressive self-states. He held and cradled patients, believing that the primary transference dimension in therapy was parental, and therefore for many patients the therapists gradually became an internalised attachment figure. Thus, the physical holding (mainly hugging and cradling) was seen by Ferenczi as potentially compensating for empathetic failures of early attachment figures (Tosone, 1997).

But Ferenczi's contribution to the development of body psychotherapy did not end with the validating and affirming touch he offered his clients, or with his willingness to engage—experientially and nonverbally—in reparative regression. Ferenczi (1926) was a firm believer in the need to observe the patient's bodily attitudes and bodily postures, as an integrated part of therapy. His unorthodox somatic attitude emphasised play and human interaction, and deeply influenced Wilhelm Reich, who admired Ferenczi's creative freedom and his uncompromising therapeutic style (Conger, 1988).

Ferenczi related the capacity to surrender to imagination and free-flowing feelings, as required in free association, to the ability to relax the muscular system (Ferenczi, 1925). He understood that increasing muscular tension could increase emotional tension and the levels of charge, and subsequently tailored his relaxation techniques, which involved muscle-relaxation and hypnosis, to overcome emotional inhibitions and facilitate surrender to the therapeutic process. This active stance, together with his own willingness to surrender to tender and loving relationships (not only the authoritative and rigid relationship) allowed for, and even encouraged, regression and strong transference love from (and to) his patients. In his most significant contribution, "Confusion of Tongues between the Adult and the Child", Ferenczi (1933) emphasised the importance of soft and gentle communication with the child (the language of tenderness), and compared the therapeutic relationship to the relationship between a parent and a small child. For reparative healing experience to take place, argued Ferenczi, the patients need to be allowed to regress to their earlier somatic, preverbal memories and only then to process them verbally within therapy. Ferenczi (1930) relayed a conversation with Anna Freud, where she jokingly remarked that Ferenczi related to his adult patients in the same way she related to the children she treated.

Ferenczi's psychotherapy was therefore more emotionally and bodily active than classic psychoanalysis. It focused on the possibility for genuine change (not merely the sublimation of drives, which was Freud's perceived therapeutic outcome)—a change that began with the inner work of psychoanalysts themselves and only later continued with their patients (Borgogno, 2004).

Based on his experience with severely disturbed patients (whom Freud considered unsuitable for analysis), Ferenczi deduced that Freud abandoned the connection between psychic pain and real life traumas too early (and here we can already identify Ferenczi's impact on attachment theory and object relations, which will be discussed in the Appendix, as well as on feminist psychology). When therapists insisted on directing their attention solely to the patients' inner world while ignoring real traumas, Ferenczi thought, the analytic abstinence could become wounding and potentially shaming, and may even repeat and perpetuate the original trauma (Ferenczi, 1933). He understood the therapeutic endeavour as attempting to stop the cycle of repetition compulsion with the help of the therapeutic relationship. According to Ferenczi, the analyst's cold and composed position, as it manifested in the principle of frustration (actively avoiding the satisfaction of needs), was not always appropriate—even though it was a central and respected principle in psychoanalysis. The analytic rule of abstinence (or principle of frustration) relates to actively avoiding the satisfaction of the patient's needs, or alternatively engaging in systematic frustration of the patient's needs for validation and confirmation of the therapist's love. This principle was meant to provide space for the patients to sense their passion and needs and familiarise themselves with those needs, a possibility that would be denied by immediate satisfaction.

However, Ferenczi argued that for some patients, the analyst's aloof position could symbolise a direct continuation of their childhood struggle with authority, thus repeating the neurotic symptoms associated with these authority figures. Naturally, just as it was imperative to look at Ernest Jones's accusations against Ferenczi as an unfinished residue of their analysis, it was also clear that Ferenczi's criticism on psychoanalysis, and his clinical and theoretical choices thereafter, were in correspondence to his unfinished analysis with Freud, which was terminated by the analyst. Ferenczi held that Freud failed to sufficiently work through his negative countertransference towards him, and was wounded by the termination (Dupont, 1994). If Freud was seen as the father of psychoanalysis, then Ferenczi's language of tenderness and his loving stance led to a frequent description of him as "the first mother of psychoanalysis" (Meyer, 2005).

Ferenczi was the first to challenge the analytic taboo against the analyst's self-disclosure. He viewed the therapeutic space as a shared human creation, an intersubjective field opening between patient and therapist (Orange & Stolorow, 1998). In so doing, Ferenczi diverted the therapeutic focus from the patient's intrapsychic experience to the emerging relationship, as it was weaved between patient and therapist, when the meaning of the relationship in the here-and-now was a fertile ground for insight development—and for reparatory therapeutic processes (Rachman, 2001; Rachman & Ceccoli, 1996).

Ferenczi's work was unique and groundbreaking, yet his significant contributions to object relations theory and relational psychoanalysis were far more familiar than his contributions to body psychotherapy. The following vignette demonstrates a body psychotherapeutic intervention which was influenced by his work.

Lilly was a small woman, beautiful and positive. She had been married for many years with no children. Lilly's eyes were mostly sparkling, full of aliveness and she was well groomed and softly spoken. Lilly came to therapy at sixty and we worked together for about six years. She was one of the most creative people I have ever known, yet when we met, Lilly was preoccupied with fears and anxiety and actively avoided many mundane and everyday activities. Her life was therefore quite limited. During her entire childhood, she was subjected to emotional and physical abuse from her mother, while her father was mostly absent—preoccupied with his multiple affairs, which bore other children too. For many years, Lilly's mum attempted to seduce the father back into the family home and in her despair used Lilly for this purpose: she tore Lilly's clothes demanding the father came back home to buy his daughter some clothes "since she has nothing to wear". Alternatively, the mother asked the father to come and discipline his rogue daughter. Lilly described herself through the eyes of her mother: "I'm a stupid unlovable little girl," she frequently said.

During our work, Lilly started daring, taking more initiative in her life while gradually differentiating from her tyrannical mother, and slowly developed compassion and understanding towards her. Transference dynamics were strong and paternal, thus much of the work was done in regressive spaces. My strong paternal feelings towards Lilly, knowing the extent of her deprivation of love and the tenderness between us, made Ferenczi's theory and practice central to our shared work, and his spirit was present in the clinical room and influenced the development of my therapeutic interventions.

It was during a period when my daughter Zohar was a baby, waking up nearly every hour, every night. Tom and I were exhausted, and I found it very difficult to function at work. I clearly recall the feeling of walking inside a cloud, struggling to sense my feet. In the clinic, I found myself frequently drifting into sleep, tired, unfocused, and operating in a trance-like state most of the time. Although I was never bored with Lilly—quite the opposite—I nevertheless found it exceptionally tempting to fall asleep, to let go and fall asleep.

Notwithstanding the erotic aspects of our transference, our relationship was markedly regressive and primarily paternal and pre-oedipal (my conceptualisation of the oedipal complex is different to Freud's and will be explicitly explored in Chapter Six), and Lilly frequently called me "Daddy Asaf", which I admittedly liked a lot. Our relationship provided Lilly with an opportunity to reconnect—as a young girl—with the father that she never had, and mourn the loss of her childhood. As for me, I was blessed with a chance to have a daughter for whom I was the favourite parent and who actively sought connection with me at a time when my own daughter was completely mesmerised by her mother and took very little interest in me, her father.

One day, during a session, Lilly asked if I was willing to hold her. It was not a rare request; physical holding formed an important part of our therapeutic work and it deepened the mutual trust and connection. We lay on the mattress and Lilly rested in my arms like a young girl; we were silent. I felt a joyous bond weaving between us, and a sweetness that I knew from connection with my daughter was spreading in my body. I surrendered to those softly pleasurable sensations and without noticing the passing time, I woke myself up with a loud snore. Apprehensively, I looked up and met Lilly's eyes, and was surprised to find her gleaming with happiness. "You fell asleep, you fell asleep," she cried with joy. "You fell asleep and you were snoring, Daddy Asaf."

During the following sessions there was a marked difference in Lilly's trust. It was as if she allowed herself to surrender to our relationship more authentically and fully. During these sessions, I learned that her father rarely slept at home; his visits were always brief and practical, and Lilly yearned for him to stay, so that she could have a real family.

Zohar's birth a few months previously shook our therapeutic relationship and threatened our alliance. Lilly had known that I had had a baby girl and my three weeks of paternity leave became a source of fear and potentially enacted a painful sense of her being the unchosen child. Lilly voiced her fear that the story of her life would repeat itself: the father who left the nuclear family and moved to another family; the father who abandoned her and chose the new girl over her. My therapeutic nodding-off (while holding her) made me the father who stayed; the father who chose Lilly as well. Lilly began to trust me and brought more of herself into therapy—becoming more loyal to our connection, and to herself. For months later we processed and celebrated the importance of this shared nodding-off and the trust that developed from it. Gradually, and alongside our father–daughter relationship (which was there all along and will always be there), Lilly grew up and matured and we have even managed to sometimes meet as two adult subjectivities.

Wilhelm Reich (1897–1957)

> It has forever been the aspiration of mankind to fly like a bird, to become a wind, a breath; and it can be done, but it is paid for by the loss of body, or the loss of humanity, which is the same thing.
>
> —Carl Gustav Jung (Jung & Jarrett, 1988, p. xix).[1]

What man is he that desireth life?

One of Freud's most brilliant disciples and certainly a most colourful figure in the history of psychoanalysis was the eccentric psychiatrist Wilhelm Reich. Reich was born in Galicia to Jewish parents, but his father did not raise him as a Jew and resented his own Jewishness. Reich was home-schooled, educated by a private tutor, and was described as an extremely lonely child (Sharaf, 1984).

Reich's early life was full of tragedies. The son of a strict and cold father, Willy was allowed to play neither with his peasant peers nor with the Yiddish speaking Jewish children. His curiosity and desperate need for connection were thus directed at the natural world. Willy was particularly fascinated by sexuality and its varied expressions. Wilhelm the boy used to drag his brother and they both stared at the mating farm animals for hours on end: while Robert was disgusted, Wilhelm was fascinated and captivated. He later stalked a household worker and peeked into her room, fascinated by her sexual activities with her lover. When nosy Reich discovered that his mother and his private tutor were having an affair, he spent long hours secretly staring at their lovemaking. This affair went on for a while, and after some time the guilt-stricken young boy Wilhelm told his father about his mother's affair.

Wilhelm's angry and jealous father confronted the mother while Wilhelm was present at the room, requested by his father to serve as an eyewitness. Wilhelm's mother, fearful of her husband's wrath and the foreseen punishment, and full of guilt, committed suicide by swallowing poison, and Wilhelm became orphaned of his mother at the age of eleven. His other significant attachment figure, the private tutor, was immediately fired and Wilhelm's life was completely ruined. Wilhelm's father, guilt-stricken, grief-bound, and furious, intentionally exposed himself to illness—he spent long hours outdoors, standing waist-deep in muddy ponds fishing until he caught pneumonia, which quickly escalated to tuberculosis. He died a few years after his wife and left the sixteen-year-old Wilhelm orphan and alone in the world.

George Atwood and Robert Stolorow (1977), both central figures in intersubjective psychoanalysis, assumed that these early tragedies paved the way to developing Reich's seminal contributions, and provided a biographical rationale for Reich's extensive (and sometimes exclusive) focus on sexuality in his theories.

Readers who are interested in the life and work of Wilhelm Reich could find fascinating accounts in David Boadella's (1976, 1985) professional reviews and in the excellent biography by Myron Sharaf (1984).

Reich meets psychoanalysis

In 1919, after completing his military service on the Austro-Russian front during World War I, the twenty-two-year-old Wilhelm began his medical studies in Vienna. He was stimulated by the "new science" of psychoanalysis, above all curious about the concept of the libido, and pursued his psychoanalytic studies with Freud, who was extremely impressed by Reich and valued him greatly. Initially, Reich directed his clinical attention to his patients' psychosomatic complaints, and thereafter turned to methodically research the bodily expressions of psychological disorders. Reich predominantly focused on the function of the autonomic (vegetative) nervous system of his patients and observed how thoughts, ideas, and emotional disturbances resulted in oscillating autonomic reactions: changes in breathing rhythms, skin colour and texture, temperature changes, and muscular contractions. These changes, he had come to realise, correlated to emotional changes and created distinctive patterns which he could then diagnose, analyse, and subsequently treat.

Reich continued to develop Freud's theory of sexual repression, which defined specific and distinct developmental stages (oral, anal, and more). Fixation during any of these stages resulted in pathology. Reich examined how different stages of libidinal fixation manifested in distinguished somatic organisation (Reich, 1933a). He conducted experiments and methodically observed his patients, examining how different neurotic positions were manifested in the body, particularly in the formation of the musculature. Reich noticed that early developmental arrests were also expressed in unmistakeably characterised muscular patterns, which he consequently termed *body armour* or *muscular armour*, a concept he later continued to develop and characterise for many years (and which will be further discussed here).

In direct continuation of Freud's early theoretical position, Reich adopted the centrality of the libido to our life and our health. For him, health and well-being were expressed in the capacity to love freely (love which also received a physical, sexual expression) and work freely, that is, to function in the world and in relationships. For him, in order to freely and authentically live we had to surrender to the vital energy which was flowing within us—the libido (Reich, 1942) (can you notice similarities with Mesmer's cosmic magnetism?). The climactic expression of this libidinal flow, and the most central dynamic for the living organism was the orgasm reflex. The orgasm reflex was a much wider concept than climax or ejaculation during intercourse, and represented a true involuntary surrender to the energy of life itself. For Reich (1960), during the full orgasm the organism became part of the pulsating universe.

Reich (1942) considered the body and mind as functionally identical: "Psychic and the somatic operate from the point of biopsychic energy, as two systems, which are unitary as well as conditioning each other" (p. 26). He correlated the Freudian drive-bound id with the autonomic nervous system which he came to understand as a highly organised system, one that deserved methodical examination (R. Carroll, 2002).

In a professional era where the body was cursed and shamed, and given his own history, Reich wished, perhaps even needed, to reclaim the body as a source for aliveness and connectedness.

Reich presented his orgasm theory at the 1924 psychoanalytic conference in Saltzburg, his first attempt to establish a cohesive scientific and methodical system for dealing with neuroses. He furthered his research and published *Character Analysis* in 1933 (1933a), receiving professional and personal validation and acknowledgement. However, his distinct views on libidinal drives and his emphasis on the bodily aspects of sexuality gradually alienated him from Freud, and at the end of the 1920s their ways separated. Reich moved to Berlin where he was still considered a respectable psychoanalyst.

Muscular armour

In 1927, Reich presented his first theory of character armour at the tenth congress of the International Psychoanalytical Association in Innsbruck, Austria. Reich demonstrated how character analysis could diagnose the muscular armour and treat it. His clinical observations illuminated how repression of aggressive drives, anxieties, pleasure, or any other powerful emotion had also a consistent muscular expression—either hypertonic (highly strung) muscular holding or hypotonic (low) muscle tone. Reich related to the character armour as a history frozen in space, a bodily expression of developmental rigidities (Boadella, 1985). Loosening these chronically contracted muscles, argued Reich, could release the frozen emotion and retrieve the free-flowing biopsychic energy.

The concept of muscular armour was central to Reich's philosophy and was certainly one of his most significant contributions. Reich suggested (1933a) that the neurotic solution for the infantile drive conflict (the conflict between drives and the social world, or in Freudian terms between the pleasure principle and reality principle), expressed itself in characterological and muscular changes that gradually habituated and rigidified to create *character*. The muscular armour was therefore understood as the organism's way of organising itself against the flow of life, with the goal of protecting the person. To reiterate: this was the first somatic expression of a defence mechanism. For example, a child whose parents rejected any expression of anger will have learned to repress the expression (and later, the feeling) of anger first by tightening the muscles used for expressing anger (for example, the jaw muscles), so the angry affect did not receive any visible muscular expression. When this experience repeated itself, a chronic bodily character was organised and muscular armour was created: this was a rigid and inflexible psychosomatic organisation.

While severe external and internal pressure could create extreme rigidities, the formation of muscular armour (rigid muscular organisation) was a human process, not merely a pathological one. Just as we could not avoid developing psychological defence mechanisms, the development of muscular armour was similarly inevitable. The muscular armour was an evidence of our political body—one that responded to familial, societal, and cultural pressures; a regulatory agent for intolerable sensations and feelings (R. Carroll, 2002, 2009), a bodily compromise for attaining the possibility for love.

Reich's theoretical and clinical contributions represented the pillars on which modern body psychotherapy was constructed. In the Innsbruck congress Reich portrayed a methodical system of psychoanalysis that included theoretical and clinical applications of working with body and with touch, with the aim of softening the muscular armour (or, in Reichian terminology, breaking the armour), in order to allow for a less defensive and more adaptive psychosomatic organisation (Boadella, 1985). Since one of the objectives of psychotherapy was melting frozen aspects of the personality, Reich offered a possible path for achieving this through disentangling psychosomatic patterns.

The idea that muscular relaxation could assist in freeing pent-up feeling was indeed not new, even in Reich's era: Ferenczi too directed his clinical attention to muscular relaxation and as we noted earlier, Janet applied deep-tissue massage to his hysterical patients. However, Reich was the first psychoanalyst to offer a methodical exploration of the somatic mechanisms involved in the processes of repression, dissociation, and other defence mechanisms, as well as offering organised and consistent methods for clinically resolving and working with those bodily mechanisms.

Reich understood that chronically tensed muscles became an inseparable element of our regulation system for repressing unexpressed emotions (Reich, 1942), and his cathartic treatment was directly derived from his theory. In his practice he encouraged patients to fully and completely express and discharge repressed feelings, thus allowing the life-energy which was at the core of every person to flow uninterruptedly (Boadella, 1988). The goal of therapy was, for Reich, assisting his patients to completely and involuntarily surrender to the force of life within themselves, as it was expressed in involuntary bodily movement and in the respiratory system (the autonomic, vegetative nervous system) (Lowen, 1975). For Reich, breathing fully and freely and being able to reach a whole-body orgasm were important markers for health.

Unless we directed our attention to the muscular armour, believed Reich, therapeutic process would be limited to insight and understanding and would fail to allow a genuine freedom from restrictive patterns of behaviours, feelings, and thoughts. Our human vitality might then be neglected and forever remain frozen in our tissues, on the immediate somatic level. When unmediated bodily techniques were practised, we could make direct contact with this life-energy and liberate the somatic aspect of the conflict, thus allowing for uninterrupted analytic work to take place, assisting patients in retrieving their self-regulatory capacities and their ability to fully experience pleasure.

Touch

Reich directly worked with the body, and also incorporated psychotherapeutic touch, while (partly) acknowledging the complexity and challenges that touch may introduce into therapy, and he integrated touch techniques with psychoanalytic theoretical foundations and psychoanalytic techniques. He used deep-tissue bodywork and muscular relaxation, working with postural reorganisation and breathwork, and furthered the exploration of cathartic work even after Freud abandoned the analytic work with catharsis. Nonetheless, as far as Reich was concerned his work was still founded on sound psychoanalytic theory and even when others no longer considered his work as psychoanalytic, Reich continued to view himself as a psychoanalyst (Boadella, 1976; West, 1994). Reich found it important to emphasise that the bodily interventions he used in analysis were categorically different from massage or physiotherapeutic manipulation (such as joint mobilisation), but instead formed an integral part of his psychoanalytic praxis.

The basic Reichian theory postulated that the muscular armour held locked-up energy and that by breaking the armour this energy could be released. It is important, however, to differentiate Reichian theory from Reich's therapeutic style which was highly confrontational, frequently aggressive, and deploying his power (and insisted on maintaining therapeutic hierarchy). Reich was attracted to working with negative transference (and with resistance) and he frequently encouraged it directly and strongly—Reich sought anger, hate, and envy. His extraverted and extreme therapeutic style was highly popular, particularly since it provided an alternative to the conservative and distanced stance of traditional psychoanalytic positioning. On the other hand, his style also planted great fears both in professional circles and the public and fuelled strong personal and professional criticisms and prejudice against him and against his methods (Boadella, 1985; C. Young, 2011a).

Reich's therapeutic strategy of "breaking the armour", which was frequently insufficiently sensitive to the patient's defences and needs, has gone through many developments and sublimations in modern body psychotherapy. Today, most body psychotherapists are more respectful of their clients' defence mechanisms (including bodily ones) and work with these creatively and from within the context of the therapeutic relationship. Chapter Ten, in the Clinical Part, expands and exemplifies working with touch in relational body psychotherapy.

Sex and politics

Reich believed that with the support of appropriate sexual education, challenging and deconstructing oppressive social structures, and appropriate psychotherapeutic work, many neuroses could be prevented. His theories were summarised and published in his book *Sexual Revolution*, in 1930. The political body is still a central shaping agent today. Consensual gender typology, consumerist and societal pressures, and religious dogma all create us as bodies that are geared to discontentedness and shame (Orbach, 2009).

Reich's eccentric views regarding sexuality and politics directly put him at risk when the Nazi party came to power in 1933 (since Reich was a Marxist, as well as a Jew) and Reich wisely left Germany. After a few intermittent breaks, Reich arrived in Oslo, where he developed a body-centred psychotherapy which he called Character-Analytic Vegetotherapy, which focused on interventions directed at changing the autonomic (vegetative) nervous system. His vegetotherapy broke two psychoanalytic taboos: touching the client, and nudity. Upon leaving Berlin, Reich also began teaching vegetotherapy in Europe, and later trained some therapists in the USA.

Before leaving Germany in 1933, Reich established a number of clinics in Berlin, which specialised in treating sexual problems. These clinics offered radical treatments for the time (and for many people, they would still be considered radical) and the clinics were successful and very popular. Reich's public sex clinics and his communist-Marxist activity attracted the wrath of many conservative middle class psychoanalysts who formed the heart of the International Psychoanalytical Association. The publishing of his book *The Mass Psychology of Fascism* (1933b), where Reich marked sexual repression as one of the political forces allowing for social oppression, infuriated the psychoanalytic mainstream who turned against him even more righteously. In 1934, following a deterioration in the relationship between Reich and the organisation, and the unbridgeable theoretical, clinical, and political gaps, Reich was shamefully expelled from the International Psychoanalytical Association.

Breathing

Around 1935 Reich began to notice that muscular organisation was highly influenced by breathing patterns. Once more, these findings were not new: breathwork has been used for centuries as a powerful tool for changing states of consciousness as well as for supporting psychological states, but these practices were outside of Cartesian cultures—in yoga, traditional dancing, Buddhism, shamanism, and more; yet Reich managed to convey the importance of breathing to the professional Western psychotherapeutic milieu. He demonstrated, for example, how children would create (consciously and unconsciously) disturbances in their breathing rhythms and use diaphragmatic tensions to deal with anxieties, and how these gradually became chronic and rigidified in the body (Boadella, 1985). Reich further deepened and characterised different patterns of breathing and types of holding the breath that correlated with specific character structures and typified a variety of ways to self-regulate and exercise control over feelings through breath. Many body psychotherapy modalities have used those clinical ideas since and further developed them. Chapter Nine will demonstrate clinical breathwork in body psychotherapy and exemplify some possible ways of working with breath.

Orgone: the cosmic energy

Unfortunately, Reich's ideas became increasingly more eccentric and less conventional and together with his radical politics, his clinical contributions drifted further apart from the psychoanalytic mainstream. Sadly, even some of his earlier significant contributions were pushed away due to his extreme later theoretical and political positions and the fields he turned to to investigate, which included esoteric subjects.

In a recent conference I participated in, a renowned Lacanian psychoanalyst spoke of Reich as psychotic; she mentioned it in passing, as if it was a known and agreed fact. It is a great shame Reich is still viewed in some psychoanalytic circles through the prejudiced and distorted historical lens. Similarly, it was not until Michael Balint brought Ferenczi's work to the UK that Ferenczi re-entered psychoanalytic thinking. The piercing words of Freud's biographer Ernest Jones, who announced without doubt that Ferenczi was mentally ill, were a character murder. Few had stopped to consider his words within the transferential context of client-therapist, an oedipal account of a client who managed to murder his father (Ferenczi, his analyst) and take his place besides the great oracle (Freud, who was Ferenczi's analyst), thus delivering a classical oedipal triumph, as unresolved as such triumph could be.

Between the years 1935 and 1955, Reich's research turned away from psychotherapy and he invested most of his resources in the physical exploration of somatic energy. Reich claimed that he discovered the existence of primordial cosmic energy that flowed everywhere in the universe, as well as within us; he called this energy *orgone*. This energy could be seen as paralleling the Chinese philosophy concept of Chi (qi), perhaps even to the Taoist Tao; and comparison to Mesmer's cosmic animal magnetism is unavoidable. According to his energetic perception, the goal of therapy for Reich changed into the attempt to retrieve energetic balance within the person—reconnecting with the orgiastic potential (the flow of orgone) of the patient, hence strengthening the patient's capacity for self-regulation and functioning. Bodywork became a concrete compass for the bodymind experience for flow.

In 1939, Reich left Europe and moved to the USA, where he built and sold his "orgone accumulator", a phone-booth sized construction, which Reich believed could accumulate this cosmic energy and release it in a controlled manner back into our bodies, thus accelerating healing and initiating rebalancing processes. At first, the orgone accumulator was but an addition to therapy, particularly when patients presented with psychosomatic symptomatology or organic diseases, or to support patients with very low levels of energy. Gradually, however, Reich argued that the accumulated energy in the orgone accumulator could weaken malignant cells, strengthen the immune system, and shrink tumours. After he publicly argued in his book *The Cancer Biopathy* (1948) that the orgone accumulator could cure cancer, his destiny was sealed. It was an unforgivable strategic mistake in this anti-Marxist and anti-communist political environment, where governing agencies were already seeking to prevent Reich from spreading his "damaging" opinions. Indeed, the US Food and Drug Administration (FDA) were quick to issue an injunction against the manufacturing and distributing of the orgone accumulator, and once Reich (true to form) violated the injunction he was sentenced and imprisoned (Boadella, 1976, 1985; Sharaf, 1984). On 23 August 1956, in New York, the FDA initiated the burning of six tons of Reich's books, papers, and articles. His physical death in jail, in November 1957—quite near his scheduled release date—was but a shadow of his ideological and professional murder a year earlier.

Aside from their clear theoretical and clinical resemblance, I find the historical parallel between Franz Mesmer and Wilhelm Reich uncanny; they both offered holistic ideas far ahead of their time. They both emerged from the mainstream, and challenged theoretical and clinical boundaries; they both miserably failed in appreciating the political maturity of the time and in the ability to contain their ideas and clinical practice; they both attracted envy attacks and wrath which created a foggy buffer, thus preventing other practitioners from professionally and objectively engaging with their important contributions. However, the ideas of both Mesmer and Reich have regained popularity and have in the last decades received increasing interest; today Reich's books are no longer burned.

In the wake of Reich

During the 1940s and 1950s Reich taught and trained many professionals. Elsworth Baker (1967) and other formal students of "medical orgonomy" continued to develop Reich's orgone experiments and formed the College for Orgonomy and the *Journal of Orgonomy*; but this group had minor influence on the development of body psychotherapy outside the orgonomy circles.

Among the second generation of body psychotherapists (who were directly trained by Reich) worth mentioning are Alexander Lowen, who together with John Pierrakos established bioenergetics, Charles Kelly who created a form of body psychotherapy called Radix, and Norwegian Ola Raknes who studied vegetotherapy and was a major influence on Gerda Boyesen, the founder of biodynamic psychotherapy (Eiden, 2011). The next chapter will discuss some of the main disciplines of body psychotherapy.

One tender touch

The following vignette demonstrates an integration of Reichian principles for working methodically with the body within a therapeutic position that was strongly influenced by Ferenczi's thinking. This case vignette highlights for me the rich therapeutic potential for working directly with embodied processes in psychotherapy, potential that both men, the forefathers of body psychotherapy, were mindful of.

Meeting Ronny for the first time was a very surprising experience for me. Ronny was a tall, strong, and impressive man and he seemed like a retired general. Physically, he looked like one of my favourite actors, Donald Sutherland. Ronny was eighty-three and it was his first time to seek therapy. During the initial conversation, I discovered that indeed Ronny had an impressive military history in an elite unit of the Israel Defense Forces; he retired as a high-ranking officer and after his retirement Ronny worked in managerial positions in big Israeli corporations. Five years earlier Ronny lost his wife, and two years later he was diagnosed with colon cancer. Following surgical complications and the subsequent chemotherapy and radiotherapy, Ronny was left with a stoma and catheter and no sphincter control (this is why he chose to keep the stoma).

Ronny described how his world fell apart during these last few years. From a powerful and fully functioning man he had become, in his words, "a depressed doormat". His daughter cared for him, bathed him, and nursed him and he spent many days in bed unwilling and unmotivated to get up, preoccupied with the sense of humiliation and castration and engaged with suicidal ideation. During these last five years not only had Ronny lost his wife and dignity, he narrated, but he also experienced physical pain on a daily basis, and required invasive medical procedures at least fortnightly. His general practitioner suggested that he sought psychotherapy to complement his antidepressants and I came recommended by a friend of his daughter. The body he brought into therapy was anything but the idealised and romanticised body of the early body psychotherapy modalities; a body that always knows and never lies, a body which is a source of pleasure and connectedness. No, Ronny's body was a body of deceit and betrayal, of pain and humiliation.

For ten sessions we tried (and perhaps failed) to understand and validate Ronny's grim and painful reality. How hard it must have been for him to sit in front of me, a then young man at the beginning of my personal and professional life. Ronny did not try to conceal his disdain for my life experience (which truly was incomparable to his), yet when I acknowledged the limitation of my experience and our age gap, and suggested to refer him to a more mature and experienced therapist, Ronny refused, dismissing the offer with: "I cannot be bothered to tell my story from the beginning, again." The first ten sessions were unpleasant and charged. Ronny sat at the edge of his chair, tense, contracted, and angry. From our very first session I wanted to reach out and touch him, allowing him to sense touch that was not invasive, hurting, or shaming. But I was embarrassed. I felt apprehensive to offer a therapeutic intervention that could portray me as soft or not masculine enough.

During our tenth session Ronny complained that "this therapy" was too difficult and exhausting for him. "We are busy sparring against one another," I suggested and Ronny nodded. I shared with him my sense that an emotional change was difficult to attain when one's body was so contracted and I offered, with great trepidations, that in the next session we could work with breathing and touch. Ronny promised to consider, and arrived to the next session willing to experiment.

Ronny lay on the massage table; his breathing was flat and almost invisible and his stomach was tense. I did not know how to approach him, too busy with my reactive countertransference to authority figures and military generals. I quietly suggested to Ronny that he tried breathing into his abdomen, and when he could not understand my suggestion, I gently placed a hand over his stomach, to demonstrate and facilitate his breathing. His own hand, which supported his stomach, inadvertently touched mine and we had a moment of soft and unplanned connection. For a brief second, Ronny hesitated whether to remove his hand or keep it there, and then his hand came back, tightening its grip on my own hand. I was so moved that I stopped breathing.

Ronny breathed, slowly and with great pain. His hand held mine with unimaginable force and we both cried (I think I also cried from the physical pain). In a moment of sharing nonverbal connection, we transformed from two fighting men to companions. The rest of our psychotherapeutic work, which lasted for just over a year, was characterised by regular hand-holding and slow breathing. Ronny's body did not transform from a body-of-pain to a body-of-pleasure, but physical contact helped in processing and tolerating the suffering.

Exercise: tracking down our breathing

(Alone or with a guiding partner)

The following exercise is based on Reich's perception regarding the central role of breathing, both in health and in ill health. This is a very basic process that could strengthen body sensations, sharpen our ability to listen to our bodies, and centre[2] ourselves. During the first practice, you may possibly experience pleasant as well as unpleasant feelings and sensations, including pain or difficulty. I recommend adopting a curious and observing attitude towards any sensation, emotion, or thought that appears, telling you about the here-and-now of your bodily experience.

1. Position yourself comfortably, sitting barefoot with your feet resting on the ground or lying down on your back with bent knees and your feet touching the ground.
2. Allow yourself to breathe quietly for a few moments, and witness your breath. Can you breathe without trying to change the breath? Let yourself notice subtleties of breath. Where is it natural and flowing? Where is it effortful?
3. Are there any body parts that feel as if they are not breathing? If so, invite breath into these parts. You can do it by imagining that with every inhale you are directing nourishment and breath to this part. You can support this visualisation by gently touching this body part.
4. What happens to the rest of the body when breathing arrives to those body parts? What happens to you? Allow yourself to pay attention to sensations, feelings, and thoughts and be mindful of different facets of your experience. Let every experience, pleasant or unpleasant, become a valuable and educating experience.
5. Repeat steps 2–4 a few times, to allow for a fuller breath, and observing the impact of this breath on all of you.

Notes

1. Reprinted with kind permission of Princeton University Press.
2. Centring is a basic concept in body psychotherapy. The second and third parts will explain and exemplify its nature. Centring relates to our capacity to sense our bodymind centre and act from it, from a place where we feel present and vital and are able to cultivate a benevolent internal and external position.

CHAPTER THREE

A roadmap to body psychotherapy modalities

> Here's my wisdom for your use, as I learned it when the moose
> and the reindeer roamed where Paris roars to-night:—
> "There are nine and sixty ways of constructing tribal lays,
> And every single one of them is right!"
>
> —*Rudyard Kipling*, In the Neolithic Age (2002)

Nine and sixty ways

Alice Miller (1981) had rejected the altruistic reasons for becoming a psychotherapist. This professional choice has usually begun with our own wound: most psychotherapists assumed a role reversal in their family—and were highly attuned to the needs of their parents. Thus, many of us have made a profession out of our pathology, and if we were lucky enough, we worked through some of these issues so they were not the *only* leading force in our working life choices. As analytic body psychotherapist Guy Gladstone (personal communications, 1999–2013) repeatedly said: "Most therapists attempted to save their mothers; the rest—were there to save their dads."

I am left curious as to the biographical forces operating when we choose a psychotherapy modality to specialise in. What is it that attracts people to train in a specific modality of psychotherapy? Are there any commonalities to those who train in a particular modality? What brings people to choose psychoanalysis or cognitive-behavioural therapy; humanistic psychotherapy or family therapy? What attracts practitioners to the field of body psychotherapy? Like many other psychotherapeutic fields, body psychotherapy attracted ambitious, creative, opinionated, and complex students and clinicians, all of whom acquired varied models of training and many sought for their own particular therapeutic and personal voice to be heard. As a discipline that attempted to integrate body and mind, the verbal and nonverbal, a discipline with wild and anarchistic roots yet one that also sought scientific grounding, body psychotherapy tended to attract individuals whose issues concern splitting and integrating, paradoxes and contradictions, complex attitudes to authority figures, embodiment and disembodiment. Appropriately, there are many modalities within body psychotherapy today—some of them hold contradictory theoretical and clinical positions. These modalities may differ in their theoretical orientations or clinical applications, in their therapeutic emphases, or the variation of tools and techniques at their disposal.

However, all body psychotherapy modalities perceive the *self* as an embodied entity. In other words, the self is understood as experienced *in* the body and *through* the body. Emotional experiences are processed in psychotherapy through conversation (talking psychotherapy), but also in unmediated bodily ways using methods such as touch, increasing sensory awareness, breathing, movement, and more (Eiden, 2011).

Most modern modalities of body psychotherapy were influenced, directly or indirectly, by Wilhelm Reich (whose ideas were described in the previous chapter) and maintained a certain dialogue with his work—just like most psychotherapeutic modalities maintained a dialogue with Freud and his work (Goodrich-Dunn, 2004); but for historical reasons, the contemporary clinical practice of body psychotherapy is mostly disconnected from its psychoanalytic roots. While the first and second generation of body psychotherapists acquired their training within the psychiatric and psychoanalytic establishment, later generations were primarily trained in the humanistic psychology streams and the "human potential" movement in the United States and Europe. Some types of body psychotherapy developed from adjacent fields, such as bodywork and spiritual or shamanic disciplines. One such example is Gerda Boyesen's biodynamic psychology, which was based on Boyesen's training in psychiatric physiotherapy (Boyesen, 1980; R. Carroll, 2002). Another example is Ilana Rubenfeld's "synergy method", which Rubenfeld created (Rubenfeld, 2000, 2001) based on her experience in music, movement, and Gestalt.

This chapter attempts to bring some order to the variety of disciplines in body psychotherapy. The chapter will explore the main orientations and submodalities in body psychotherapy. Readers who are interested in deepening their exploration of body psychotherapy modalities will enjoy Nick Totton's review in his excellent book *Body Psychotherapy: An Introduction* (2003). Readers who are interested in a comprehensive review of dance and movement therapy are invited to look at Helen Payne's book (1992) on the subject. This chapter is largely based on the structure suggested by Totton. The websites of both the United States Association for Body Psychotherapy (www.usabp.org) and the European Association of Body Psychotherapy (www.eabp.org) provide comprehensive information about the variety of body psychotherapy modalities, as well as hundreds of accessible professional papers about body psychotherapy. Choosing which disciplines to cover and review here, and to what extent, was directly influenced by my own theoretical and clinical orientation.

In addition to reviewing some categories of body psychotherapy, I have also chosen to mention some bodywork modalities that are not psychotherapy but adjacent to psychotherapy (such as "rebirthing"). In so doing, I wish to acknowledge some of the historical sources of body psychotherapy, which were created and further developed outside the psychotherapeutic milieu. These bodywork methods are "close relatives" of body psychotherapy. Additionally, some bodywork modalities become, over time, body psychotherapy methods. When practitioners of a deep bodywork modality become more aware of transference dimensions and integrate such understandings in their practice, it comes closer to psychotherapeutic practice and deserves to be noted (an excellent example is Rosen method bodywork). In my opinion, for a therapy to be considered psychotherapy it needs to demonstrate a unique and cohesive philosophical model (theory of mind, developmental theory, ethics, and more), a clear diagnostic stance (including psychopathology), and applicable translation of these principles into therapeutic interventions (techniques and therapeutic skills).

In presenting this road map to body psychotherapy modalities I used two main sources, both categorised body psychotherapy in ways I found useful. The first is the doctoral dissertation of Stephanie Rauch (2005). Rauch looked at the difference between body psychotherapists and traditional counsellors and created an impressive mapping of the field. The second source, which I have already mentioned, is Nick Totton (2003), one of the most fertile and influential writers and clinicians in the field of body psychotherapy, whose contribution to the field uniquely transcends body psychotherapy. Totton is one of the few body psychotherapists who regularly appears in psychoanalytic journals and books (1998, 2006) and is therefore a significant ambassador of the field to the broader psychotherapeutic milieu. Totton's own clinical modality, embodied relational therapy, will be expanded upon towards the end of this chapter.

The division offered in this chapter is predominantly based on Totton's, although I removed one of his categories (integrative body psychotherapy), added another (relational body psychotherapy), and changed the inner organisation to better fit my own theoretical understanding while also drawing from Rauch and other sources (Eiden, 2009; Smith, 1985; C. Young, 2011c, 2011d).

The variety of body psychotherapy categories and the multitude of modalities within them do not contradict the common base they share, which will be presented in the theoretical and clinical Parts. Among other reasons, this versatility also results from the fact that body psychotherapy has been vitally alive and developing for many decades. I have divided body psychotherapy modalities into six categories: Reichian body psychotherapy, personal development and human potential treatments, body psychotherapy for trauma work, process oriented body psychotherapy, expressive body psychotherapy, and relational body psychotherapy.

Reichian body psychotherapy

Wilhelm Reich trained many practitioners in Europe and the US, and a large number of body psychotherapy modalities remained faithful to the theoretical and clinical foundations he laid, some of which were presented in Chapter Two. The concepts of energy, muscular armour, and inner vitality are still central in most of the Reichian and neo-Reichian psychotherapeutic modalities. According to Nick Totton (2003), all Reichian psychotherapies share the following four assumptions:

1. We are understood as comprised of pulsating energetic fields.
2. Flow and pulsation represent health, while obstructions to pulsation and flow represent ill health.

3. We are in our nature full of vitality, love, creativity, and productivity.
4. Social and familial oppression is the primary reason for disturbances in our natural and organic capacity to flow.

Another characteristic aspect of Reichian body psychotherapies is the centrality of bodily techniques: particularly working with charge and discharge, grounding, touch, and breathwork. In Reichian and neo-Reichian (which took aspects of Reich's work and constructed as separate theoretical and clinical modality) therapies, both therapist and client usually expect touch to be a part of the therapeutic process. The question *whether* touch will be used or not is typically less prevalent than the questions of *when* to use touch, *what type* of touch would it be, and *which* processes will be most suitable for working through them with touch (Kertay & Reviere, 1998). Many of the Reichian modalities maintained basic principles and emphases from Reich as well as kept a dialogue with psychoanalytic developments. At the end of the chapter, a clinical vignette demonstrating Reichian therapeutic intervention will be presented as well as an exercise based on Stanley Keleman's (1985) "formative psychology". Below, I shall briefly describe some of the major Reichian modalities.

Medical orgonomy

Created by Reich and his students in 1948, medical orgonomy was one of the first branches of body psychotherapy (Baker, 1977). Orgonomists were all medically trained before attaining further Reichian education. Orgonomists worked with seven patterns of muscular and emotional tension (Chapter Seven will expand on Reichian body segments). After Reich's death, Elsworth Baker (1967) became the main leader of the orgonomy movement, which religiously observed Reichian concepts (Sharaf, 1984). The therapeutic goal of orgonomy was the release of bodily-trapped feelings, particularly anxiety and anger. To achieve this, practitioners used deep touch, breathwork, and movement (Goodrich-Dunn, 2004).

Bioenergetics/bioenergetic analysis

In the world of body psychotherapy, Reich's most important developer was undoubtedly Alexander Lowen who, together with John Pierrakos, developed bioenergetics. Both men were medically trained doctors who studied with Reich for years.

Unlike medical orgonomy, Lowen and Pierrakos created a different model to Reich's both in terms of theoretical emphasis and in terms of clinical accessibility. They have narrowed Reich's emphasis on the orgiastic potential, thus making bioenergetics less sexually threatening. They have also differentiated Reichian clinical work from orgone research. Lowen developed therapeutic exercises, which moderated Reich's confronting style and turned bioenergetics into a highly popular modality. Pierrakos later left Lowen to create, together with his wife Eva, a more transpersonal system of work ("core energetics") (Sharaf, 1984).

Lowen (1974) defined bioenergetics as the study of personality in somatic terminology: the study of psychosomatic organisations. He furthered Reich's theoretical ideas (Lowen, 1958) by expanding developmental aspects of character structures, but also—and perhaps mostly so—by developing and fine-tuning therapeutic techniques. Lowen believed that therapy that was solely insight-based might fail without the emotional and bodily charge required for creating change. He offered many therapeutic techniques aimed at releasing bodily tension and reorganising psychosomatic forms (Lowen, 1965, 1975). Another important contribution in bioenergetics, which is still being expanded and developed today in modern practices of bioenergetic analysis, was the concept of grounding: our capacity to experience our bodily and unmediated connection with the ground, drawing strength and support from it.

Totton (2003) asserted that the difference between the therapeutic systems offered by Reich and Lowen parallels the difference between classic Freudian psychoanalysis and ego psychology. While Reich's emphasis was the unconscious processes and drives, thus focusing on the id and autonomic nervous system, Lowen emphasised ego strength which was the interface between will and capacity for mindful decision-making—and external reality.

Lowen's significance, aside from the popularity of his work, was also in his prolific creativity and writing, which contributed to the exposure of body psychotherapy to both professionals and the public. His clear writing helped the normalising of Reichian vegetotherapy and to retrieve body psychotherapy from the exile it suffered following Reich's personal and political prosecution (C. Young, 2011a).

Contemporary bioenergetic analysis is fundamentally different from Lowen's technical and exercise-like practices, and is highly informed by analytic developments. Some of these developments have integrated relational concepts (Eichhorn & Hilton, 2012; Hilton, 2012a; Sletvold, 2012). Readers who are interested in learning more about contemporary developments in bioenergetics can visit the website of the International Institute for Bioenergetic Analysis at www.bioenergetic-therapy.org.

Formative psychology

Formative psychology was developed by Stanley Keleman, who was a student of Reich and colleague to Pierrakos and Lowen. At the heart of formative psychology is the assumption that every mental, emotional, and bodily state has an organisational-somatic expression, and that by increasing our consciousness to this organisation we can introduce movement and choice into the system, thus liberating the organism. Keleman has thoroughly researched the field he called "emotional anatomy", which examined connections between feelings and their somatic organisations (Keleman, 1985). Keleman has further developed a cohesive and encompassing terminology unique to somatic psychotherapy and based on embodiment.

Keleman holds a truly positive outlook for the possibility of change through exercising mindful embodiment. He writes (2012): "A few of us know how to participate in giving shape to our tissues and the organism's pulsatory organising waves within us that connect us to the vast ocean of life both in and around us, without losing our personal formed identity" (p. 56).

My own clinical thinking was strongly influenced by Keleman's work and Part II (Theoretical) (Chapters Four to Seven) will expand my understanding of psychotherapeutic organisation which I developed from Keleman's work.

Biosynthesis

David Boadella is one of the most important clinicians and theoreticians in body psychotherapy today, and biosynthesis, the model he developed and founded is a central body psychotherapy modality which is widely learned and developed. For many years, Boadella was the editor of the most influential body psychotherapy journal *Energy and Character*. Boadella's biosynthesis added pre- and perinatal research (influenced by Frank Lake and Francis Mott) to Reichian thinking (Boadella, 1976, 1987).

Much of the work in biosynthesis is structured around three foetal developmental layers and stages. The endoderm, which later became our visceral organs, was seen as connected to the quality of centring and regulating the autonomic nervous system. The mesoderm, later becoming the muscular system, bones, and vascular system, was seen as connected to the quality of grounding and muscular regulation. Last, the ectoderm, later becoming the skin and nervous system, was understood as relating to facing (meeting, being with)—and the ability to balance external and internal influences, and mediating different aspects of the self (Rauch, 2005).

Functional analysis

Created and developed by Will Davis, functional analysis is a body oriented depth psychotherapy based on Reich 's functional understanding of the body and mind as two forms of the same thing just as ice, steam, and water are three forms of an underlying reality. It is the meeting place between psyche and soma. The specific themes identified in functional analysis are the emphasis on the inward movement of the pulsation—the instroke, the role of connective tissue in the defence system, the gentle touch technique of points and positions, non-activation of the defence system, and an emphasis on the relation to the self as the primary relationship that is then engaged in relations to others. As a result this non-invasive, self-oriented approach is especially suited to working safely and respectfully with early disturbance.[1]

In relation to trauma work, Davis recognises that since splitting off the traumatic experience was lifesaving it would be dangerous to charge or push the expressive outstroke that leads back into the world of catastrophic memory which the body still holds—or in other words, to retraumatisation. The function and effect of the instroke is meant to be the opposite by centring and gathering the self-organising desire to stay in existence on a level before the differentiation of body and mind. Davis considers the self and not the other as the primary *organising agent* of experience, and is informed and influenced by Rogers's client-centred position (Davis, 2008a).

Will Davis has made significant theoretical and clinical contributions to the field in understanding early developmental injuries in general, and the schizoid (fragmented) character position and trauma in particular (Davis, 2008b).

Biodynamic therapy

Biodynamic psychology was developed by Norwegian Gerda Boyesen, who integrated physiotherapy with her experience as an analysand of Reich's student Ola Raknes and her psychology studies to create her therapeutic system. Boyesen expanded Reich's concept of muscular armour and added the tissue armour, believing that bodymind rigidities were not limited to the muscular system. Boyesen softened Reich's attitude of "breaking the armour" into "melting the armour".

Boyesen's biodynamic psychology placed great importance on peristaltic movements, the rhythmic intestinal pulsation. Biodynamic massage, one of the major tools in biodynamic psychology, utilised a stethoscope for listening to intestinal sounds (borborygmi) which, according to Boyesen, marked somatic-emotional shifts and facilitated both diagnosis and appropriate intervention.

Malcolm Brown integrated biodynamic psychology and Reichian principles with humanistic psychology to create a humanistic body psychotherapy called "organismic psychotherapy". Influenced by Boyesen, organismic psychotherapy emphasised emotional and metabolic regulation and is focused on strengthening the body's inner capacities for self-regulation. Many of the techniques employed here were aimed to provide a soft, containing and comforting environment to the client (M. Brown, 1989).

Bodynamics

A body psychotherapy modality developed by Danish psychotherapist Lisbeth Marcher who has for years researched child development and a variety of bodywork modalities, bodynamics emphasised body-awareness as an important means for strengthening ego functioning. Marcher (Marcher & Fich, 2010) offered an impressive somatic mapping of the psychological functions of specific muscles and bodynamics psychotherapists were trained in this elaborated system. The psychotherapist used the body map to establish which muscles (and their respective psychological functions) were tightly held (hypertonic) or underdeveloped (hypotonic), allowing for a better muscular balance which further supported bodymind balance (Macnaughton, 1998). Bodynamics has been known to be highly efficient with clients who experienced severe trauma or torture (Goodrich-Dunn, 2004).

Integrative body psychotherapy (IBP)

Founded by Jack Lee Rosenberg, integrative body psychotherapy is theoretically influenced by Reichian and neo-Reichian approaches, as well as transpersonal psychology (viewing the therapist as channelling healing energy), traditional healing, spiritual disciplines, and object relations theory (Rosenberg, Rand, & Asay, 1985).

In the clinical setting, IBP places great importance on breathwork and bodywork, as well as seeking meaning—including spiritual meaning (Rauch, 2005). The therapist searches for disturbances in breathing, movement, or boundaries and helps the client in regaining balance and flow, grounding, and embodied presence—both psychologically and spiritually.

Postural integration

Developed by Jack Painter, postural integration (PI) integrates Gestalt with very deep (and sometimes painful) Reichian bodywork, closely related to the deep-tissue massage method

Rolfing (Rolf, 1977). Theoretically, PI is based on Reichian and bioenergetic character structures, but adds some humanistic and spiritual elements to it (Painter, 1984).

Out of all the modalities mentioned in the Reichian body psychotherapy section, PI is the closest to bodywork and some practitioners offer it as a creative therapeutic method, which is not psychotherapy, that is, as bodywork with psychotherapeutic aspects to it. Body psychotherapists who work with PI help the client strengthen body awareness, self-awareness, and awareness to others within the therapeutic relationship. Postural integration emphasises working with breath and touch, body reading, somatic transference, and personal responsibility.

Personal development and human potential treatments

The personal development and human potential movements developed as political, humanistic, and existentialist trends in the 1960s. They operated as a part of the humanistic psychology wave (Maslow, 1943; Rogers, 1951), which boldly challenged the psychoanalytic emphasis on the diseased, pathological, neurotic, and distorted on the one hand, and the reduction of human motivation into conditioning as was offered by behaviourism on the other. Humanistic psychology, which was referred to as *the third force* in psychology (Goble, 1970) focused instead on the human potential, health, and capacity, emphasising an active avoidance from labelling and pathologising the client (the shift in describing the recipient of psychotherapy from *patient* to *client* is also a result of the humanistic movement and its effort to de-medicalise psychotherapy).

As a part of this movement, some methods for personal growth (and group work) developed, which did not wish to consider themselves as psychotherapy modalities but instead as personal development and growth methods. The resistance to the psychotherapeutic label was originally a rigorous political declaration discontented with the medical model of psychotherapy, the hierarchical tone it carried, and the power trips it was predisposed to. Some of the methods developed herein were highly impactful and effective, while most placed great emphasis on regressive work, where the client moved through deep primal emotional and bodily experiences and states, allowing for cathartic expression for these processes.

Under safe facilitation, these methods are among the most powerful for healing potential. However, like other powerful therapeutic methods (such as past life regression, Osho's active meditation, and more), without clear boundaries and responsible training and practice, this work may become explosive.

Although these methods are not identified with the label of psychotherapy, and some actively resist being described as psychotherapy, they do combine important bodymind principles and practices and are thus closely related to body psychotherapy. Furthermore, I strongly believe that the loose boundaries and somewhat irresponsible reputation, which these methods are frequently associated with (New Age trash culture), is not immanent to humanistic thinking—or to the methods themselves, but is instead an unfortunate side-effect of the democratisation of and pluralisation of personal growth work. In my opinion, this price (some charlatanism and unprofessional conduct followed by inclusive and democratic provision of personal development) is still, in many cases, a better compromise than the compartmentalisation of therapy and hierarchical academic and classist training system which, in effect, allows only those from elite socio-economic backgrounds to train as psychotherapists, and significantly limits those who can therefore receive therapeutic services without shame or great financial losses. Humanistic psychology and philosophy have politically chosen to place themselves outside the mainstream medicalisation of psychotherapy and their avoidance of using analytic and medical terminology was not due to lack of rigour but instead to a humanistic stance.

Primal integration

Primal integration is a deep and rigorous developmental process, which fosters exploring primal experiences, and assumes responsibility for a fuller, more authentic life. The process was developed by William Swartley at the beginning of the 1960s and is mostly done in groups, with minimal facilitation but while maintaining some ground rules. The primal integration process emphasises self-direction, self-regulation, and self-responsibility and is not psychotherapy (J. Brown & Mowbray, 1994).

Swartley was influenced by humanistic psychology, Gestalt, and Reich's work, and incorporated cathartic and bodily processes in his system. The method resembles Stanislav Grof's (who was friends with Swartley) holotropic breathwork. Primal integration practitioners Juliana Brown and Richard Mowbray (1996), from the Open Centre in London, describe four central elements in primal integration: "(1) This is a personal development process working in an educational rather than medical model; (2) early life experiences are central to our development, including prenatal and perinatal ones, which could be remembered and worked through; (3) working through these memories is sometimes cathartic and involves deep bodily and emotional expression; (4) the process takes place in an unstructured framework, respectful of the individual's personal pace and emphasising self-regulation and self-responsibility."

Holotropic breathwork (or holotropic therapy)

Czech psychiatrist Stanislav Grof was renowned for his controversial use of hallucinogenic drugs in psychotherapy, particularly LSD. He claimed that non-ordinary states of consciousness (NOSC) were highly significant for personal growth and trauma recovery (Grof, 1975, 1980). However, LSD psychotherapy suffered increasing public and professional criticism, following which Grof made two major adjustments to his work: the first was a gradual abandonment of LSD and searching for other means of working with NOSC; the second was redefining his system as non-psychotherapeutic. Training in holotropic work was therefore open to the public as well as to psychotherapists from different modalities.

Holotropic breathwork incorporated shamanic trance techniques, drumming and rhythmic movement, cyclical breath (close to hyperventilation), and bodywork (Grof, 1988; Grof & Bennett, 1993). The holotropic therapist accompanied the client with little intervention and the work was usually done in a group setting, while encouraging controlled surrender to bodily rhythms and altered states of consciousness. This was done by incorporating intensive breathwork (an element integrated into holotropic work following Reichian orgonomy), pressure points, and appropriate external stimulation, methods which closely resembled those of Mesmer and Charcot, which were described in the first and second chapter.

Holotropic work encouraged early regression, particularly to prenatal stages. Many neuroses and associated pains, believed Grof, were rooted in those prenatal traumas. By accessing our early psychobiological patterns (which Grof called basic perinatal matrices—BPMs), we could release some pent-up bodily and emotional energy and live more fully. The basic perinatal matrices were one of Grof's important contributions to both body psychotherapy and transpersonal psychotherapy (Boroson, 1998).

Rebirthing[2]

Rebirthing is a unique breathing technique aiming to heal repressed emotions (particularly birth traumas), with the aid of deep circular breathing cycles. The method was developed by Leonard Orr in the 1970s out of an eclectic spiritual practice drawing from Christian esoteric traditions, Eastern philosophies, and yoga (Orr & Ray, 1977).

The main technique in rebirthing is continuous breathing cycles, without stopping between inhaling and exhaling, so that gradually breathing becomes intensified and takes over the breather, who is called to surrender to breathing. Orr (2002) describes rebirthing as "learning to breathe from breath itself" (p. 6). This method tends to be highly cathartic, both physically and emotionally, allegedly assisting the breather to re-experience and process painful birthing experiences. Hyperventilation has been traditionally used to create altered states of consciousness for eras, both in shamanic practices (Keeney, 1994) and in hypnosis (Baykushev, 1969), and can sometimes occur spontaneously without intervention, either as a result of anxiety or extreme emotional states. Rebirthing is a deeply regressive work that can be transformative and requires appropriate support and holding.

While rebirthing is not psychotherapy, it could be a powerful experiential tool within psychotherapy. Nick Totton (2003) places rebirthing "perhaps part-way between a psychotherapy, a form of yoga and a religion" (p. 103). For me, rebirthing technique represents both the potential of the New Age wave, as enabling growth, development, awareness, and freedom from limited beliefs, and at the same time the pitfalls and danger associated with New Age culture: lack of boundaries, lack of containment, and retraumatisation. In terms of rebirthing, what differentiates the potential from the risk is not the technique in itself, but the facilitators and assistants, and the context within which rebirthing takes place.

Deep memory process

Developed by Jungian analyst Roger Woolger, deep memory process is a therapeutic regressive method, incorporating both biographical regression (to earlier developmental stages) and past life regression. Two aspects of his work mark Woolger's therapeutic system as relevant here. First, Woolger relates to past lives symbolically—not necessarily as truth but as a useful structure for working with bodymind material (Woolger, 1988). Second, the process itself synthesises Jungian theory with Reichian and shamanic practices. Theoretically speaking, Woolger interpreted and developed Grof's philosophy from a Jungian perspective. Clinically, the practice integrates psychodrama, breathwork, Reichian touch, and an interpretive, processing stage where the experiences are integrated and given meaning.

Trauma-based body psychotherapy

I was born
With fear in my throat.
How could I ever trust my voice?
I could not sing.

I was born
With fear in my lungs.
The feeling I have drowned.
And could not breathe.

I was born
With fear in my mind.
How could I not know?
This fear was never mine!

I was born
With fear in my heart.
Until one day it healed,
Giving me a fresh start.

—Dorothy Oger (2012, p. 29), "I Was Born"

Trauma happens when the organism is exposed to an experience that threatens (concrete or experienced threat) the life, health, or safety (bodily and/or mentally) of the person or those close to him or her. Traumatic stress is therefore a normal and natural response to an abnormal or extreme life event (such as an accident, rape, assault, war, etc.), although it can also result from continuous threatening conditions. Post-traumatic stress disorder (PTSD) includes a myriad of responses to an event that was perceived as traumatic by the person and continues to limit his or her functioning even after the traumatic stimulus has long gone. PTSD is an extreme anxiety disorder, as it seriously limits the lives of those suffering from it and may significantly impair the quality of their lives, health, functioning, and relationships.

The post-traumatic response is a survival reaction that might have saved the person from stronger physical or emotional pain yet it ruptured a deep aspect at the core of the sufferer's being: PTSD sufferers continue to respond to the world as if the traumatic event has not stopped, long after they were safe. Different psychotherapy modalities have tried for many decades to find therapeutic solutions for those suffering from post-trauma.

When French philosopher Simone Weil (1947) wrote: "The false god changes suffering into violence; the true God changes violence into suffering," (p. 122) I believe she spoke of trauma. Dealing with intolerable suffering usually involves a choice between two qualitatively different responses: severance or surrender. When we cannot tolerate pain, we dissociate from it—a split that may save our physical or psychological life. The severance involves a splitting, thus it is an act of violence, even when it is necessary. Analytically speaking, therapy wishes to assist clients in processing their lives' material without the necessity to dissociate from them; to remain present in their own lives and grieve the pain they had to be exposed to (Rolef Ben-Shahar, 2012b). When the pain is great, the process is slow and gentle.

Research in neuroscience indicates that unprocessed trauma is directly expressed in somatic processes. Additionally, many researchers show that the most effective models for healing PTSD include and integrate somatic interventions (Lopez, 2011; McFarlane, Atchison, Rafalowicz, & Papay., 1994; Ochberg, 1991; P. Ogden, Minton, & Pain, 2006; Rothschild, 2000; Schore, 2002; Sinason, 2002; Van der Kolk, 1996).

Indeed, somatic methods for trauma therapy are largely responsible for increasing the awareness and embracing of body psychotherapy by the larger psychotherapeutic milieu. Some of the therapies mentioned below are not psychotherapy, although they are mostly practised by skilled practitioners and psychotherapists. There are many similarities between these trauma therapy methods and they mostly differ in their emphases. There is ample literature regarding body psychotherapeutic interventions for trauma healing and recovery.

Somatic experiencing (SE)

Somatic experiencing is a usually short-term therapeutic modality developed by Peter Levine following his many years of research in animal physiology and psychology. Levine observed that although animals in nature were frequently exposed to life threatening situations, they rarely experienced post-traumatic symptoms. He recognised that animals used physiological response patterns, such as shaking (which released neural residues), for regulating the accumulated energy. This somatic regulation enabled the animals to return to activity while maintaining relatively low levels of neural arousal (Rauch, 2005). Thus, Levine perceives the trauma to reside in the nervous system—not the event, defining trauma as an event which overwhelms our nervous system.

According to Levine, humans also possess those physiological capacities for monitoring and regulating trauma, but we have lost spontaneous access to those healing agencies. This is exactly what SE is attempting to reclaim. SE uses a variety of skills for identifying neural charge and allowing discharge without emotional or neural flooding (i.e., processing without retraumatisation) (Levine, 2005; Levine & Frederick, 1997). SE also incorporates psycho-education elements to help clients understand the somatic and emotional mechanisms for dealing with trauma, to reduce the associated shame, and normalise and contextualise post-traumatic symptoms.

Somatic trauma therapy

In many ways, Babette Rothschild's somatic trauma therapy resembles Peter Levine's somatic experiencing. Both methods, argues Totton (2003), are based on neurological studies and both were affected and influenced by Lisbeth Marcher and bodynamics. The main difference between the two methods is in Rothschild's emphasis on slow pace, based on her belief that trauma work requires "frequently applying the brakes" (2004), that is—systematic and frequent breaks in the therapeutic narrative flow to avoid flooding and retraumatisation. Rothschild also places great importance on the therapeutic relationship as a safe container.

Somatic trauma therapy views clients' defences also as resources for dealing with and containing traumatic material. The therapist is therefore respectful of them and cautious in challenging these defences. Through body awareness and strengthening of regulatory capacities, the client is assisted in better utilising the necessary resources for recovery (Rothschild, 2000). The therapist helps clients retrieve control over their bodies and lives by reducing traumatic symptoms and through building and cultivating safe places both within them and outside them. While somatic trauma therapy does not require remembering, it does offer means of dealing with traumatic memory. Therapy can be both short and long term.

In addition to her important contributions to trauma therapy, Rothschild also researched and has extensively written about and worked with secondary trauma—the effects of trauma on surrounding others, including on the therapists. Today, it is widely acknowledged that psychotherapists working with PTSD are exposed themselves to post-traumatic symptoms (secondary and vicarious traumatisation) (Cerney, 1995; Figley, 1995; Pearlman & Mac Ian, 1995). One of Rothschild's significant contributions to the field is in applying body psychotherapeutic skills to support therapists who work with trauma, helping the helpers regulate the impact of their work on their bodies and minds (Hadad & Rolef Ben-Shahar, 2012; Rothschild & Rand, 2006).

Sensorimotor psychotherapy

Sensorimotor psychotherapy was developed by Pat Ogden as complementary bodywork to Hakomi (a type of body psychotherapy that will be described later). Ogden differentiated between trauma therapy and recognising and working with developmental trauma, arguing (as it is widely recognised today) that PTSD and developmental traumas or attachment disorders are highly interlinked (Liotti, 2004; P. Ogden, Minton, & Pain, 2006; Rolef Ben-Shahar, 2012b).

Sensorimotor psychotherapy is focused on attending to movements and sensations through emotional and cognitive processing, with the view of developing self-awareness and body awareness and by paying attention to micro-movements, breath, postures, and slight tremors characteristic of traumatic responses. Therapy is thus slow and gentle to allow for increased tolerance to traumatic material without hyperarousal.

Tracking body sensations, however, is not a goal in itself in sensorimotor psychotherapy. Ogden believes that sensorimotor psychotherapy contributes to the field of trauma therapy by providing cognitive and emotional processes that can facilitate the processing and integration of traumatic material in addition to the somatic and neural processing (P. Ogden & Minton, 2000; P. Ogden, Minton, & Pain, 2006).

Eye movement desensitisation and reprocessing (EMDR)

EMDR is arguably the most familiar, most researched, and most acceptable therapeutic method today by psychiatrists, psychologists, and researchers in the field of trauma-focused therapy. EMDR is a structured method developed by Francine Shapiro in the late 1980s (2001), which combines principles and methods from psychodynamic psychotherapy, cognitive-behavioural therapy, humanistic approaches, and body-oriented practices. EMDR provides some useful and applicable clinical protocols; the most basic includes eight stages.

At the heart of EMDR is a simple technique of bilateral stimulation, usually a visual one. While processing traumatic material, the EMDR therapist moves two fingers from side to side while the client follows the movement without turning his or her head.

As early as while conducting trauma evaluation, clients are requested to scan their body and attend to the sensations that accompany images and traumatic material. Sensory symptoms become a crucial diagnostic marker throughout therapy. Furthermore, the central curative aspects of EMDR (desensitisation and reprocessing) are achieved through somatic stimulation of both sides of the body (visual, auditory, or tactile stimulation). This process assists clients in connecting the fragmented traumatic experience with narrative thinking. Throughout therapy, both client and therapist monitor for hyperarousal through body sensations, foster sensory awareness, and support the gentle discharging of the traumatic experience (F. Shapiro & Maxfield, 2002).

Even though EMDR is not described as a body-oriented therapy, and unlike the previous three methods it does not identify itself as such, it utilises many somatically based processes. From the initial stages of body diagnosis (body scan) through to somatic intervention (bilateral stimulation), EMDR demonstrates how trauma-healing is facilitated by working through and with the body.

Process oriented body psychotherapy

> And thus the sailors sing aloud:
> The world is but so wide,
> It has some flowers and some thorns
> There's land, and there's high tide
> It has some waves, and some safe shores
> There's silence, there is storm
> Of thousand things of beauty, voyaging's the epitome.
>
> —The Voyaging Song, Lea Goldberg (1949)

Process oriented body psychotherapy places greater emphasis on processes (emotional, bodily) and lesser emphasis on states; the voyaging—the movement and dynamic journeying—is a highly important principle for the therapeutic work of these modalities. Since the only experiential time is the present moment, those methods work with the here-and-now experiences, and are less concerned with the past, not because the past is not important, but drawing on the assumption that change requires affective processes, and these only exist in the present moment; to the extent that our past is alive in the here-and-now, it will arrive in therapy too. Psychologist and researcher Daniel Stern (2004) phrased this beautifully: "The only time of raw subjective reality, of phenomenal experience, is the present moment" (p. 3). The invitation to surrender to the present moment strikes great similarities with Bion's (1962) concept of reverie, a state of open receptivity to the other, an unmediated presence which embodies a leap of faith into unconscious processes, without continuous attempt to intellectualise.

The therapeutic methods described below do not ignore rigidities in bodymind states (such as symptoms or psychopathological conditions); however they choose to focus on flexibility and mobility more than on fixation: the *how* rather than the *why*.

Gestalt therapy

Gestalt therapy is widely known but not always recognised as body psychotherapy. Its roots, however, as well as many of its principles, are strongly grounded in Reichian tradition. It was developed in the 1940s and 1950s by Fritz and Laura Perls and Paul Goodman. Fritz Perls attended Reich's seminars in 1933 and was deeply influenced by his work (he also was his client for a while).

Gestalt therapy integrated Reichian principles with Taoist and Buddhist influences (Smith, 1985) and was deeply reliant on experiential learning. Perls emphasised body awareness (1969) and the language and practice of Gestalt therapy involved sensory-embodied terminology as well as using Reichian concepts such as self-regulation, charge, and contact. Gestalt therapy worked with different aspects of the self (parts, or self-states), to facilitate better organisation and reintegration. The therapy was structured to support clients in discovering how they did what they did, encouraging greater flexibility and adaptability. Perls was less interested in the origins of trauma, and more in the capacity to respond in the here-and-now.

As a modality of body psychotherapy, Gestalt therapy focused on flow and vitality, on retrieving our spontaneous and authentic responsiveness to life. The therapist encouraged her clients to express their experiences authentically in the present moment, daring to bring different aspects of themselves (including shadow aspects) into the clinic, through verbal communication, movement, somatic expressions, and role play. Thus, clients developed self-awareness and insights through doing, moving, and relating and not necessarily through understanding cognitively. Perls was one of the first clinicians to abandon the therapeutic attempt to focus on the *why*, and emphasised the commitment to introduce change and movement. For him, when there was sufficient self-awareness and body awareness, the organism could discover its freedom to think, feel, create, and act in the world (Zahm & Gold, 2002).

Process-oriented psychology

Jungian analyst Arnold Mindell developed process-oriented psychology (also known as process work) in the 1970s, while synthesising work with non-ordinary states of consciousness with the energetic body, which Mindell termed dreambody. Process-oriented psychology was rooted in shamanic traditions, and it involved conscious entry into altered states of consciousness to support the client and the community (Audergon, 2005). Mindell's later work further incorporated principles of quantum physics into the therapeutic work (Mindell, 2004).

Mindell (1982) described the dreambody as commonly experienced in dreams, meditation, and recreational drug use, where we experienced our dreambody as an energetic field: "The dreambody frequently appears as an out-of-body field intensity, as a total gestalt moving with relatively vague extremities in a sort of magnetic field" (p. 31). The dreambody was released in profound experiences where boundaries of time and space lost their rigidity. According to process-oriented psychology (like Freudian analysis), it was possible to work with symptoms, pain, and disease exactly as one worked with dreams: by directing our attention inwardly we could retrieve their meaning and liberate ourselves from their grasp. Thus, the principles of process-oriented psychology bore a similarity to Gestalt.

Although process work was not defined as body psychotherapy, its theoretical and clinical reliance on somatic processes justify its inclusion here. Furthermore, Mindell's description of the clinical work with the dreambody is remarkably close to the relational psychoanalysis understanding (which is expanded on in the Appendix) of the intersubjective entity: "Understanding the dreambody requires a feeling for the field in which the body exists, or, formulated less classically, understanding the body requires experiencing the field of which the body is a part" (ibid., p. 17).

Hakomi

Hakomi was developed in the late 1970s by Ron Kurtz, bringing together many therapeutic fields within a process-oriented framework. Hakomi was influenced by Reich and Lowen, Gestalt therapy and bodywork such as Feldenkrais (a movement-based bodywork method for expanding self-awareness and body awareness) and Rolfing (structural deep-tissue bodywork). Other influences include focusing (which will be explored here later), and Ericksonian hypnosis. (Psychiatrist Milton Erickson developed strategic psychotherapy, which made extensive use of improvisation, trance, working with metaphors, and storytelling. Erickson influenced many types of psychotherapy, including hypno-psychotherapy, systemic therapies, and short-term psychotherapy. My PhD dissertation (Rolef Ben-Shahar, 2010c) looked at the common grounds between Ericksonian psychotherapy, body psychotherapy, and relational psychoanalysis.) Another influence was neuro-linguistic-programming (NLP, a therapeutic modality that was created out of a search for models of excellence in psychotherapy. Founders of the approach, John Grinder and Richard Bandler, researched the therapeutic brilliance of some leading therapists, including Virginia Satir, Milton Erickson, Fritz Perls, and Gregory Bateson, attempting to deduce models and linguistic and emotional patterns, which they turned into therapeutic procedures and protocols). Additionally, Hakomi was developed from Buddhist and Taoist philosophy and accordingly emphasises principles of loving presence, mindfulness, and organicity.

In Hopi (the language of the Hopi people from Arizona), Hakomi has two meanings: the first is "How am I positioned with all dimensions for life?" and the other is "Who am I?"[3] Both these questions are central to Hakomi clinical work.

Hakomi psychotherapy involves "experiments", in which the therapeutic dyad partakes in exploring, in order to increase the client's awareness of behavioural, cognitive, bodily, and emotional patterns. These experiments are based on narrative listening but also on attention to postures, movements, and sensations (Rauch, 2005). The therapeutic position involves mindfulness with soft and non-judgmental presence; these create soft, non-violent, and containing psychotherapy.

Rubenfeld synergy method (RSM)

Ilana Rubenfeld developed her synergy method in 1977, following her enthusiastic experience of Alexander technique (a somatic-education system for acquiring better postural, motoric, and bodily habitual forms), which made huge improvements to Rubenfeld's physical health, as well as her positive experience of psychotherapy, which eased her psychological pains. Rubenfeld sought to create an integrated field and trained in Alexander technique and Gestalt therapy (with Fritz Perls), before creating her synergy method. Rubenfeld synergy method (RSM) is a gentle and attentive therapeutic modality. While clients sit or lie down, the therapist attentively accompanies them—through touch and conversation, in a voyage of shared discovery (Rubenfeld, 2001).

Inspired by Gestalt therapy, RSM places great importance on self-awareness and body awareness, personal responsibility and the here-and-now, with an additional facet of embodied spirituality, and a technique of bodily reflections (e.g., "Did you notice that when you talked about your partner you stopped breathing?"). Some other tools include trancework, guided visualisation, and gentle touch (Rubenfeld, 2000). A similar therapeutic modality that does not, however, define itself as psychotherapy is Rosen method bodywork, which incorporates deep somatic listening to processes that emerge from the relationship between clients and their bodies through deep touch, attuned connection, and focused conversation that continuously encourages clients to listen to their body.

Focusing[4]

Focusing is based on the work of philosopher and psychologist Eugene Gendlin (1978). In his research he found that clients who succeeded in therapy were those who not only talked about their problems, but rather those who paused regularly and took the time to sense the bodily felt experience of a situation. Gendlin coined the term "felt sense" to describe special characteristics of this meta-sensation, the bodily felt experience. Most times, the felt sense is vague and unclear at first, yet with cultivation the implicit becomes consciously known.

Focusing has been applied in many different ways; as an additional method in psychotherapy, as a self-help technique in everyday life, and as a programme for community wellness. Focusing has contributed to fields as varied as education, medicine, business, art, creativity, bodywork, movement, and more (M. Hendricks, 2001).

Focusing oriented psychotherapy (FOT) is a further development of Gendlin's philosophy and its experiential psychotherapeutic application (Gendlin, 1998).

Some examples of the principles embedded in FOT are:

The body is not an object or a mechanical machine, but rather a living organism that interacts continuously with the outside world and responds to these interactions. When the felt sense is attended to, it unfolds into a felt meaning and novelty emerges naturally. Thus, the healing process happens from inside-out.

Clients are taught to mind the ongoing bodily experience in their inner space, developing a compassionate inner observer. Clients are also encouraged to pause regularly in the session and tune-in to check appropriateness of interventions against the felt sense, which serves as a compass for the healing process.

The FOT therapist listens to the client's experience beyond content, words, and thoughts. The therapist listens to what is implicit without yet knowing the meaning of it. She is able to use different skills to help the client experience a felt sense even when the process is blocked or stuck. The client is trained to attend to the hidden aspects in the body's wisdom, thus "coming home" to oneself.

Expressive body psychotherapy

While dance and movement psychotherapy clearly fits the broad definition of body psychotherapy, it is often not recognised as such, perhaps because most types of movement psychotherapy were historically developed outside the spheres of body psychotherapy (or psychotherapy at all); perhaps because expressive psychotherapies are currently widely acknowledged as distinctive modalities in psychotherapy.

Expressive therapies work with images, metaphors, and symbols that are encountered through creative and expressive processes. The engagement in creative processes opens a new channel through which one can (re-)connect with inner and outer worlds. At times, words cannot describe, express, or contain nuances of sensual experiences and emotion, and expressive therapies provide alternative languages for their expression. This enables people with different expressive styles (more visual or tactile/touch or through movement, etc.) or disabilities (such as Alzheimer or traumatic muteness) to express themselves in therapy in an affective and authentic manner. The creative processes in therapy have the potential to affect people in ways that are not possible through conversation alone. The forming and transforming nature of art modalities and materials have great facilities for representation and for working with inner process. Clients have the opportunity to be active participants in their therapy and use imagination, play, and art in order to encounter and work with/through their issues. This kind of engagement stimulates and awakens all bodily senses; hence the client enters a deep process of self-exploration, including exploring parts which are inaccessible through words alone.

This engagement can also be helpful with creating new and healthy attachments and patterns of inter-relations through sensual interactions, movement, and activities involving touch. The use of senses and the body can reconnect one to primal situations, when words have not yet become the dominant mean of communication; this offers the opportunity to construct new patterns of attachment and relationships in the brain (Zack, 2013).

Not all expressive therapies fit within body psychotherapy, but some place a greater emphasis on the body. Like many body psychotherapeutic modalities, expressive arts pay attention to the emotional charge carried by words, and to the way they are used. The capacity to work through embodiment, movement and dance, music, or through clay facilitates therapeutic work which is at times without words and without the kinds of thinking related to verbal language. Experiences which were nonverbal can be reflected more easily and in unmediated ways. The therapeutic functions of the arts stem from their use of images, metaphors, symbols, colour, sound and voice, taste, smells, touch, and movement—all of which are primary and subsymbolic languages which speak of the unconscious and from the unconscious, allowing the clients to express their inner worlds by forming and re-forming them in the external one (ibid.).

It is important to stress that despite the emphasis on nonverbal processes, verbal communication and language are vital to the expressive therapies and help deepen, contain, understand, and give meaning to the therapeutic material. Language is also utilised as part of the creative process itself (such as in drama psychotherapy) (ibid.).

Dance movement therapy (DMT)

Dance movement therapy (DMT) has its roots in two disciplines: the art (of dance) and psychoanalysis. This therapy developed from similar assumptions to body psychotherapy: the inseparable links between mind and body, and the endeavour to widen our possibilities of movement between the two, as well as between ourselves and the outside world. DMT works with the connection between motion and emotion. Things that are difficult to say become evident in movement, as do unconscious processes. Movement reflects personality, including psychological developmental processes as well as psychopathology and interpersonal patterns of relating.

DMT was developed by Marian Chase in the 1940s. Chase, who was a dancer and dancing teacher, discovered that many of her students came to her solely for personal development and growth, which they indeed gained through movement. Chase studied psychodrama and integrated structured and improvised movements within therapy to facilitate the integration of cognitive, social, emotional, and bodily processes within a group framework (Payne, 2006).

Chase developed her concepts of treatment working with schizophrenic and psychotic patients before the advent of psychiatric medicine (Chaiklin & Wengrower, 2009). Chase's patients worked in a circle, while using movement and rhythm to communicate with each other and with Chase. One of Chase's most famous techniques was the mirroring technique: she would acknowledge the patient's movement by repeating it and letting it resonate in her own body (Malchiodi, 2007). This enabled her to create deep emotional communication with the patients, even with the most disconnected ones among them (ibid.).

DMT is one of the most appreciated and accepted forms of expressive psychotherapy. All DMT's pioneers were dancers, performers, choreographers, and teachers; they were mostly women with diverse psychological backgrounds. Mary Whitehouse, Trudy Schoop, and Joan Chodorow are three DMT pioneers who continued to develop this therapy, each in her own way, while refining its techniques and making it available and useful for different populations, as well as for dyadic therapy.

Yona Shahar-Levy, an Israeli DMT pioneer, has created the "Emotorics" (emotion, motoric): a system for evaluation and observation of movement which leans heavily on the foundations of DMT theory (and practice), and psychoanalysis (Shahar-Levy, 2004). Shahar-Levy argues that every movement and posture is a bodily phenomenon as well as a story of feelings, relationships, memories, personality, and experiences. She sees these expressions as externalisation of our inner worlds, mirroring and resonating our internal subjectivity (ibid.). Shahar-Levy perceives bodily postures, movements, and structures as materialisations of our primal attachments, our developmental processes, and as evidence of our intersubjective relationships (Zack, 2013).

Traditional body psychotherapy, and particularly the theories of Reich and Lowen, have influenced and been incorporated in DMT throughout the years. The place for improvisation and nonverbal interaction, and the potential for mutuality alongside transference dynamics turn DMT into a vital and moving sphere, which perfectly matches contemporary relational thinking and practice.

Pesso Boyden system psychomotor

Created in 1961 by former dancers Albert Pesso and Diane Boyden-Pesso, Pesso Boyden system psychomotor (PBSP) is a therapeutic modality that begins by tracking the clients' motoric impulses and allowing their expression through movement. Therapy takes place in a group setting: once a client has expressed her feelings and experiences in movement, the other group members are invited to "respond" with their own authentic movements to the first person's expression. Therefore, PBSP combines movement with psychodramatic role-play, allowing for symbolic dramatisation in movement, enacting relationships and traumatic scenes from the lives of the clients. With the support of the group, this dramatisation fosters curative processing of traumas and finding alternative expressions and experiences in their lives (Rauch, 2005).

Continuum movement

Emily Conrad, who developed "continuum movement", was also a dancer. During a five-year stay as a choreographer in Haiti, Conrad was captivated by the oceanic movement, which characterised local dancing. Her method began as a dancing training and developed into body psychotherapeutic practice.

Continuum movement integrated breathing techniques and releasing bodily micromovements by expressing these, in order to discover the body (and mind) as a part of eternal flow—a wider field, instead of a fixed and rigid form. We can appreciate the resemblance to Keleman's formative psychology, and the spiritual approach, which characterises Mindell's process-oriented psychology. Continuum movement proved particularly effective in working with physical problems (including paralysis), which were unresponsive to conventional medical or psychotherapeutic treatments (Totton, 2003).

"One aspect of the entire human system," writes Conrad (2008), "is a vast communication network beginning within our own bodies. Continuum uses movement, the dexterity of breath, the resonance of sound and the value of meaning to amplify and refine this far-reaching communication within ourselves, with others and with our world." Unlike the previous two methods, continuum is not presented as psychotherapy in itself.

5Rhythms®

Another form of dancing practice that is not strictly psychotherapy, but worth mentioning here is 5Rhythms. 5Rhythms is a simple, powerful meditation practice based on movement and dance. Created by Gabrielle Roth in the late 1970s, 5Rhythms is a highly popular movement-meditation practice today, involving distinct rhythmic patterns of moving between five different musical and bodily rhythms.

5Rhythms is practised in group settings, and it draws from shamanic and ecstatic traditions as well as from Gestalt, human potential, and transpersonal psychology. The five rhythms are flowing, staccato, chaos, lyrical, and stillness and when these are danced in sequence they create a *wave*, which provides the basic platform for personal development, spiritual growth, and interaction (Moving Centre School, 2013).

Relational body psychotherapy

> The eyes you're longing for
> listen now—
> the eyes you see yourself in
> are eyes because they see you.
>
> —Antonio Machado (1983, p. 149)[5]

What goes around comes around

As the first two chapters demonstrated, the main streams of body psychotherapy emerged from psychoanalysis, yet body psychotherapy was then expelled from mainstream psychoanalysis. Consequently, body psychotherapists sought and found a welcoming home in humanistic psychology, personal development, and human-potential movements. Only a few therapeutic modalities, such as medical orgonomy and bioenergetic analysis, as well as dance movement therapy and in general expressive therapies, maintained connection with their analytic roots (at the expense of maintaining contact with the broader body psychotherapy community), but the majority of body psychotherapy modalities gradually distanced themselves from psychoanalysis. Parallel to that, psychoanalysis carefully and consistently differentiated itself from bodywork and body psychotherapeutic modalities.

Many body psychotherapists began their practices as bodyworkers and through exploration with touch. Sensitive bodyworkers quickly become aware of the psychological, ethical, and transferential complexities inherent in therapy, whether they are verbally discussed or not. Some therapists and practitioners seek to further train in psychotherapy to ground those complexities in a theoretical, clinical, and appropriate ethical framework.

Relational psychoanalyst Muriel Dimen (1998) writes: "Body matters are so weighty, so deeply important, they often cannot be spoken. Untellable, they can only be shown—like much that happens in consulting rooms" (p. 66). The therapeutic exposure to complex transference dynamics and the potential for misinterpretation drive many body psychotherapists to feel ill at ease with the gap between the psychodynamic approach and a bodily practice that does not take into account relational challenges. Sadly, many practitioners subsequently choose to stop working with touch; some altogether withdraw from relating to the body in psychotherapy.

And so, history repeated itself and yet again the potential split between body and mind manifested, not unlike the unravelling scene at the dawn of psychoanalysis, only this time the dilemma was found in the centre stage of body psychotherapy. Few possible solutions to this conundrum were found. Flooded with this psychodynamic complexity, some psychotherapists (Shiraz, 2013) actively elected to move the complexity of the therapeutic relationship to the background in order to allow space for the traditional bodily-therapeutic work, with breathwork, movement, and touch. Such a position did not reduce the importance of the therapeutic relationship, but instead acknowledged that intensive work with the therapeutic relationship in general, and transference dynamics particularly, limited the liberty of using bodily interventions and required greater complexity. On the other hand, other psychotherapists felt it was impossible for them to turn a blind eye to the therapeutic complexities and therefore chose to let go of working with potentially highly charged interventions like bodywork and catharsis. This stance, too, did not deem catharsis and touch as ineffective or non-therapeutic, but was based on the argument that it was too difficult to retain relational complexity when there were surpluses of highly charged interventions, which created transference distortions.

Relational body psychotherapy is a relatively new development in body psychotherapy, flourishing mainly in Europe and the USA, which represents a determined effort to maintain the bodily focus of body psychotherapy, including somatic intervention, without reducing the complex tapestry of the therapeutic relationship: an attempt to hold the paradoxical polarities rather than choose one over the other. The dialogue with contemporary psychoanalytic thinking allows the relational body psychotherapist to participate in deeply affective interventions while still grounding her interventions in the therapeutic context.

This pulsation, between separation and integration, between polarisation and reconnection, echoes through the history of humanity and parallels the intersubjective tension (Benjamin, 1990) which is discussed throughout the book, particularly in Chapter Five. On the one hand, we yearn for symbiotic enmeshment; we crave to surrender to a wider mind, which could offer our bodymind a resting place, a momentary relief from our isolated, individual self. On the other hand, we fight against such surrender with all our might, both due to our wish to retain our separated subjectivity, and because of our wish to subordinate the other to our own world: using the other as a part-object. I oscillate between wanting to relate to you as a separate individual and wanting to see you as an extension of my own universe.

This tension manifested in manifold splits and dissociations throughout history, whether it was the Cartesian body–mind split, the Christian splitting of divinity and the exclusion of the devil from the Holy Spirit, or the Western modern split between I and thou. It is probably inevitable, that from the relational body psychotherapy attempt to hold together thesis and antithesis, a new split will also be created, and we shall continue to pulsate in spiralling cycles, inwardly and outwardly, between surrender and distinction, individualism and community.

As relational psychoanalysis became more popular (the Appendix discusses relational psychoanalysis and its relevance to body psychotherapy), it also proved willing and open to dialogue with and be influenced by other psychotherapeutic modalities. The relational approach is a psychoanalytic model with an affective emphasis, which can integrate well with theoretical and clinical principles of body psychotherapy. Many body psychotherapists and humanistic psychotherapists found validation of their affective work in relational psychoanalysis, attachment theory, and object relations. Thus, after many years of segregated practice, body psychotherapists could resume the connection and dialogue with psychoanalytic thinking without giving up the body and without losing their professional identity, which included bodily interventions. While relational psychoanalytic thinking provides a fertile theoretical dialogue to the keen body psychotherapist, relational body psychotherapy can offer psychoanalysis practices that translate relational conceptualisation into practice. Thus, the two disciplines can mutually enrich one another.

Relational approaches in body psychotherapy acknowledge the fact that introducing the body (and bodily interventions) into the therapeutic dialogue may challenge and complicate matters for the therapist, the client, and the community. Regressive transferences, dependency, power dynamics, high emotional charge, disturbances in symbolising processes, and amplification of erotic transference—all these might happen in the body psychotherapeutic field. Nevertheless, working with body and with touch could also deepen the connection, strengthen blurred boundaries, foster deep understanding, insight, and empathy, support the creation of therapeutic attachment, and potentiate immediate and unmediated work with the intersubjective body (Bar-Levav, 1998; Torraco, 1998).

Relational psychoanalytic concepts provide the body psychotherapist with tools for dealing with the powerful affective and emotional charge that takes place in an embodied practice, which raise questions such as: how important is the therapeutic relationship in body psychotherapy?, how weighty are transferential dynamics in the work?; what is the place of the therapist in the therapeutic relationship?; what complexities enter therapy when clients lie down on a massage table or a mattress, and may take off some of their clothes?, and what happens to the therapeutic relationship when touch is a possibility?

The relational body psychotherapist aspires to ground insights and bodily interventions within a vital and dynamic therapeutic relationship, which takes part in dialogue with (among other material) transferential fields, complexities of touch, power imbalances, the movement between satisfaction and frustration, gender and sexual dynamics, and the paradoxes which are inherent to the therapeutic relationship. At best, relational body psychotherapy is not a set of somatic interventions but a *dance*: an alive, pulsating, and breathing dance of presence and mutual emergence, realising the intersubjective field, and embodying it thoroughly.

Today, body psychotherapists who choose to use bodily and cathartic intervention can no longer resort to the naïve and spontaneous stance, which characterised the first few decades of body psychotherapy; they need to be willing to hold the paradoxical tension between complexity and simplicity and make a choice, be willing to position themselves authentically and responsively with their clients, and take responsibility for their clinical interventions: with the potential and risk these may hold.

Before we review three modalities of relational body psychotherapy, I wish to present some of the historical sources of relational body psychotherapy. One such source, and a personal inspiration for me is British body psychotherapist Nick Totton, whose writing, politics, and clinical position shaped my therapeutic thinking and practice (Rolef Ben-Shahar, 2013e). Totton initially trained in Reichian body psychotherapy and gradually acquired psychoanalytic education which influenced both his therapeutic position, and his writing and ability to engage and enter into dialogue across different modalities. In their succinct way, Totton and Priestman (2012) phrased the essence of relational body psychotherapy: "We need relationships with others to survive and thrive … One could equally, if less literally, say that our need for relationship requires us to have bodies, as the vehicle for our relating" (p. 35). In a similar vein, Robert Hilton (Eichhorn & Hilton, 2012), another important contributor to the field, claimed: "Our longing needs to be embodied. We need to allow it to find expression in our eyes, mouth, face, and arms" (p. 4).

Another important agent for advancing relational body psychotherapy was the Chiron Centre in England, which during the 1990s became an important centre for relational body psychotherapy. The clinical work, teaching, and writing of Chiron trainers, such as Shoshi Asheri, Roz Carroll, Michael Soth, Tom Warnecke, and others brought analytic and relational richness into the training of generations of body psychotherapists, all the while conversing with other therapeutic positions and deepening their familiarity with body psychotherapy. In 2009 the Chiron Centre published an edited book (Hartley, 2009) presenting its body psychotherapy and allowing a peek into the historical, conceptual, and clinical development of relational body psychotherapy.

At the Open Centre in London, Silke Ziehl further developed Jack Painter's "postural and energetic integration" into a body psychotherapeutic modality that combines Reichian bodywork with relational thinking. I would also like to argue that Stephen Gilligan's "self-relations psychotherapy" should be considered as a close relative of relational body psychotherapy. All these approaches made a significant impact on my theoretical thinking and clinical work.

In the last European Association of Body Psychotherapy (EABP) international congress in Cambridge, an entire day was dedicated to relational body psychotherapy (Asheri, Carroll, Rolef Ben-Shahar, Soth, & Totton, 2012). It was an important acknowledgement and validation of this modality, which gradually becomes central in body psychotherapy, influencing training, practice, and literature. The discussion panel, which included Nick Totton, Shoshi Asheri, Roz Carroll, Michael Soth, and myself, examined different facets of relational body psychotherapy, such as the place of Reichian character in relational thinking, enactment, the somatic nature of intersubjectivity, self and mutual regulation, improvisation, and paradoxes in therapy. The first published edited book about relational body psychotherapy (C. Young, 2012) further strengthened the centrality of this modality.

The therapeutic body

> "What is REAL?" asked the Rabbit one day, when they were lying side by side near the nursery fender. [...] "Real isn't how you are made," said the Skin Horse. "It's a thing that happens to you. When a child loves you for a long, long time, not just to play with, but REALLY loves you, then you become Real."
>
> "Does it hurt?" asked the Rabbit. "Sometimes," said the Skin Horse, for he was always truthful. "When you are Real you don't mind being hurt."
>
> —Margery Williams (1922, p. 10), *The Velveteen Rabbit*

The placenta is a living somatic dialogue between a foetus and its mother; the nipple as an expansion of the dyadic immune system (via milk); arms grasping and a baby is held; a couple unite as one and redefine their separate subjectivity in the act of lovemaking: these are all examples of our ontology. Like the velveteen rabbit, we emerge as real from a loving connection, we are created in relationships and by relationships, and at the same time partake in their creation. And these relationships are first and foremost bodily events.

When we examine bodily processes through relational eyes, we might understand these as means of bridging the gap between self and other (Greenberg & Mitchell, 1983). We learn to know the world through intricate relationship between body, mind, and environment. As psychotherapists, suggests psychologist Yorai Sella (Keet, Sella, & Ziv-Beiman, 2013), we attempt to find ways of crossing the interface between one person and another without collapsing the space—neither reducing the therapeutic act into a solely cognitive exercise, in the hope that consciousness will materialise into connection, nor merely operating in a concrete intervention in the hope that this collapsed interface will transform into consciousness. Thus, relational body psychotherapy relates to the body both as an object, but also—and more so—as a part of a dialectic dance between somatic events, cognitive organisations, and relational constellations—as a subject in relations. Your body and mine are created in the act of conversing with another and with the world around us; a dialogue which our bodies express and so, time and again, we are created anew. In a similar vein, relational body psychotherapist Robert Hilton (2012b) poetically wrote: "As my clients and I have faced our limitations, we have discovered that our mutual caring has made us real to each other and ourselves. We are still crooked trees, but we have discovered that even crooked trees, given the proper care, can blossom in the spring" (p. 91).

While this entire volume is dedicated to relational body psychotherapy, I would still like to specify some of the differentiating qualities you will encounter in this book. What is it that makes relational body psychotherapy different from other bodywork or body psychotherapy modalities? The book is interspersed with vignettes, which demonstrate some of the applications of relational body psychotherapy. Nonetheless, below you can find some important features in relational body psychotherapy: relational therapeutic terminology, the centrality of the therapeutic relationship, two-person psychology, attention to the three bodies in the room (the therapist's body, the client's body, and the intersubjective body), and last—the emphasis on working with paradoxes.

Therapeutic terminology: Relational body psychotherapy is influenced by psychoanalytic thinking and developments. Relational body psychotherapists are therefore able to express their therapeutic understanding, theoretical stance, and clinical intervention in a terminology that is understood by other therapeutic languages. The therapeutic language is both psychodynamic and yet grounded and embodied. Clinically speaking, the work of the body psychotherapist may look very different to that of the relational psychoanalyst, yet they both share similar understandings.

The centrality of therapeutic relationship: The therapeutic dyad and two subjectivities therein—the client and the therapist—are all central to the therapeutic process and therapeutic enquiry. That is, therapeutic interventions stem from the client's needs as well as the needs of the therapeutic relationship, and are mindful of the influence they might have on the client, the therapist, and the relationship. While some therapeutic interventions may carry a technical proficiency (e.g., bodywork technique), it is the therapeutic relationship and the therapeutic process that dictate their use and not the other way round.

Two-person psychology: Relational psychotherapists attribute great importance to working with transference and countertransference, which they use in their work. The therapist is not perceived as an external spectator assisting the client's change, but an active participant in a process of change that takes part in the therapist as well. By recognising that her presence impacts and creates change, the psychotherapist converses with her clients and discusses issues of influence and power with them rather than ignoring or avoiding such important matters. Somatic transference and countertransference are openly and appropriately examined and discussed as part of psychotherapy. Notwithstanding the inherent asymmetrical nature of the therapeutic relationship, the relational body psychotherapist endeavours to allow authentic presence and mutual influence, partnership and mutual validation.

The three bodies in treatment: The body in relational body psychotherapy is not only seen as a separated object but also a shared process of bodies-in-relation. Nick Totton (2005) writes: "To be a body is to need other bodies" (p. 169), hence any vertical (intrapsychic) therapeutic work is understood as partial and complemented by horizontal (interpersonal, within the therapeutic context) work—and vice versa. The relational body psychotherapist relates to her own body as part of the therapeutic dyad, the intersubjective body. The three bodies (and their kaleidoscopic multiple manifestations)—the body of the client, the body of the therapist, and the intersubjective body all receive therapeutic attention.

Risk and potential—holding paradoxes: The quality of relational work is challenging for therapist and client alike. Both enter intersubjective fields, both risk changing. Since intersubjectivity is understood here as profoundly embodied, it requires spontaneous responsiveness instead of therapeutic protocols, improvisation, and appropriate self-disclosure. Relational body psychotherapy recognises the potential and risks in psychotherapy, and the fact that every therapy involves oscillating between these two polarities.

Under the category of relational body psychotherapy I shall present three modalities of body psychotherapy that were developed from psychodynamic, analytic, and post-Reichian principles. These three approaches preserve the dialectic tension between body and mind, simplicity and complexity, splits and integration, and other dualities.

The Chiron Centre's body psychotherapy

The Chiron Centre in England was an important brewing platform for integrative body psychotherapy, integrating bodymind psychotherapy with psychodynamic and relational thinking. Although the centre no longer offers training (since 2010), its contribution to bridging interpersonal trends in psychotherapy (attachment theory, object relations, relational psychoanalysis) and body psychotherapy was highly valuable.

The Chiron Centre was named after the centaur (half man/half horse) Chiron (Χείρων in Greek), who was accidentally wounded by Hercules. Chiron was one of the most experienced and valued healers, but he could not heal himself. The (Jungian-based) concept of the wounded healer was inspired by Chiron's myth. The centre was established in 1983 by Bernd Eiden, Jochen Lude, and Rainer Pervöltz—three German body psychotherapists who trained with Gerda Boyesen and were further influenced by the work of John Pierrakos, David Boadella, and Jack Lee Rosenberg (whose respective works were described under Reichian body psychotherapy). The three wanted to offer a holistic training, minding the whole body, as well as integrative—which takes neo-Reichian body psychotherapy into account, alongside humanistic, Gestalt therapy, and psychodynamic understanding.

According to the Chiron approach to body psychotherapy, whether bodywork techniques were used or not, the therapist's awareness to somatic processes was central to the work, and part of what defined her as a body psychotherapist. Therefore, bodywork could be a focus for exploration in psychotherapy but it was not a therapeutic goal in itself (Eiden, 2009; Hartley, 2009).

Over the years, and especially from 1992, some teachers at Chiron became increasingly mindful of potential problems in body psychotherapy. The deeper understanding of the therapeutic relationship shattered the initial idealisation of the body and bodily processes, which was amplified the further body psychotherapy moved away from psychodynamic work and manifested in generalised statements such as "the body always knows", or "the body never lies".

This understanding pointed at potential complications in body psychotherapy methods that ignore the complexity of the therapeutic relationship. Among such dangers is the tendency to get pulled into idealised positive transferences (which are more convenient), including the saviour fantasy, and avoid working with negative transference. When these foggy illusions overtake therapy, the body psychotherapist can easily be seen as offering something "more real and authentic" than the psychodynamic (or any non-body) therapists, because she is willing to bodily attend to the primary oral needs of the client, including the need for touch. It is ever so much easier to remain in a relationship where the therapist is good and kind, and not having to deal with frustration, anger, hate, envy, and the undercurrent power struggles that flow in body psychotherapy as in any other therapeutic relationship. Additionally, there is a potential danger for collusion and enmeshment with the client. This is an understandable mixing up of empathy and over-identification, which seduces the therapist into symbiotic spaces in order to avoid the pain associated with separateness, thus failing to hold the necessary complementary position of separateness. For example, a therapist who complies with her client's request for touch without any consideration, and instead of allowing the client to grieve for his unmet needs, colludes with the client's saving fantasy, may easily "drown" in oceans of repetition compulsion, enactment, and retraumatisation. Other risks in working with bodywork techniques in psychotherapy without holding complexity in mind include emotionally flooding of clients and therapists, breaching appropriate therapeutic boundaries, premature breaking of protective defences resulting in breakdown, and perpetuating the saving fantasy of "the good therapist". These understandings brought emotional unrest to the Chiron Centre. To survive those complexities and paradoxes, training at the centre became increasingly analytical and relational (Eiden, 2009; Soth, 2009).

The next developmental stage at the Chiron Centre was paradoxical. A divide was created in the centre between teachers who leaned more towards bodywork and worked directly with the body, and those who, under psychoanalytic and psychodynamic influences, chose to focus on the therapeutic relationship. Therapists and students tended to take sides similarly. What made the Chiron Centre special was the attempt to deal with this divide transparently and while remaining in dialogue regarding the differences. After all, choosing to focus on the relationship while abandoning the body or choosing to focus on the body and ignoring the relationship are two sides of an ever echoing process of dissociation and connection (or, intersubjectivity).

Relational body psychotherapy is, for me, an approach that currently allows both bodywork processes and therapeutic relationship their due place. Somatic interventions are viewed under their prism of therapeutic relationship, and relational interventions are encouraged to find embodied expressions. Thus, relational body psychotherapy provides a synthesis between polarities (without reducing them to a single, new solution), marking a new and blessed developmental stage for body psychotherapy.

In addition to the Chiron's significance to forming a relational body psychotherapy model, the centre was also important in increasing general awareness of body psychotherapy in the wider psychotherapeutic milieu. The Chiron Centre collaborated with important therapeutic centres from other modalities, such as the Bowlby Centre, the Minster Centre, and extensively worked within the United Kingdom Council for Psychotherapy (UKCP).

It is interesting to note that similar historical processes to the ones the Chiron Centre went through occurred in other modalities of body psychotherapy. One example was the transition from bioenergetics via bioenergetic analysis to relational somatic psychotherapy (Hilton, 2012a), or the incorporation of psychodynamic thinking within Hakomi (and the refined Hakomi method). Silke Ziehl's deep bodywork is yet another example of further development of Jack Painter's postural and energetic integration and integrating it with contemporary psychoanalytic thinking. This wave, between a necessarily naïve and open approach, through awakening of awareness to complexity and disillusion, to finding a human and balanced holding of paradoxes, is not only characterising the history of body psychotherapy, but also of the therapeutic process itself.

Embodied relational therapy (ERT)

Embodied relational therapy (ERT) integrates Reichian body psychotherapy, contemporary (mainly relational) psychoanalytic thinking, process-oriented therapies, earth-based spirituality, with socio-political and eco-psychological thinking. It was originated by Nick Totton and Em Edmondson in England.

"As human beings," writes Totton (2005), "we are integrated body–mind-spirit, and that on the whole, we find this condition hard to manage. Our nature seeks to express itself freely, while at the same time protecting itself, sometimes in conditions of great difficulty. This double task of expression and protection makes us often subject to contradictory pulls, and offering double messages about what we feel, want and need" (p. 169). ERT provides a possible platform for (partial) disentangling of this human paradox, to allow greater flow and vitality within the person and between persons.

Nick Totton is one of the leading forces in body psychotherapy today as a writer, clinician, and trainer. As a writer, not only has Totton contributed significantly to the field of body psychotherapy in editing and writing both introductory and advanced texts (Totton, 2000, 2010; Totton & Edmondson, 1988; Totton & Jacobs, 2001), but he also wrote and published papers and books about body and body psychotherapy to psychoanalytic and psychodynamic readerships, and by so doing made a great impact on the legitimisation of body psychotherapy in Europe (Rolef Ben-Shahar, 2013e). Until 2012 Totton also edited the important *Psychotherapy and Politics International* journal which he had established.

Clinically speaking, ERT managed to maintain deep and authentic connection with body, touch, and bodily expressions (i.e., to stay in touch with its Reichian roots and its connection to the human potential movement), yet was also mindful of the complexities of therapeutic relationship and integrated somatic interventions with relational and analytic consideration. The therapeutic relationship is seen as central in ERT: the therapist is understood as a subject, and an important part of the therapeutic dyad, and the work with transference dynamics is immanent in bodywork too (Priestman, 2013; Totton, 2005). Today, ERT training includes one year of "wild therapy", Totton's newest development which reflects ERT's eco-psychology and politically minded focus.

Totton (2003) writes about ERT: "Embodied-Relational Therapy redefines Reichian work as centred on breathing and relationship. It explores the odd-sounding but fundamental question: *how can I breathe and relate to someone at the same time*?" (p. 100). To allow for this tension between inside and outside, self-expression and self-preservation, between apart from and a part of to exist, the psychotherapist might use a variety of skills: among them are conversation, body expression, breathwork, and bodywork. However, faithful to relational thinking, the therapist is primarily there, responding to the clients, to their needs and communication, and to the connection that emerges from the therapeutic alliance. Therefore, ERT uses techniques but it does not emphasise technique; instead it focuses on therapeutic positioning, improvisation, and authentic presence.

Totton (2005) summarises: "Human beings are self-regulating and self-healing ... our job as therapists is to support what is already trying to happen" (p. 181).

Integrative mindbody therapy (IMT)

Integrative mindbody therapy (IMT) is the youngest psychotherapy modality presented here. It was developed by me in the late 1990s and received its relational edge in the mid-2000s. Therapy is structured around three clinical axes: body psychotherapy, trancework, and relational psychotherapy. Common to all these strands is close work with affective processes, which encourage the creation of intersubjectivity—a field where the self is both separate and a part of a broader process at the same time (wider mind, a concept clarified in Chapter Five). The therapeutic toolbox is rooted in Reichian and hypnotic traditions, yet interventions are made while in dialogue with analytical and relational theoretical and clinical models (Rolef Ben-Shahar, 2013a).

In constructing IMT, I was influenced by Reichian body psychotherapy, and particularly the works of Stanley Keleman, Nick Totton, Guy Gladstone, and Silke Ziehl, but also by Ericksonian hypnosis and psychotherapy, mainly Stephen Gilligan's self-relations psychotherapy (S. Gilligan, 1997; 2012; S. Gilligan & Simon, 2004) which will be expanded on in Chapter Four. Both these directions emphasise working with embodied processes on the one hand, and altered states of consciousness (generative trances) on the other. My psychoanalytic influences include attachment theory, object relations, and intersubjective and relational psychoanalysis (Rolef Ben-Shahar, 2008a).

In IMT the organism (and the shared dyad) is understood as forever moving between form and flow, between states and processes. The ability to adaptively organise and remain in the spaces between organisations (Bromberg, 1998) is seen as a mark of health. In fact, IMT examines how we organise ourselves—inside our body, in our emotional-mental-linguistic structures, and within relationships. The psychotherapy process is less concerned with "fixing" difficulties or pain and instead focuses on improving relationships between internal and external levels of organisation. The therapeutic relationship becomes not only a transferential platform for previous relational organisations, but also a microcosm of internal levels of organisation, and change in the relationship is understood as an inner change, paving paths for reorganisations. The concept of trance (the space in-between) is therefore crucial to the therapeutic work.

Psychotherapeutic interventions in IMT, whether bodily or otherwise, are secondary to the therapeutic relationship, are in constant dialogue with it, and are brought back into the relationship. IMT style combines yin and yang—a masculine therapeutic style (archetypally penetrative and initiative) and a feminine style (archetypally containing and waiting). Among the contributions of IMT to the body psychotherapy field are exploration of touch as relational affirmation (King, 2011), body psychotherapy work with dissociative disorders (Rolef Ben-Shahar, 2009; Rolef Ben-Shahar & Wood, 2009), and the flow-form cycle presented in this book.

Training programmes in IMT are offered in Israel (the Relational Body Psychotherapy Programme at the Israeli Centre for Body–Mind Medicine) and the UK, and IMT workshops are regularly given across Europe. The training emphasises positioning and therapeutic orientation, alongside experiential and introspective work.

Should I stay little? A Reichian vignette

For months on end I have tried to understand with Meredith why she was so scared of confronting her partner. Meredith was fifty, a senior journalist, connected and intelligent, and has been married to Derek for fifteen years. In comparison with her strong body and powerful personality, her voice was almost inaudible, and I needed to make a real effort to hear her well.

Meredith wanted to experiment with liberating her breath and sound, and we opted to do some bodywork. I asked Meredith to breathe fully and accompany her exhale with sound. While she breathed I began to press against her diaphragm: it was an invitation to safely confront me through the diaphragm—to push me out so that she could breathe. The strong pressure on her diaphragm disrupted her breathing, and in order to retrieve her rhythms she had to be very active—both in terms of breathing, and by creating muscular tension and responding to the pressure.

At first, Meredith struggled to breathe or make a sound; it was too embarrassing for her. But soon the exploration became pleasurable for her, and her breathing deepened and became more charged; her voice got correspondingly louder. Meredith looked at me and started pushing me with her diaphragm, with increasing amplitude and strength.

Suddenly, while Meredith was pushing with her body and voice, her eyes seemed full of fury and wrath. I was both excited to witness her power, and admittedly a bit frightened too from the sheer power of her presence; within seconds her facial expressions changed and she softened, and all of a sudden seemed placating and weak. "What happened?" I asked. "I could finally see how powerful you are." "I know it makes no sense, but I was really scared that you'd leave me if you saw my anger," she said. We processed this experience over a few sessions, as Meredith realised that her parents (particularly her father) were unable to tolerate her anger or her enthusiasm. Meredith was highly attuned to her father's fear ("I was too much for him"), which she saw in my eyes too when she embodied her power, and kept herself little in order to keep his love.

We would have probably reached the same insight without the bodily intervention; I am not even certain that it would have taken longer. But there was something in the immediate nature of those experiences, and the vital and real transferential enlivening that allowed Meredith and me to understand, not just conceive, her transferential trap, and my part in it. We kept on working with this material for long months to assist Meredith in changing those patterns of fear and self-reduction.

Exercise: one step forward two steps back

(Particularly useful as a therapeutic process)

The following exercise is based on Stanley Keleman's (1987) accordion exercise, with some alterations from Gestalt and NLP. The basic premise of this exercise is that every emotional state has a somatic form. Sometimes, it is easier to change painful and rigid emotional states through working with somatic organisations, which provide another door into change and greater flexibility.

1. The psychotherapist invites the client to speak about a stuck emotional experience (or state) and encourages him to associate with the feelings and sensations involved in this experience by asking sensory-based and affective questions, which direct the client to sensations and embodied emotions without attempting to reach understanding, track the emotional source of pain, or bring about insight. These are questions that enquire about the *what, how, when,* and *where* and not the *why* or *where from*. The client is invited to think and speak in the first person and in the present tense. For example, he might say: "… and then I had to speak in the group and I suddenly froze." Therapist: "So you have to speak in the group and suddenly you freeze. Where do you first sense the freezing in your body?"
2. Once some affect is built (please exercise clinical judgment regarding the volume needed) and the client is *in* the experience (without being flooded and dissociated), the therapist asks the client to show her what this feeling looks like: to sculpture himself in order to illustrate the inner feeling of this stuck place (i.e., to give it somatic form). If bodily changes are minute, the therapist can ask her client to amplify his somatic form.
3. When the client embodies the stuck form, the therapist asks the client to find a symbol, image, or voice to represent this place (a beginning of symbolisation). A deeper exploration is possible here, by examining the beliefs and thoughts that condition this form, when and from whom this place was learnt, etc.
4. The therapist guides her client out of the stuck bodily form, and asks him to gently shake his body while thinking of the opposite of the stuck place, even if it is in a completely different context ("stuck" might be in speaking to groups, "flowing"—in gardening). The therapist encourages the client to amplify the dialogue about this opposite sensation, by asking sensory-based and affective questions, and speaking in the first person and in the present tense.
5. After affect for the new, flowing state is created—that is, after the client was able to bodily and emotionally experience this flowing state, the client sculptures this state too in his body, to illustrate it through posture, gesture, and movement. If changes are minute, the therapist could ask the client to amplify the form. Here too the client is asked to think of an image, a word, or a sound to represent the flowing state, then shakes off the form and returns to base position.

6. The therapist guides her client in once more organising the stuck state somatically, but slightly less amplified (say, 80 per cent), then to gradually move to the flowing form. When the client reaches the flowing form, he is once more asked to return to the stuck form, basically creating a dance between flowing and impasse.
7. Therapist and client continue with the last stage until there is a flowing motion between the polarities and then the therapist asks the client to slow down and stop shortly after the stuck place. This is the first stage to change. What does it feel like? What information is revealed in the body? What would it take to move from the stuck place to this first step? What beliefs and values helped the client? What word, image, or touch might help to strengthen this place and remind the client of it when needed?
8. Complete the exercise and process together.

Notes

1. I wish to thank Will Davis and Theresia Mestmäcker for their help in conceptualising functional analysis.
2. I wish to thank Neta Shaked for her illuminating comments on rebirthing.
3. I wish to thank Keren Tzarfati, Dr Ido Semion, and Michal Barnea for their help in describing and clarifying Hakomi.
4. I wish to thank Dr Atsmaout Perlstein and Bilha Frolinger from the Israeli Focusing Centre for their contribution and help in writing this section.
5. Excerpt from Antonio Machado, "Moral Proverbs and Folk Song", from *Times Alone: Selected Poems of Antonio Machado*, translation ©1983 by Robert Bly. Reprinted by permission of Wesleyan University Press.

PART II

THEORETICAL

I rested in the arms of my arms
I no longer slept
It was night in the summer, winter in the day
An eternal shivering of thoughts
Fear love Fear love
Close the window open the window
You'll see you'll see
The hummingbird motionless as a star.

—*Dora Maar*, "I rested in the arms of my arms" (1942–1943, p. 82)*

I once knew a uniquely talented Chinese doctor, who was almost equally cynical. The concept of *Chi*, which describes life-energy and is central in traditional Chinese medicine, was merely a metaphoric construct for him. "I don't believe in Chi," he used to teasingly say to his fellow practitioners. One day, when I asked him why he had chosen to practise Chinese medicine and not Western medicine, when he was clearly not "a believer" he replied: "Western medicine relates to the body as if it was a biological machine; traditional Chinese medicine relates to it as poetry." He continued: "People respond differently to poetry than to mechanics, and I personally find it more aesthetic."

In his excellent and extremely relevant (yet depressing) book *Brave New World*, Aldous Huxley (1932) related to the consequences of this very choice my friend has described: "God isn't

*Dora Maar's poem is reprinted with permissions of © ADAGP, Paris 2013 and English translator Mary Ann Caws.

compatible with machinery and scientific medicine and universal happiness. You must make your choice. Our civilization has chosen machinery and medicine and happiness" (p. 214).

Part II (Theoretical) presents some theories and concepts from the world of body psychotherapy. We shall examine different levels of self-organisation, the theory of mind in body psychotherapy (which in body psychotherapy becomes bodymind); we shall further examine some developmental theories, conceptualisations, and terminology used by body psychotherapy. To say that our body expresses feelings and thoughts is, of course, a metaphor—not "truth". On the other hand, the unconscious, mind, psyche—these are also metaphors. We use language to describe something that is not from language, and hope that the other person will understand. In so doing we both limit communication and enable it.

I find the metaphors of body psychotherapy aesthetic and relevant to therapeutic thinking and to human interactions, and I invite you to check whether you can relate to these metaphors as well. Perhaps, when we agree to pay the price of giving up objective truth, we might find and co-create beautiful and meaningful poetry together.

CHAPTER FOUR

Form and flow: three levels of self-organisation[†]

> I said to my soul, be still, and wait without hope
> For hope would be hope for the wrong thing; wait without love
> For love would be love of the wrong thing; there is yet faith
> But the faith and the love and the hope are all in the waiting.
> Wait without thought, for you are not ready for thought:
> So the darkness shall be the light, and the stillness the dancing.
>
> —*T. S. Eliot* (1940, p. 188), Four Quartets—"*East Coker*"[1]

Introduction

What is it that defines body psychotherapy as a distinct modality of psychotherapy, which could be distinguished from other psychotherapy modalities? Is it the tools and skills used in body psychotherapy—the use of touch, breathwork, and movement? If that is so, then body psychotherapy includes such variegated modalities within it, each using different therapeutic tools and operating different clinical judgment and justifications (sometimes contradictory to one another) for the use of these therapeutic tools or avoiding their use, that it would become difficult to gather all these under the same umbrella of a unified field. Additionally, some therapeutic modalities, which are clearly not psychotherapy, incorporate touch, breathwork, and movement too. Furthermore, some psychotherapy modalities, which are not body

[†]This chapter is partially based on a paper previously published in the *USA Body Psychotherapy Journal* (Rolef Ben-Shahar, 2011a).

psychotherapy, utilise somatic interventions as well. Why would body psychotherapy deserve this distinct modality definition?

Body psychotherapy attempts to address the pain resulting from body–mind splits, yet at the same time—as psychologist Yorai Sella (Keet, Sella, & Ziv-Beiman, 2013) pointed out—by maintaining its name it also perpetuates it, as if there were a psychotherapy that did not include the body. Nevertheless, many of those who seek therapy bring with them pain and suffering that manifest both in body and mind, and psychotherapists who offer to work with the body encounter complaints that tend to be seen as irrelevant outside the somatically oriented framework. Body psychotherapists are lucky enough to have backaches and migraines, muscle pains and period pains, chronic and acute physical pain, enter the clinic alongside the emotional and cognitive suffering. To deal with such suffering, body psychotherapy proposes a unique therapeutic position, which involves somatic curiosity. The body psychotherapist is attentive to somatic processes that take place within the client, the therapist, and the therapeutic relationship. Could this special positioning be the distinguishing mark of body psychotherapy?

But today, many psychotherapists from other modalities (including within psychoanalysis) maintain an active explorative attitude towards somatic phenomena both in the client and the therapist. For example, Didier Anzieu's seminal work *The Skin Ego* (1989) describes a very meaningful and deep approach to bodily clinical curiosity. Renowned psychoanalyst Joyce McDougall (1989) also illustrates body-to-body dialogues taking place between therapist and client. The work of psychoanalyst Wilma Bucci (2001, 2008, 2011) places a crucial emphasis on the emotional-somatic communication, demanding of the therapist not only to be attentive to somatic phenomena, but also to communicate with those—sometimes in nonverbal language. Susie Orbach (2004c, 2009) too, invites the psychotherapist to seriously examine her own body and that of her clients. Could it possibly mean that the age of body psychotherapy is over? Perhaps the growing psychoanalytic and psychotherapeutic awareness to the place of the body in therapy, and the incorporation of somatic interventions into psychotherapy make body psychotherapy redundant? Perhaps there is no justification to maintain the field as a distinct and distinguishable modality? Indeed, there are clinicians—even within body psychotherapy, who ponder this question. As for me, I think differently.

Body psychotherapeutic tools are of immense value, and I hope the clinicians among you will at some point acquire body psychotherapeutic skills for working with the body through breath, somatic attunement, movement, and touch. The therapeutic positioning of the body psychotherapist is also noteworthy and unique, having been developed and fine-tuned over many decades of bodymind theory. This historical context, which was expressed in the last three chapters, relates to the point I wish to make here.

Both positioning and the therapeutic techniques and skills are applied in context, and are a product of a long professional history. Body psychotherapists are trained to methodically observe somatic organisations, backed with decades of theoretical and clinical research in the field. While the orientation of the psychotherapists might differ, as well as their chosen technique, there is a huge difference when a technique is applied from a cohesive and organised theoretical and clinical position. The combination of the skills and techniques, the unique positioning, and the historical and theoretical context—these are the elements that create a distinctive therapeutic identity. Such identity is coherent enough to allow for variety and differentness within it on the one hand, while on the other hand it can still be recognisable and distinguished when compared with other psychotherapy modalities.

The theory of mind in body psychotherapy and the body–mind dialectics with which the discipline struggles, the body–mind developmental organisation, and the perception of character structure as a primarily embodied process, all these provide the body psychotherapist with a sound theoretical base from which her professional identity crystallises and forms. It is the same base that would later be translated into the therapist's clinical skills, and from which stem both her therapeutic positioning and her therapeutic intervention. In my opinion, body psychotherapeutic theory, which is the source of its therapeutic positioning and clinical intervention, is distinctive enough to maintain its separate identity as a unique therapeutic modality. The body psychotherapist occupies a cohesively distinct professional identity, incorporating therapeutic positioning, therapeutic skills and techniques, and a solid theoretical base. However, I can also sense the danger for this distinct organisation becoming rigidified. The movement between distinguished identity (with its predisposition to splitting) and flexible flow (with its potential for charlatanism or indecision) invites us, as a discipline, to announce our separate identity yet be willing to deeply challenge its necessity.

This chapter and the two following ones will present three theoretical axes around which the identity of the body psychotherapist is organised: the organisational structure of the self (and the place of the body within it), the theory of bodymind, and the bodymind character structure. In these theoretical chapters I do not pretend to present a consensual body psychotherapy theory, but instead unravel my own theoretical position as a relational body psychotherapist. I hope that psychotherapists from different modalities (including body psychotherapists) would be willing and able to examine their own work through this theoretical and clinical prism.

This chapter will explore three levels of developmental organisation and the dynamic movement between those three. The theoretical conceptualisation in this chapter is my own amalgamation of relational thinking, Stephen Gilligan's self-relations psychotherapy, and Reichian theories. The structural organisation explained in this chapter forms a platform for understanding the concepts explained in the next chapters.

Psychologist and founder of self-relations psychotherapy Stephen Gilligan (1996) described three functional fields comprising together the self: a somatic field (the somatic self), a cognitive field (cognitive self), and the field of relationships (the relational self). The self, for Gilligan, was expressed in the movement (the relationships, the patterns which connect) between those levels of self. To reiterate, the self is seen as *a relationship* between somatic and cognitive aspects. The relational field inside us parallels, for Gilligan, the relational field that opens when we enter a dialogue with another person. Gilligan, who is influenced by anthropologist and philosopher Gregory Bateson, understands *mind* as a process that is not merely located within the individual, but also in the system in which the individual partakes. According to this view, the mind has another dimension; the mind is not exclusively ours, but instead becomes part of a broader relational context: we partake in a *wider mind*, on the basis of which relationships are constructed. This view challenges two paradigms regarding the self: that the self is a limited object/subject, bounded within our skin (static), and that the self exclusively belongs to us.

When we let ourselves open to a relationship field, we enter a shared space much broader than ourselves, a mind that includes us but is not limited to us or excludes the other. As we shall discover in the next chapter, this understanding of a *wider mind* is extremely similar to the relational psychoanalytic conceptualisations of intersubjectivity (T. Ogden, 1992, 1994a), and is also influenced by Kohut's description of transmuting internalisation (Kohut, Goldberg, & Stepansky, 1984; Osterville, 1995), and in general by Kohut's concept of selfobject. Relational psychoanalyst Stephen Mitchell (2000), for instance, followed the thinking of interpersonal psychiatrist Harry Stack Sullivan (1953), and asserted that mind was a *transpersonal phenomenon* and therefore that intersubjectivity had a spiritual dimension.

This chapter sets the scene for understanding the concept of bodymind, presented in Chapter Five. In this chapter I shall present the "form-flow" theory, a synthesis of varied theoretical sources, from body psychotherapy, modern physics, relational psychoanalysis, and spiritual traditions.

Shiva and Micky

> Everything is in flux. Only after we have been stunned by the infinite diversity of processes constituting the universe can we understand the importance of the organizing principle that creates order from chaos. [...]
>
> —Fritz Perls (1948, p. 571)[2]

Like the Hindu deity Shiva, the creator and destroyer, all organic matter pulsates between form and flow, organisation and deconstruction. The dance into assuming organisations, deconstructing these, and reassuming forms exists on all levels of nature. Life is continuously revealed in the process of distinction and differentiation.

As part of nature, we too organise our reality through forming and deconstructing. The same organised reality, in turn, characterises and shapes us. When a toddler takes her first steps, for example, every stumble and fall assists her in developing and calibrating her proprioception. Her musculature organises appropriately to the force required to lift her leg and remain stable and erect, to fall forwards (in her taking a step) and re-stabilise her position. This type of bodily organisation dictates a certain mutual relationship with the environment and managing gravity, which in turn impacts and influences the toddler and her development. If, for example, the toddler learned to walk in a carpeted house, or on a beach, or on grass, her walking would be categorically different to the walking of a toddler who learned to walk on a tiled floor. These different walking styles will shape the development of her muscular organisation, her bodily relationship with gravity, and her bodily capabilities. The toddler thus creates (organises) a walking style, and this walking style shapes and organises the toddler in return.

Here is another, therapeutic example. Christina experienced her father as weak and helpless, while her mother was described as powerful and dominant; and Christina despised her father's physical and emotional softness. Time and again, Christina chose men who seemed physically and emotionally strong and powerful as partners, only to discover within a short while that they were weak, incapable, and very passive. Christina's way of understanding masculine power was in constant dialogue with the power-model (passive-active, weak-strong) in her family, and the polarity she was attracted to continued to shape her by "finding herself" in the same type of relationship, increasingly persuaded that no other types of relationships are possible for her.

Adopting a form, the organising process, is thus a dialectic process. We are created by assuming forms through the process of making distinctions. We impose models of reality on the world and actively shape our reality, which in return shapes our thoughts, feelings, and actions. Life could therefore be understood as a movement through patterns of reality-making in the creation of which we partake (a series of steps) (Rolef Ben-Shahar, 2001b). This, in my understanding, is the essence of Freud's developmental model and the rationale behind Reich's character analysis.

I use the term *form* to describe an organisation (structure, the noun) and *flow* to represent the process of deconstruction and emergence, the in-between space of flux (the verb, of becoming); yet these two phases are forever in continuum. At each given moment, some aspects of our reality are organised into form while others undressed of theirs; the terms flow and form are therefore metaphoric approximations, describing pulsatory rhythms.

In his call to allow space for the flow, the yet unformed, the emergent rhythm, relational psychoanalyst Steven Knoblauch (1999) advocated surrender to flow: "By shifting from noun, place, and state to action, attention is focused on an unfolding, continual process" (p. 44). For Knoblauch (1997), this resonant interaction was both verbal and nonverbal, hence requiring the therapist to remain attuned to bodily interactions without hastening to interpret these and instead "suspending judgment until a meaning emerges" (p. 496). Knoblauch recognised that giving form to emergent moments too early (in the form of interpretation) might disturb the musicality and efficacy of the therapeutic act.

At the heart of the claim that life unfolds as an organising principle, lies the assumption that both reality and self are continually pulsating. According to this view the universe pulsates, and we share in its pulsation. Movement is therefore at the base of reality—this is a basic stance in expressive psychotherapies and body psychotherapy. We might argue that the universe has not fully emerged out of *tohu bohu*, the biblical state of pre-creation: undifferentiated chaos is still within our midst, but in the process of creation we give *tohu bohu* shapes. And creation itself is temporary, forever in motion and constant movement.

My friend Micky Gerber offered the metaphor of the ocean and waves to better illustrate this pulsation. Human beings, she said, could be understood both as an ocean (the universe we are a part of) and as individual waves (the individual selves that we all are). On a certain level, our existence as individuals could be distinguished; on another level, speaking of individual waves is meaningless outside the wider context of the ocean. The essence of the ocean is in the paradoxical holding of both truths—in its movement. The water is not the same water; it evaporates only to transform and return from the rivers; the landscape too keeps changing; but the inherent and immanent movement of the ocean remains, the currents and undercurrents, the unifying flow of the ocean's aliveness is always there. It means that the person as an individual (as emphasised in Western philosophies) and the person as a part of a larger relational context (as emphasised in Eastern philosophies) are two faces of the self, forever in tension with one another, yet also complementing each other. The next chapter will demonstrate how the concept of bodymind in body psychotherapy is integrated with this eternal movement.

This idea of universal flux relates to and is informed by the Buddhist notion of emptiness (Preece, 2000; Sumedho, 1992) and is also connected to Taoist philosophy (Lash, 1989). The pulsating universe also relates to the theories of philosophers like Immanuel Kant (1781), Arthur Schopenhauer (1818), and Maurice Merleau-Ponty (1962), and to those of certain psychoanalysts, such as Ronald Fairbairn (1952), Harry Stack Sullivan (1953), and of course, to the work and research of Wilhelm Reich (1942). This perception of flow helped in crystallising a theory of developmental bodymind structures (the character structure), which is an important tenet in body psychotherapy theory.

Our dynamic reality within this flux therefore depends on the temporary forms we assume (and create) and on the guiding principles of these organising processes. What kind of waves are we becoming? What is the quality of land we chose to step upon, and what kind of steps do we take? Our subjective existence, short-lived as it may be, bittersweet as it is, is transient and can only be captured in the here-and-now. Using theoretical concepts and clinical vignettes, I hope to demonstrate in this chapter the importance of the *flow-form* cycle to the body psychotherapeutic process.

Form and flow in three levels of self-organisation

I am suggesting here that three primary channels assist us in organising the kaleidoscopic matrix of self: the somatic channel (bodily aspects), the linguistic channel (cognitive aspects), and the relational channel (organising relationships). These are three axes that will be further explored and presented here. Through those organisational channels, we create distinctions (artificial and organic ones) that allow us to cross the divide between inside and outside, mediate between fantasy and reality, between you and me. Body psychotherapy presupposes that within every human organisation, and along the cognitive channel, each one of these channels is expressed: that every emotional-mental event will have a bodily expression and will also be expressed in (internalised or external) relationships, and vice versa.

Somatic organisation

> The basis of our psychic life is the construction of bodily states, gestures, and ways of moving which have social and emotional meaning.
>
> —Ian Grand (1998, p. 172)

In each given moment, we take shape, making somatic organisations on cellular, histological, muscular, neural, and structural levels. These organisations mediate between inside and outside. From our conception, our bodies are preoccupied with distinction and differentiation, grouping and unification. Amoebas define themselves through their flexible membranes, which create boundaries and maintain a fluid dialogue with these membranes: what comes in and leaves uninterruptedly; what is actively taken in or actively pushed out; what belongs and what does not. To an extent, each and every cell of our body does the same, and to a certain degree we are active participants in this process on much more complex levels as well. Creating somatic organisations is necessary for survival: we need somatic organisations to breathe, digest, think, and act in the world. For instance, it is of utter importance that certain cells develop and function as liver cells and not as muscular fibres, that the muscular contractions of the heart attain a certain steady frequency and intensity. It is important that the quadriceps (an important group of muscles in the thigh) maintain a more-or-less steady rhythm of contraction when we walk, lest we fall backwards or forwards with each step.

But these somatic organisations require a degree of flexibility, too, for us to successfully respond and adapt to our changing external and internal environment. The less mobility and flexibility a form attains, the more likely it is to become rigidified and maladaptive when environmental pressures change. Should the heart muscle, for example, contract at a regular pulsating pace and unchanging intensity even when a person begins to jog, oxygen supply to the musculature will be insufficient, the blood pressure will drop, and the person will faint.

When muscular and skeletal forms become rigid, they express what Reich termed character armour, or muscular armour (a concept expanded on in Chapter Two). Part of Reich's work (1933a), which was developed by researchers and clinicians such as Lowen (1958), Boadella (1985, 2011), Keleman (1985, 1987), and Carroll (2002), involved characterising and mapping patterned bodily organisations and correlating these with different developmental stages. Somatic typology, including character structure, is far less dogmatic today than it was in the days of Reich. Today, we recognise that these generalisations are useful only to the extent that we, as clinicians, remember to first and foremost remain in a dialogue with the person, not a typology. Nevertheless, the shapes of our somatic organisations (functional and psychopathological) and the knowhow of reorganising somatically are among the most important contributions of body psychotherapy to the wider field of psychotherapy. Chapter Six will expand the discussion on somatic organisation through examining the bodymind character structure.

The following vignette[3] will demonstrate focused therapeutic work with patterns of somatic organisation.

Owen was a fifty-four-year-old insurance broker, lean, intelligent, and anxious, who was referred to me by his general practitioner (GP). Owen was reluctant to commence psychotherapy and preferred medication, but his GP persuaded him to attend three therapeutic meetings. For many years, Owen suffered from debilitating panic attacks and severe insomnia. Recent change in work (an unsolicited promotion) brought with it great distress and Owen felt anxious, under pressure to preform, and flooded by new demands and managerial obligations which he resented. Furthermore, he experienced his immediate boss as a tyrannical bully. From what little information Owen was willing to provide, I learned that his father was physically abusive to him. Owen described himself as struggling against depression for as long as he could remember, but reiterated his disinterest in long-term psychotherapy.

One of the most striking features in Owen for me was connected to his physical appearance, or more specifically, his jaw. Compared with his thinness and hypotonic structure, Owen's face seemed powerful and strongly held, and his jaw was disproportionately muscular and powerful. Looking at his face, I imagined a volcano about to erupt. The muscles in Owen's jaw were irregularly developed, and I was curious about the dissonance between his loose body and strong face. Interestingly, my own jaw started aching from the moment we faced each other in our chairs. Such a strong and dense jaw may indicate to the body psychotherapist a possible muscular holding, which if released might bring other organisations (emotional, mental, and relational) to the surface, thus allowing the therapeutic dyad to explore and possibly work with these.

I would usually refrain from offering such body intervention so early on in therapy, but Owen only came for a few sessions. I offered him to do some bodywork together, and to my surprise he readily agreed. Perhaps the immediacy and tangible nature of my offer were more appealing to Owen than the thought of psychotherapy or speaking about his pain (or the medical model more appealing than a potential relationship): I am not sure. After some warming up of the area, I applied strong pressure to the masseter muscles and waited.

Owen's face became crimson red almost immediately, and he got up and started pacing the room up and down like a caged wild lion. "I'm furious," he said. I handed Owen a racket and a big cushion and, without much ado, Owen started hitting it and shouting loudly. It was as if the cushion was changing faces before our eyes: at first it was his boss, then other bullies from his life, and in the end, his father. It was as if this small tense muscle held a historical array of subordination.

True to his word, Owen came to see me three more times, and reported great improvement both at work and at home. He assertively confronted his boss and co-workers: "I am no longer everybody's doormat," he told me proudly.

In my opinion, Owen would have undoubtedly benefited from long-term psychotherapeutic process. In many ways his life was rigid and limited, but he was uninterested in—or not ready for—embarking upon such process. Our brief work together merely opened the door to a new somatic organisation, long enough for something to change, and for that particular context, it was a good enough change.

This type of therapeutic intervention was geared towards challenging and changing somatic organisations, and many forms of somatic interventions (particularly in traditional body psychotherapy) tended to operate on this level. I would like to emphasise that this type of bodywork was not a panacea; it simply allowed for somatic reorganisation, which required work—sometimes a lot of cultivation work and over a long period of time—to be successfully internalised and integrated. However, sometimes the very possibility of experiencing the world and yourself different to how you were used to could be a significant and meaningful change in itself.

Linguistic organisation

> Language is a tool for imposing distinctions upon the world.
>
> —Bradford Keeney (1983, p. 25)[4]

Cognitive processes are presented here as interactive processes of distinction-making through symbolic means, including language. By imposing these distinctions we create our world and at the same time limit it with this very creation. Let me illustrate this statement with an example. When Zohar was four she listened to a story about Smurfs,[5] and heard how Brainy-Smurf told Papa-Smurf that he recognised over thirty-five hues of blue. Zohar thought for a moment then said: "I don't know so many blues." The concept of *blue* enabled Zohar to organise her world in colours, but also created generalisations that limited her sensitivity to the infinite variety of information. Our thoughts and our beliefs, language, and other cognitive schemas that we use create artificial impositions, which interface the infinite experiential information and our capacity to contain and tolerate this information. Neuro-linguistic-programming (NLP) relates to three qualities of impositions: generalisations, distortions, and deletions (Dilts & DeLozier, 2000). Zohar's shades of blue and the Smurfs exemplify *generalisations* (as are, "Men are all the same, they are all after one thing," "I never get what I want," "Everybody knows it's never gonna happen," etc.). *Distortions* allow us to change our perception to better match it to our worldview. For example, a Jewish colleague of mine treated a young Muslim man who was dreaming of joining Al-Qaeda and becoming a suicide bomber. After some deliberation, she decided to disclose her religion to him. For weeks on end, he argued with her that she must have been wrong, and in the end concluded that she was "Jewish with Muslim blood", that even if she was not aware of it, she had Muslim blood flowing in her veins. The youth distorted the reality to fit his world view. *Deletions* are simple acts of selectively ignoring information that disturbs our habituated reality-organisation; selective-hearing is a classic example of deletion.

Just as our somatic organisations provide us with a bodily container (both real and imagined at the same time) for our experience, so does our language equip us with a similarly real-and-not-real psychic container. Thanks to our linguistically based cognition, we are able to engage in continuous reorganisation of meaning: we reorient ourselves temporally, between past and present, and position ourselves in space and in relation to others (Fangarette, 1963).

To illustrate linguistic organisation, let us look at Preston, a thirty-eight-year-old single man, who sought psychotherapy following repeated depressive episodes. I had a great difficulty understanding Preston's speech, which was highly associative and jittery, and moved from one subject to another without proper grammatical structure ("Yesterday was a difficult day at work because the noise—can you close the window—struggle to focus—maybe better to change jobs?"). This fragmented language made it extremely challenging for me to communicate with him or relate to him. Preston's mum was depressed and alcoholic and was diagnosed as schizophrenic, and he himself presented with symptoms that bordered on schizophrenia (he underwent two inconclusive psychiatric assessments), with periods of excessive paranoia and a somewhat amusing affinity for conspiracy theories.

Preston's sense of self was very fragile, and he struggled to fully differentiate his feelings and thoughts from those of others. He was absolutely certain that he could read everybody else's mind and, at the same time, he felt transparent—and believed that others too could read his every thought and feeling. We spent long sessions in which Preston got angry with me for thoughts I supposedly had about him (he was mostly, but not always, wrong). Preston was angry with me for wasting his time asking questions instead of tuning in and directly and uninterruptedly reading his mind.

Curiously, in his speech, Preston rarely spoke in the first person, and regularly omitted the word "I" from his sentences. For example, instead of saying "I'm not sure that I'll be able to come next week," Preston would say: "There's a problem coming next week." Instead of saying: "I wasted all my weekly salary on someone I mistakenly thought was interested in me," he would say: "Someone said she wanted to go out, somehow all the money was spent." Just as Preston struggled to maintain a continuity of himself, he also found it difficult to maintain therapeutic continuation, and I therefore encouraged him to write me an email between each session. Even in the emails he made little use of the first person or the word "I". His written language was even more robotic than his spoken one: "Good to write difficult at work wanting to make redundant tomorrow there's date—stressful."

Preston's social life was expectedly very limited, and a large portion of our psychotherapy was dedicated to supporting him in building social skills, increasing his capacity to understand social situations, and daring to feel and sometimes express his feelings in a safe and secure manner. Three years into psychotherapy, with mostly somatic interventions (primarily touch), and without any specific or direct focus on his language, Preston's speech began to show pronounced changes. His language became more coherent, and his sentences became fuller with first-person pronoun use; his "I" began to appear in his spoken and written language: his reality changed alongside his language, both strengthening each other and informing one another.

Interpreting linguistic organisations as a crucial aspect of human development is based, among other sources, on the philosophy of Ludwig Wittgenstein, who in 1921 stated: "The limits of my language mean the limits of my world" (p. 148). Other contributing sources for linguistic organisation are Noam Chomsky's transformational grammar (1957), systemic thinking (Bateson, 1972; Keeney, 1983; Korzybski, 1924), and, as mentioned here before, NLP (Bandler & Grinder, 1979; Dilts, Grinder, Bandler, Bandler, & DeLozier, 1980).

Relational organisation

> The infant organises its feeling-experience relative to the feeling states of others, and there is a clear interactive learning process between the infant and others right from the beginning.
>
> —Franklyn Sills (2009, p. 53)

When all is well (and this is not always the case), our lives emerge from deep symbiosis. In the warm and protective uterine environment, many of our needs are satisfied without us experiencing desire. We are fed and nourished without eating; oxygenated without inhaling; protected by an immune system without having a completely operative immune system of our own. Even gravity has a lesser hold over us in the uterus thanks to the amniotic fluid, which also acts as shock absorber and mediates between us and the world. And then, abruptly, we are thrown into an unknown land of infinite unrealised possibilities and (since it is so unknown) potential great fear.

Within moments of our emerging from the womb, both the respiratory and the digestive systems begin to operate more-or-less autonomously, and the mother–baby symbiosis takes its first turn (of course the womb experience is not only symbiotic). Any newborn is faced with a dramatic experience and huge demands for self-regulation and survival, long before the organism is consciously capable of trusting and of submitting willingly to the care of others. According to some clinicians (e.g., Grof, 1988; Lake, 1979), any later surrender (and any letting go) is saturated with the terror and potential which characterised our decent from the birth canal, the necessary exile from the uterine heaven en route to becoming conscious human beings (heaven, for me, in its essential lack of consciousness, is not fully formed, waiting for movement). In order to survive this extreme transition the infant requires a container—an embodied wider mind, which could regulate the newborn and contain it. The newborn needs to be a part of a larger system, which is one of the first roles of its attachment figures.

Researcher Colwyn Trevarthen, who spent many years studying infants, termed this preliminary symbiosis between the newborn and its mother *primary intersubjectivity* (Trevarthen, 1993; Trevarthen & Aitken, 2001). This primary wider mind was characterised by ultimate surrender, yet one which was (mostly) lacking consciousness or real choice (at least on the newborn's behalf). The ability to form intimate relationships later on, to consciously submit into a wider mind (what Trevarthen called *secondary intersubjectivity*), relied on that primary symbiotic connection from which we emerged. To reiterate: connection with others was possible because it was our most familiar position, we knew it from inside; in connecting we re-established the most familiar state we have ever known in our body. Our primary identity in the world was dyadic *alongside* our individual identity: we were mother–baby parallel to our being a mother and a baby (an ocean and a wave). An important factor to note about this dyadic entity was that it was first and foremost of the body.

Relational theories (as well as attachment theory, which informed relational approaches) perceived the self as forever organised in a dialogue with another. We emerged out of a union with the mother and the self was initially primarily dyadic in its essence; a separate subjectivity developed much later. We were created as separated individuals only thanks to our earlier relationships (S. Mitchell, 2002; Sullivan, 1940).

Throughout life, one major way of organising our identity relates to tectonic shifts in relationships: entering them, engaging with them, and leaving relationships. The qualities of our identity-formation and our ego-strength largely depend on our capacity to be open to different orders of dyadic-self (the couple that we are), familial-self (the family that we are), or organisational and societal selves. Our early forms of relational organisations (attachment relationships) become the matrices through which we engage in connections in adulthood, and which later become our reality (Bowlby, 1988). Heinz Kohut (Kohut, Goldberg, & Stepansky, 1984) described the process of structuring the self as based on internalisation of parental figures; according to Kohut, the self was created out of the dialectics between real child–parent connection and internalised child–parent connection.

Our character, personality, and identity are therefore engaged in ongoing dialogue with our real and internalised attachment figures (Whitaker, 2000). Unless we actively learn to identify these relational forms, it is doubtful that we can ever have significant relationships other than those we have always known: we need to claim our identity and consciously shape our relatedness to truly become separated yet connected human subjectivities.

This view shares great resemblance with Stephen Gilligan's self-relations psychotherapy which was presented in the beginning of this chapter. Dyadic forms of consciousness (or wider minds) are deeply challenging to Western-indoctrinated philosophy, where the self is seen as localised within clear bodily boundaries and is sharply distinguished and separated from its environment (we live in our skin and we are separated from others). Here, relational thinking asks of us to reconsider this stance and relate to the individual also as a partial system, a partial self. Bodies and minds touch one another, create each other, and become one against the presence of another.

The following example presents a clinical vignette demonstrating therapy with relationship organisation.

Roland came to therapy because of what he called "my temper problem". Roland was a busy and successful family doctor, married and a father to two young children, who told me of a happy, harmonious, and successful marital relationship, which was only challenged by his angry temper. Over the last two years, Roland reported, and without any justifications, he was experiencing waves of fury and violence inside him, which were mostly directed at his wife. These violent and angry outbursts were mostly verbal, but after he "found himself" shaking his wife, Roland was alarmed by his expressed violence and decided to start psychotherapy.

For a few weeks, as part of building our therapeutic alliance, we tried to validate the tensions in his life, which Roland dared not name. We noted the sexual frustration he felt with his wife who was exhausted from bringing their two sons up and his anger with the financial burden which, mostly, rested upon his shoulders. I enjoyed being in Roland's company, and delighted in his eloquent expressions, his emotional openness, and his true willingness to work. I also enjoyed our sessions because *our* relationship was calm and collected; when Roland spoke of his rage, it was as if he spoke of another person. Inside me, I was scared of meeting the violent Roland, and perhaps I cultivated this charming and calm quality of Roland, as to not rock our (and my) own boat too much.

Until one day I cancelled a session. About three months into our psychotherapeutic work I had to cancel a session—a pressing family matter. Roland cancelled the following session at the last minute, and when I insisted he came that week at an alternative time, he barged into the clinic irritable, sweaty, and angry. He started a verbal onslaught and blamed me for my lousy, expensive therapy, for wasting his time, since "nothing changed anyways". I was scared when he yelled at me at the top of his voice, when suddenly I felt a (metaphoric) kick in the pit of my belly. Hey, I know this response!

As a boy, my mother was ill for many years. Although she had recovered since, when people around me are ill (a simple cold will do the trick) I get furious, erratic, and impatient. The boy who nearly lost his mummy tends to emerge without my adult control, certainly unable to express his helplessness. I shared my sensations and feelings with Roland, and he went white as a sheet, and sat beside me.

When he was seven years old, Roland nearly lost his mother who struggled with cancer. His mother survived and died many years later, when Roland was thirty, but the first round of cancer left an unforgettable mark on Roland. The life after his mother's illness was never the same. His father struggled to support the family and function emotionally, and was far less available to the two children. Everybody walked on eggshells near mum.

"I'm a doctor," said Roland, "but really, when my own family members are ill I am the most obnoxious person I know. I never made the connection with mum." Two years ago, when the angry outbursts started, his younger son was seven. The possibility for repetition was painfully near—too much to tolerate. "Perhaps something in you cannot forgive your wife for the mere possibility that one day she would leave you and your boys like your mother did," I offered. Roland thought for a long while. "Perhaps," he replied.

Therapy with Roland continued for a few more years. The outbursts stopped quickly after this discovery, but Roland still felt angry and terrified when his wife or sons were ill. Nevertheless, he was better able to identify it, and recognise that under the anger there was a scary and helpless boy. Knowing this allowed Roland to show some compassion to this young self, and made his wife's life easier too. My self-disclosure—exposing my vulnerability to Roland—allowed us to move between binary distinctions (weak-strong, bad-good, angry-loving) and open to a third, which Lewis Aron (Aron, 2013) might have called "an undecidable"—this mutual vulnerability normalised and neutralised the shame with which Roland's pain and fury were associated, also by preventing him from merely using me as an object. As he was able to recognise me as a human being, he was also able to relate to himself more kindly, more compassionately.

Dancing between form and flow

To sustain physical and mental health we need to maintain an appropriate degree of flexibility: balancing form and flow and challenging our somatic, cognitive, and relational habitual positions, so that we may play. Without movement and flexibility we lose our responsiveness to an ever-changing environment and our aliveness is compromised; we become rigidified, and life becomes rigidified for us.

Health is not solely about our capacity to assume more adaptive forms (better job, fitter body, closer relationships), but also connects to our willingness to cultivate transitional spaces of flux and flow. As Winnicott (1971a) identified and noted, these transitional spaces—the play zones—were frightening and threatening, but they also held immense potential for growth.

When we are unable to tolerate flow, and need to quickly find a new organisation (a new boyfriend, the newest iPhone, a new addiction, something new to occupy ourselves with), we would in all likelihood assume our habitual organisation, even if the new form looks like the complete opposite of the old one.

Stanley Keleman (1985) depicted the need for fluid movement most beautifully in writing: "The state of liquidity reveals the state of human life. An embryo or an infant is somewhat liquid-like, fragile yet flexible. Growth makes an organism more dense, stringy, solid" (p. 56). Keleman (1987) further regarded symptoms as resulting from not knowing how to organise and disorganise ourselves. According to him, many of us require retraining in forming ourselves in the world; in forming an embodied life (Keleman, 2012). Body psychotherapy invested a great deal of effort in learning how to somatically organise and reorganise, and in imparting this knowledge "in the first person" to the client. Body psychotherapists consider direct intervention with somatic organisations as a legitimate entrance-portal to change and enquiry, paralleling other therapeutic portals, such as conversations, dream interpretation, free association, or relational exploration.

A basic premise in body psychotherapy concerns the immanent life-seeking quality of our organism. We believe that uninterrupted, each and every one of us is naturally capable of self- and dyadic regulation. We are organically geared to maintaining a homeostatic relationship between inside and outside, between being a part of and merging with another, and being apart from and distinguishing ourselves from the other.

This human organisational process could be compared with the structure of scientific revolutions as described by Thomas Kuhn (1962). The process begins with a specific adaptive organisation, an appropriate form for a particular situation. For instance, "When I am hungry, I cry → mum hears me, comes and feeds me." As situations change, the particular organisation becomes increasingly maladaptive until it is obstructive for the system. To follow the above example: "I am bigger now. I sit at the table and cry with hunger → mum gets upset with me and puts me in my room." At this stage, great pressure is operated on the system to change. Alongside this pressure, there is also an investment in preserving the status quo; our desire to stay the same strengthens when change approaches. Therefore, as the form begins to deconstruct, an intense period of uncertainty and not-knowing follows. I call this stage *flow*. To continue with the example: "I no longer cry when I am hungry, but what am I to do?" Through trial and error (sometimes quickly, at other times slowly), a new form emerges out of flow, and depending on the conditions of its creation it is more or less adaptive to the new situation. "I am pointing at the food and making funny noises → mum understands, smiles, and gives me food."

This cyclical movement described here is not a process that simply happens to us: we are active participatory agents in its unravelling creation. Psychoanalyst Thomas Ogden (1985) wrote: "The dialectical process moves toward integration, but integration is never complete; each integration creates a new dialectical opposition and a new dynamic tension" (p. 131). Body psychotherapy utilises this natural phenomenon: as psychotherapists we seek to create the necessary and sufficient conditions to remobilise impasses and reconnect with the movement between flow and form. One of the greatest contributions of body psychotherapy resides in its willingness to work with somatic expression and somatic impasse in the same language with which these were offered—not translating the body to a symbolic language and then therapeutically working with the symbolic, but speaking directly with bodily structures "in their own tongue": through touch, movement, breathwork, and somatic attention.

Loosening rigid forms and surrender to flow

Many people seek therapy because of an outdated form. Common examples are vows we have unconsciously made as children, representing the best we could have done at the time—but no longer relevant to us today. These old organisations, which might have been appropriate then, could become obstructive (e.g., "I shall never cry again," "I will never let anybody know how I feel") or self-limiting (e.g., "Nobody can love me unless I sacrifice myself and my integrity").

These bodymind organisations—however outdated or harmful they have become (illness, pain, self-hate, perversion)—deserve our respect and caution. They all had their contextual use—they have emerged from a systemic and honest attempt to foster self-regulation and systemic regulation (e.g., my sacrifices kept the family intact—in reality or in my perception). Even the most painful and harmful organisations might be seen as testimonial evidence for what we were willing to sacrifice for love.

Surrender to flow can be frightening; it carries a risk in its midst, and nobody knows for certain what organisations, if any, will arise from flow. Under the appropriate facilitative and supportive circumstances, the ability to loosen forms could bring with it health, joy, and increased flexibility, but premature or mindless surrender to flow could also be dangerous (Fellows, 1986).

Psychologist Wilson Van Dusen (1958) acknowledged both the terror and the potential in what I call here *surrender to flow*: "At the very center of psychotherapeutic experiences there is an awesome hole" (p. 87). Van Dusen continued: "The state is characterized by total uncertainty. One doesn't know answers, one doesn't know solutions. Even the problems besetting one may be unclear. This uncertainty can be painful" (p. 93). However, the way out from the void emerges not from actively seeking, but through surrender: "It is chaotic with possibilities. One feels helpless and waits. It is central that one's own will can no longer find a way out" (p. 93).

Body psychotherapist Ilana Rubenfeld (2001) echoed this voice in saying: "We cannot experience with new, nonhabitual behavior unless we experience the discomfort of our old ways breaking apart. We cannot change without first falling into what I have called 'the fertile void'" (p. 20).

According to the model offered in this chapter, all psychotherapy modalities involve assisting clients in loosening rigid forms and encouraging their organic capacity to surrender to flow. Different modalities apply different theoretical constructs, techniques, and other tools to facilitate the process. Psychoanalysis, for example, places an important emphasis on tolerating the unknown, as analysts do not rush to provide or suggest alternative forms. Other therapies may focus more on providing adaptive organisations, and less on surrendering to flow. However, as noted by psychologist Efrat Even-Tsur (in Rolef Ben-Shahar, 2013a, p. 129), the psychoanalytic setting in itself is an important and highly structured form. The body psychotherapist's willingness to come into direct contact with somatic organisations, and not only engage with cognitive or emotional forms, can sometimes allow the unfolding of qualitatively different connections. In his lecture on the body as a base for creation and provision of meaning, psychologist Yorai Sella[6] (2003) expanded:

> As clinical psychologists we are accustomed to witnessing the long line of clients passing through our clinic, leaving behind a captivating and painful story—or a captivating and painful silence—yet after a session or two they never come back, leaving behind them shadow and fog. Should we conceptualise the riddle of their appearance-disappearance, we may understand that it concerns a feeling that accompanied us when faced with their presence-absence—which was also our own presence-absence for them: we did not shake their hand; something in the "energy" of the room did not match. There was a sense of un-clarity, un-conceivability, and fog. [...] Analytic, narrative, and verbal therapy might be experienced as lacking in continuity, space, direction, and clarity—and therefore—could be experienced as meaningless.

Family therapist Douglas Flemons (2001) compared the psychotherapeutic work to jazz improvisation, encouraging "freedom within form" (p. 236). Relational psychoanalyst Knoblauch (2000, 2011–2012) had also consistently compared the therapeutic act with musicality and rhythms. Therapeutic work, for him, could be seen as a jam session—both verbal and nonverbal, whereupon interactive rhythms "constitute the kind of holding (Winnicott, 1954/1975) or selfobject dimensions of transference (Kohut, 1971) that make possible a loosening of the vertical split, initiating an undoing of dissociative lockups [...]" (p. 423). Thus, Knoblauch was echoing Donnel Stern's (2010) conceptualisation of dissociation as shared defence from connection. By attending to the changing rhythms of the therapeutic dyad, including "the subtle shifts in vocal tone, rhythm, and turn-taking" (Knoblauch, 2005, p. 814), we stand a better chance of embodying our experience and making shared sense of the mutual interaction, or—in Knoblauch's (2011) words, to the possibility that "where dissociation was, embodied signification becomes" (p. 425).

Approaching the same phenomenon from a different angle, Wilhelm Reich saw the goal of therapy as attaining the capacity to fully give in to the involuntary pulsation of breath (Gilbert, 1999). The sometimes concrete nature of interventions in body psychotherapy was structured to meet not only cognitive-linguistic organisations and relational organisations, but also somatic ones. In discussing relational body psychotherapeutic approaches to crying, body psychotherapist Liron Lipkies (2012) suggested that "There are moments where words do not serve us well, and the language of the body is the most appropriate one to use" (p. 53). As body psychotherapists, we endeavour to initially speak with somatic processes in their own language, rather than forcing these into symbolic cognitive terminology, since such a transition incurs a loss of a qualitatively meaningful aspect of the conversation, one that belongs in the bodily realm.

Now that we have examined somatic, emotional, and relational organisation we can turn our attention to the concept of bodymind in body psychotherapy, which is presented in the following chapter.

Exercise: dance me to the end of love

(Particularly appropriate as a therapeutic process)

The following exercise utilises Gestalt therapy skills to flex somatic organisation through the use of somatic language. It can certainly be incorporated as a therapeutic process.

1. When the client (or therapist) recognises a stuck feeling (a rigid bodily, psychological, or mental organisation that has some somatic feature), the therapist invites the client to focus on the feeling. The conversation directly addresses the pattern with which we like to establish connection.
2. To facilitate the process, the client is asked to amplify the somatic expression of this stuck place with the help of muscular contraction, exaggerating body posture, or limiting the breath.
3. The therapist checks: is there a sound that matches this place? An image? A sentence or two?
4. (To avoid shaming the client, the therapist can actively participate in the process.) The therapist asks the client to move around in a way that expresses the stuck feeling.
5. The therapist asks the client to "dance the stuck feeling". What happens when movement is introduced? Is there a place for novelty in this organisation? Can something new be created there?
6. Client and therapist share and process together. If there was a novel element, how was it translated to sensations and thoughts? If there was not, what was it like to stay with the unsolvable?

Notes

1. Excerpt from "East Coker" in *Four Quartets* by T. S. Eliot. Copyright 1940 by T. S. Eliot; copyright © renewed 1968 by Esme Valerie Eliot. Reprinted by permission of Houghton Mifflin Harcourt Publishing Company and by permission of Faber & Faber. All rights reserved.
2. Reprinted here with permission of the Association for the Advancement of Psychotherapy.
3. An earlier version of the vignette appeared in the *USA Body Psychotherapy Journal* (Rolef Ben-Shahar, 2011b).
4. The quote, taken from *Aesthetics of Change* is reprinted with permission of The Guilford Press. Copyright Guilford Press.
5. Readers who are unfamiliar with Smurfs are strongly advised to ameliorate this shameful ignorance and check out http://www.schlumpf.com/en/.
6. I wish to thank Yorai for his generous sharing of a transcript of his lecture.

CHAPTER FIVE

Theory of bodymind in body psychotherapy*

> Our bodies are us as process, not us as thing. Structure is slowed down process. As life builds structure, it builds itself in.
>
> —*Stanley Keleman* (1981, p. 29)

Introduction

Body–mind relationships are at the theoretical and clinical core of body psychotherapy. Naturally, we were not the first to grapple with the body–mind problem: exploring the connection between physical phenomena and psychological ones is as old as humanity, and as demonstrated in Part I (Historical), psychoanalysis itself began from studying body–mind interactions (as they manifested in hysteria). To this day, neuroscientists, linguists, anthropologists, sociologists, psychologists, and other clinicians are trying to decipher the mysterious connection between body and mind.

Body psychotherapists presume that Descartes was wrong, and that his *cogito* offered a limited and partial description of human identity. The heart of our ontology (existence) is not seen as our disconnected thoughts but instead our embodied presence (including our embodied thoughts): "I am embodied, therefore I am." Relational body psychotherapy adds yet another facet—it is not merely my own existence as a bodymind that indicates my being, but the interaction with other embodied beings (and the world) is how I am created ("I am a bodymind among bodyminds, therefore I am").

*The chapter is partly based on a paper previously published in the *USA Body Psychotherapy Journal* (Rolef Ben-Shahar, 2010b).

All streams of body psychotherapy reject the equation of self with the thinking-self: the belief that *I* am first and foremost a *thinking I*, and perceive our bodily existence (I am a body) and our thinking existence (I am mind, I am psyche) as maintaining a tight, dynamic, contradictory, and complementary intertwined relationship.

If body and mind are indeed interlinked, then where does the mind reside? Are the mind and psyche but complex expressions of neural activity? And what is the relationship between mind and brain? How do neurotransmitters conducting messages between nerve cells relate to feelings, thoughts, and sensations? What is the quality of the relationship between the endocrine and biochemical systems, secreting bodily hormones and enzymes—and cognitive and mental processes? Is it true, for example, that emotions are located in the right cerebral hemisphere and cognition in the left? Do specific areas in the cerebral cortex create (rather than correlate with) different feelings, different thoughts? And should psychotherapy seek biological and scientific answers to the body–mind dilemma? After all, refusing to accept this causal subordination of psychotherapy to the physiological-biological paradigm raises concerns for swinging to the other extreme: a spiritualised theory, turning the mind into an ethereal object at which we cannot look critically at all.

Let us suppose for a moment that the mind-body affinity is indeed causal and hierarchical, or as Freud (1912d) clearly asserted: "Anatomy is destiny." If that is indeed the case, then how exactly is the mind *in* the body? Is it like the Holy Spirit in the Holy Grail? Like a princess captivated in a fortified palace? Perhaps like gas in sparkling water, or like two different expressions of the same phenomenon? For instance, could body and mind be like yin and yang in Chinese philosophy? Perhaps there is a distinct hierarchical connection between the two, like the relationship between notes and symphony, or bricks and a house? Perhaps we are looking in the wrong direction and we should explore causal connection between body and mind—like the relationship between an architect's blueprints and the final building, or between still shots on a speedily moving film and the final projected cinematic experiencing? Or maybe the relationship between body and mind is like the connection between computer hardware and software?

The way we perceive the interconnection between body and mind is not only reliant on philosophical stance or phenomenological experience, but also on the values and beliefs which guide us in our lives. Since human heterogeneity and variety are "irreparable" (thank goodness for that) and human beings operate out of a huge number of beliefs, the differences in how we understand body–mind connection are not bound to disappear. This chapter has no pretence of solving the body–mind dilemma. Instead, I shall present here a few possible attempts to look at body–mind interaction and connection, through exploring neurological models, as well as discussing three phenomena: embodiment, intersubjectivity, and emergence.

Embodiment and disembodiment

> Life is chaotic and unexpected—and people do their best to remain present to the flow of experience. Attending to narrative alone and disowning body sensations narrows down our capacity to be present in our lives, limiting our ability to cope, to enjoy, and to feel satisfied.
>
> —Noa Oster (2011, p. 4)

Disconnection from bodily sensations (disembodiment) is, by and large, an indication of dissociative processes at place, splitting from one of the multiple aspects of self, a difficulty in identifying my body with myself, and perceiving the body as an object that is different to me: "This fat stomach is not me; it's just my stomach"; "This tormented and painful back is a foreign object"; "This aroused penis might possibly belong to me, but it is certainly not me". Embodiment is an act of self-validation, establishing aspects of my somatic-self as a part of me. Embodiment expands my identity field to include my bodily experiences—"Perhaps this is not all of me but it is part of who I am"; "When my leg hurts, I am hurting"; "When the stomach is fat—I am fat"; "When my penis is aroused, I am currently aroused".

When we experience the world, we do so through our body; without connection to our body we become lost and homeless (Judith, 1996). Carl Jung (Jung & Jarrett, 1988) expressed it with poetical beauty: "It has forever been the aspiration of mankind to fly like a bird, to become a wind, a breath; and it can be done, but it is paid for by the loss of body, or the loss of humanity, which is the same thing" (p. xix). Relational psychoanalyst Donnell Stern (2010) proposed that enactment in itself was a relational dissociation, and that dyadic embodiment was necessary to disentangle and reclaim connectedness. The exercise at the end of the Chapter One demonstrates practical embodiment skills.

Embodiment is one of the basic concepts in body psychotherapy, indicating how our lived and felt experiences are alive in as much as we are bodies—in somatic fields. Stanley Keleman (1981) writes about embodiment: "To be embodied is to establish a living body—not just to be *with* your body, or in relationship to it. Your living body created your relationships" (p. 29).

Throughout the book I use the term embodiment in two ways. The first, which is examined in this chapter, signifies *a phenomenon* whereby our entire existence is a priori embodied; all of our experiences, since it is us who experience them, are experienced through our bodyminds—it is about our being with our body—with its sensations, postures, structures, and boundaries. The second way of using the term is as *a skill* of strengthening and cultivating the relationship between the bodily and the psychological aspects of our being, as exemplified by Keleman's quote in the previous paragraph.

As I mentioned in Chapter One, Freud (1923b) believed that the ego was "… first and foremost body-ego […] ultimately derived from body sensations, chiefly from those springing from the surface of the body. It may thus be regarded as a mental projection of the surface of the body" (p. 16). Winnicott (1988) too coined the oft-quoted phrase "the psyche indwelling in the soma" (p. 44), thus paraphrasing the Freudian mind-body connection in a less biological and more psychological terminology.

Body psychotherapists use skills for enhancing somatic attention, in order to deepen our awareness of ourselves as bodies. Both therapist and client turn their attention (also) to sensory and bodily experiencing, cultivating mindfulness—an inner witness of sorts, attentively listening to our sensory responses even before these are organised as emotions or thoughts (or as language). We learn to inhabit our bodies with ourselves and inhabit ourselves with our bodies. The starting point of body psychotherapy assumes that the act of attending to the body creates a dynamic bridge. We assume that by embodying our experiences, we stand a greater chance of liberating our rigid psychological and bodily patterns: we acquire a somatic language in addition to our emotional, cognitive, and affective ones, with which we can play and communicate, with which we can bring about movement and change.

Embodiment is a bodymind position (a state of being) and a bodymind action, and body psychotherapy is unique in its work with embodied positions and actions. We may assist clients in building bridges between somatic expression and symbolic cognitive and linguistic language, and thereafter process the experience together through verbal interaction. We may, however, also consent to speak without translators; to directly converse with our clients through our own body, without attempting to symbolise the expression. Our bodies, if we dare use them fully, are a rich source of communication that can be used in psychotherapy. While contemporary psychoanalytic writers, like Nitza Yarom (2013), attempt this very task, I daresay that body psychotherapy has been doing it for decades, and it would be worthwhile to engage in dialogue with the body of our work too.

The main skill in body psychotherapy is therefore not about one therapeutic intervention or another, but about willingness to remain somatically curious and playful, to actively engage (in a theoretically and clinically grounded way) with somatic processes that take place in the therapeutic field, the client, and within the therapist.

The shared bodymind and mirror neurons: I have a body, I am a body, I belong to a body

Before assuming a biological perspective on body–mind connection, let us momentarily adopt a psychological angle. From a psychological perspective we may ask, for example, who does the placenta belong to—the mother, the foetus, perhaps to both? Putting aside the biological answer to this question, we could possibly look at the placenta as a living bodily dialogue between mother and baby. The placenta regulates the needs of the foetus, who in turn communicates its changing needs to the mother and shapes its uterine environment, the endocrine system—the mother. A foetus and mother shape and create one another already in the womb.

Like Winnicott's (1971a) transitional space, which exists thanks to the relationship between baby and mother (or environment), the placenta is a somatic-biological climax of primary relationality. From our very first moments in the world (i.e., our conception), we share a wider self with our mother. Through the placenta we concretely and metaphorically partake in a distinct dyadic being: our bloods are shared and transfused, we are separated and connected at the same time; life pulsates inside us and between us: we are one, and at the same time we are two. "Even if viewed from a purely biological point of view," wrote Margaret Mahler and John McDevitt (1982), "the newborn infant is only a partial system: between the distress signal and the relief of need, there must be a mother" (p. 828).

And later, the nipple. Here is a nipple, and the baby latches onto the nipple and is nourished by the breast and protected by the breasts; antibodies flow through the stream of milk. The baby's needs are expressed in the duration of feeding and the intensity of sucking, which influence the flow of lactation, as well as affect the milk production and its quality. Perhaps we can understand the nipple (and milk) as an expansion of the immune system to a dyadic immune system? Here, the hands are holding a baby, and a baby is held. We are created in relationships and by relationships, and at the same time we partake in their creation. And these relationships are first and foremost created as bodily events.

Phenomenologist Maurice Merleau-Ponty (1962) claimed that the experience of our body results from the dyadic process of sensing the other, and the other sensing us. To reiterate: our body is created and develops through sensing some-body else and being sensed by some-body else. However, it is not only the personal other which shapes us: we are also created through discourse, norms, societal values, differentiating conception (race, gender, class), etc.

Current developments in neurosciences have demonstrated how our somatic organisation and our mental and emotional organisations communicate with one another and condition each other (e.g., Kandel, 2005; Schore, 1994). Accordingly, recent studies on trauma, attachment, and brain support the efficacy of body-based interventions for the healing of trauma (P. Ogden, Minton, & Pain, 2006; Rothschild & Rand, 2006). Body psychotherapy modalities specialising in trauma work utilise such research. In the last decades, these scientific studies have attracted clinicians and clients alike to experience body psychotherapy, and aroused professional interest in psychotherapists from other modalities (e.g., Rappoport, 2012).

If we looked at the placenta as the heart of our earliest shared self, representing the first intersubjective organ, then mirror neurons could be perceived as the nervous system of this wider mind (a concept expanded upon later in this chapter). Mirror neurons were discovered in the mid-1990s (Gallese, Fadiga, Fogassi, & Rizzolatti, 1996), when a group of Italian scientists researched the motor neurons responsible for grasping in monkeys. The researchers accidentally discovered that certain motor neurons, which were activated during grasping objects, were also activated when the monkey *observed* its operator taking a raisin. This was a groundbreaking discovery: the same motor neurons which were activated when the monkey picked a raisin were activated when the monkey merely looked at somebody (its operator, the researcher) picking a raisin to eat.

This discovery led to widely spread research on this startling phenomenon, whereby one person's (or monkey's) activity affected someone else's nervous system, simply by observing the activity. Researchers have since attempted to understand a myriad of phenomena through a mirror neuron lens—from looking at contagious yawning (Platek, Critton, Myers, & Gullup, 2003) to explaining mirror neurons as the biological mechanism for enabling empathy (Kaplan & Iacoboni, 2006).

What was it that activated such neural activity by observation alone? Apparently, in order for a mirror neuron to be activated, the neural stimulus needed to be affectively meaningful for the observer (Gallese, 2001). Once more, we encounter a similar argument which guided Mesmer's clinical work in the late eighteenth century: an affective charge was required in order for mental change to take place (Gezundhajt, 2007).

For an electrical stimulation of a mirror neuron, we need to be affectively and emotionally activated by observing the other: something that is taking place in the other directly impacts physiological mechanisms inside our own bodies. We are not separated from our environment—to a certain extent even without any conscious or informed choice (I would argue, a very large extent—this is the very basis of the effectiveness of advertising). Mirror neurons are therefore iconoclasts of solipsistic fantasies, according to which only the subject exists or is truthfully knowable. Communication expert and interdisciplinary scholar Ann Marie Barry (2009) argues that mirror neurons break the walls between us, allowing us to identify with one another and feel the other through our own bodies.

I would like to offer a more radical claim, that the boundary (or wall) between us and the other never really existed, that we always had two types of body. Our first body is the skin-bound body, the body that we identify as our own (either as an object or subject); a body which is a closed system capable of communicating with its environment; a body that is knowable to us without having to relate to another person. The second body is a partial body, a half-body, a body that is fully realised only in connection with another person (or the outside environment). This is the body of the wider mind, of the dyadic self, a body that is never whole and complete in and by itself. This body comes to life and is activated by attachment and connection, a connection which psychiatrists Lewis, Amini, and Lannon (2000) termed *limbic resonance*. We may consider this half-body of ours the essential component that allows our first body (us as body) to perform the impossible, cross the divide, and create an interface between you and me, between one person and another. In essence, I am proposing that self as a closed system and self as an open, partial system are complementary and dialectic processes.

This structure may provide a certain explanation for our constant search for connection and contact (object seeking) on the one hand, and our need for individuation on the other, which is an attempt to balance the complementary and contradictory needs of these two bodies of ours, these two complementary nervous systems. I believe that intersubjectivity is first and foremost bodily, and therefore, when I am attentive and attuned to sensations and bodily experiences within an affective, emotional relationship, it is not merely my own body that I am feeling, but instead (also) our shared body, the body we created and that made us alive. We do not only have a body and are a body, but we also belong to a wider body. This position will be further discussed in this chapter and amply demonstrated in Chapter Eleven of Part III (Clinical), when elaborating on resonance—a phenomenon which represents for me the most important clinical application for working with the intersubjective body.

Between body–mind and bodymind: splitting and uniting

The last section described research in neuroscience, which demonstrated how our somatic organisations were in direct relationship with mental and emotional organisations; indeed, there is an accumulated body of knowledge in the fields of trauma research, attachment, and brain research which supports the efficacy of therapeutic methods incorporating somatic interventions. The increasingly shared understanding that body and mind are inevitably interlinked and that successful therapeutic intervention should ideally involve both, is a welcome development, which has contributed to the growth of psychotherapy, science, and medicine in the last few decades. But neuroscience and medicine relate to the body only as a biological entity, while "The body as means of expression, the body as I-me, is easily forgotten" (Svensen & Bergland, 2007, p. 44). When body psychotherapy attempts to understand and explain the body, it relates to the body–mind dilemma not just from a biological point of view. The holistic approach (from Greek *holos*—whole), which sees the person as a whole (bigger than the sum of its parts) is different *in principle* from the medical or neuroscientific model of the body–mind.

According to the holistic approach, the person represents a bodymind whole which cannot be reduced into merely somatic language or a psychological one. In traditional therapies and Eastern philosophies, body and mind unity is a given, understood a priori as belonging to a unified and undifferentiated whole. In traditional Chinese medicine, for example, emotional and bodily expressions are not separated or differentiated from each other (Connelly, 1994). However, unlike those traditional and Eastern views, body psychotherapy developed at the heart of Western civilisation from a Cartesian–Newtonian starting point, saturated with, and unable to deny its paradigmatic splits. Therefore, the body–mind unity (the bodymind) cannot be taken for granted. We are required to "earn" our bodymind unity, which is not culturally acceptable. Winnicott (1987) phrased it gracefully: "I heard it said that it is in the newborn that physiology and psychology are one […] This is a good start. Psychology is a gradual extension from physiology" (p. 36). This means that holistic Western philosophy is principally different from Eastern philosophies or medicine where the conceptual splits did not take place; we are called to choose the body–mind connection, but do so with a long history of body–mind splits, which has conditioned our thoughts and understanding.

Reich suggested that a functional identity existed between somatic and psychological processes, and this functional identity contained a historical and cultural contradiction, which we have all inherited from dualistic philosophy. The culture from which we emerged no longer permits us to hold a naïve position regarding bodymind unity. Thus—in the West—the concept of embodiment already includes immanent splitting and differentiation. We might speak of unity and integration, but we do so from a divided starting point, from an inner knowing of our expulsion from the harmonious heaven. Post-exile Adam and Eve cannot but carry the pain of consciousness as they yearn to return to their preconscious state.

The impossibility of naïve bodymind connection is at the heart of our Western dissociative suffering (as argued by Erich Fromm, 1942, 1957), but at the same time this impossibility enables theoretical and clinical maturity (through bereavement), and more so—the possibility for intersubjective experiences, since the tension between body–mind and bodymind expresses similar dynamics to the tensions between I and thou (and us), between subject and object, an individual and the cosmos (and the Jungian *unus mundus*—one world, Jung, 1934). When bodymind unity is not a given, it requires of us an act of submission, of surrender—and allows us to exercise a unique act of choice. In *The Fear of Freedom*, Erich Fromm (1942) wrote: "The dynamic quality of love lies in this very polarity: that it springs from the need of overcoming separateness, that it leads to oneness—and yet that individuality is not eliminated" (p. 225).

Perhaps, alongside the suffering that those splits caused, we have also gained a real possibility for reclaiming ourselves and our connections—both to ourselves, to others, and to the world around us. As illuminated by Fromm (1957): "In the act of loving, of giving myself, in the act of penetrating the other person, I find myself, I discover myself, I discover us both, I discover man" (p. 24). The power of body psychotherapeutic work also rests in holding the complex tension between splits and unions: we choose to relate to the bodymind, notwithstanding the historical and conditioned culture of body–mind, which is inevitably alive in us too. The bodymind concept is therefore discussed here in light of other relevant splits and integrations.

The philosophical arguments for bodymind connections, which were posed by Edmund Husserl and Maurice Merleau-Ponty, paved the way back into the reunion of body and mind in Western thought (a parallel movement could be found in feminist thought which argued against these delusional splits) as well as contributed to the theoretical and clinical development of body psychotherapy, even if their influence was not always direct. Husserl claimed that it was impossible to perceive the world other than through our body (Carman, 1999). Merleau-Ponty (1962) presented a more radical view: not only were we conscious of the body via the world and conscious of the world through our body, but moreover we *were* bodies and "[T]he body is a natural self and, as it were, the subject of perception" (p. 206). This dialectic position presented the relationship between body, mind, self, other, and environment as conditioning each other; this was the organisation of a culture. Relational body psychotherapy indeed related to cultural organisations (intrapsychic, interpersonal, intersubjective, and societal/ecological) as necessary contexts for the therapeutic work (Appel-Opper, 2010).

Hence, body psychotherapy is neither monistic nor dualistic. According to *monistic* philosophy, the union of all aspects of being is at the heart of existence and is the ultimate truth. Body and mind are but two faces of the same thing. We are never separated, and examining these as separated is faulty. An example for monistic philosophy is Taoism, according to which the entire world is an echo of the Tao, the single unity of all things (Lash, 1989; Seaward, 2005). *Dualistic* philosophy of body and mind views the two as belonging to two distinct fields of knowledge—the cognitive field (or the psychological) on the one hand, and the bodily field on the other. Descartes's philosophy, which was mentioned in Chapter One, is an example of a dualistic philosophy.

As an example of the dualistic approach in Western culture, consider the following example. One day a client failed to show up to her session, without any prior notice or contact. I was anxious about her, since she was actively suicidal and had previously attempted suicide. During the period preceding this disappearance she was depressed and indifferent. I managed to get hold of her only after two days and later the same day developed a severe full-body rash, painful and very itchy, which did not leave me for three weeks. When I told the GP about the emotional circumstances leading to the rash, as I believed it could have been connected, he looked at me shocked: "This has nothing to do with your condition," he said with authority, "you simply have a strong allergic reaction."

As individuals who grew up and developed in Western culture we can no longer hold a monistic view—we were all expelled from paradise, we have eaten from the forbidden fruit. Our perception of body–mind unity is therefore different. Even if you disagree with my GP's irritated reaction, his view is alive in us all and has conditioned our thinking and feeling. We have developed in a culture which rested on such views and created its therapeutic modalities in accordance with them (medicine for the bodily machine, psychotherapy for the psyche, and religion for the spirit and soul)—or in opposition to them, but with these dichotomies in mind. The holistic approach in body psychotherapy is characterised by holding the tension between the partial truths of both these positions together (Rolef Ben-Shahar, 2001a, 2001b). Western holistic approaches are not ready made, but a product of active choice in unity; an active and mindful stance—and not a starting position.

This stance carries significant consequences for the clinical work of the body psychotherapist. Body psychotherapists regularly elect to use tools and techniques which are not usually found in talk therapies, but at the same time use psychotherapeutic tools and techniques of conversation, attempting to understand the client, exploring the client's world, the therapeutic relationship, and transference dynamics and more (in accordance with the therapist's clinical orientation).

Body psychotherapy perceives human beings as psychosomatic systems. Wilhelm Reich (1933a) suggested that: "It would be wrong to speak of the 'transfer' of physiological concepts to the psychic sphere, for what we have in mind is not an analogy but a real identity: the unity of psychic and somatic function" (p. 340). Later, he added: "The psychic and the somatic operate from the point of biopsychic energy, as two systems, which are unitary as well as conditioning each other" (1942, p. 26). Reich therefore identified body and mind as holding a twofold relationship: on the one hand as complementary aspects (body–mind), and on the other as functionally identical (bodymind).

Wider mind and intersubjectivity

While the last two sections dealt with the tension between body and mind and bodymind, this section will portray the tension between the individuals and the relationships created by them, within which they are created. We shall examine the theory of mind through the systemic thinking of Gregory Bateson (who influenced, among others, body psychotherapists Nick Totton and Ron Kurtz and the therapeutic modalities they respectively developed (Kurtz, 2007; Totton, 2005)), as well as considering contemporary psychoanalytic approaches and other philosophical sources.

Gregory Bateson was a rare modern image of a renaissance man: he contributed to fields as varied as cybernetics, psychiatry (particularly to understanding schizophrenia and its sources in familial mixed messages, the double-bind theory), and anthropology. It is his theory of mind, however, that deserves special attention here. Mind, according to Bateson (1979), was a dialectic system. It was constituted not only by intrapsychic relationships (between body, emotions, and thoughts—for example) but also from interpersonal connections. Mind was relationships between patterns—the patterns which connect.

This concept is worth expanding on. According to Bateson (1972), when I am walking in the woods, mind is not just the mind of the walker—my own mind as a separate and distinct individual. Instead, mind is comprised of the organism that I am and the trees that are around—from the woods and the relationship we form. In fact, Bateson translated the understanding that the whole is larger than the sum of its parts into our very ontology—our being: we are more than just us. Bateson's description of mind as a system of connections and relational patterns is closely related to the shamanic perception of the mind (which will be further discussed in Chapter Eleven); and indeed, Bateson's first wife, renowned anthropologist Margaret Mead dedicated many years to studying the perception of mind in shamanic cultures.

At the core of Jung's collective unconscious (1934) rests the *unus mundus*, the singular and united principle of existence—which is a wonderful platform for understanding the wider mind: *unus mundus*, one world, is a space that connects us; a field that requires us to surrender into it and then allows deep connections to interpersonal, collective, and spiritual resources. Jungian analyst Steven Joseph (2007), who studied the relationship between Jungian thinking and Kabbalah argued: "While there may be no Archimedean point outside of the psyche from which to perceive and understand ourselves objectively, there is such a point inside, within the deep centre of the psyche" (p. 324). Joseph continues by quoting Jung, who in a letter to Victor White related to this sense of self: "The Divine Presence is more than anything else ... This is the only thing that matters" (ibid.). Coming back to Bateson, the following description astutely portrays the bodily, intersubjective, and transpersonal aspects of the wider mind. Bateson (1972) wrote:

> The individual mind is immanent but not only in the body. It is immanent also in pathways and messages outside the body; and there is a larger Mind of which the individual mind is only a subsystem. This larger Mind is comparable to God and is perhaps what some people mean by "God," but it is still immanent in the total interconnected social system and planetary ecology. [...] A certain humility becomes appropriate, tempered by the dignity or joy of being part of something much bigger. A part—if you will—of God. (pp. 467–468)

Yet this perception of mind and self was not only present in shamanic cultures: it was also deeply rooted in Jung's analytic psychology and drew inspirations from Jewish philosophy, dialogic philosophy, and the Hassidic movement. Martin Buber's (1958) *I–thou*, for example, expressed a similar idea to the wider mind concept: "I become through my relation to the Thou; as I become I, I say Thou" (p. 11). Buber distinguished the relationship between *I* and *it*, which represented an interaction with an external object, to the *I–thou* affinity: "I do not experience the man to whom I say Thou," wrote Buber, "but I take my stand in relation to him, in the sanctity of the primary word" (ibid., p. 9). I–thou connection was, therefore, a spiritual stance of unity: "Spirit in its human manifestation is a response of man to his *Thou* [...] Man lives in the spirit, if he is able to respond to his *Thou*" (ibid., p. 39). Buber further recognised that the separate consciousness was created by and from the wider mind and not the other way round: "The person becomes conscious of himself as sharing in being, as co-existing, and thus as being" (ibid., p. 63). Therefore, there existed a constant tension between the individual and his wish to preserve himself as such, as well as to gain knowledge (which was only possible in I–it relations, because the experiencing self could not also understand—understanding already implied moving away from experience), and the wish to surrender to a wider mind and become through and from it. Similar to Bateson and relational psychoanalysis, Buber viewed the solution in tolerating the paradoxical position of the two: "But a moment comes, at it is near, when the shuddering man looks up and sees both pictures in a flash together. And a deeper shudder seizes him" (ibid., p. 72).

The Kabbalistic concept of *Tikkun* (repair), according to which a person could heal an entire world with properly directed attention and inner work, rested on surrendering to the wider mind as well (external and internal, both my own unconscious and that which was bigger than me) (Fine, 2003). Jewish philosopher Frantz Rosenzweig presented a similar view: affinity and connection (like Bateson's *patterns which connect*) were essential aspects of being, of existence: the triangular affinity human-god-world was mutually creating the three elements which were in relation to one another, as well as being created by them. Philosopher Samuel Hugo Bergmann explained: "We cannot, says Rosenzweig, speak about God without building a 'bridge' from him to the world and to man. [...] God would have not been God if he did not create the world and revealed himself to man through his love" (1974, p. 220). For Rosenzweig, the dialogue between God, human, and world was a dialectic process of continuous becoming (or emergence) and of eternal genesis (of human, of the world, and of God): "It is as if the world, which has previously been a cosmos sunk into itself, is now waking up to acknowledge its creation. First it was whole and complete within itself and by itself, now it had lost wholeness and has turned to be world-in-becoming" (ibid., p. 235).

In a similar vein, the influential Rabbi Abraham Isaac Kook (1990) described our psyche as forever seeking to unite with God, cultivating divine devotion, to surrender to this wider mind. For Kook, this devotion (or adherence) was the deepest desire of humanity, transcending and elevating the soul—saturating it with wholeness and unity. According to Kook: "Love in its purest form spreads into our souls, which are comprised by and are surrendered by the loving soul. The loving soul is forever broader and bigger than the loved soul" (p. 406). Kook's concept of *the loving soul* is in essence what Bateson called *wider mind*.

In all the above descriptions, the psyche was seen as a dance: an ongoing movement between belonging and individuating, form and flow, statics and dynamics. Like Rosenzweig's world, the dynamic mind awakened to acknowledge its own creation: previously it was whole and complete in and by itself; presently it has become compromised and lost its wholeness turning into a mind-in-becoming.

Let us turn to look at this understanding of mind in the clinical setting. When a therapist and client sit together in the clinic, mind is neither merely an object, nor simply a separated subject; instead, *mind is an intersubjective process*, inclusive of the therapist and client, the processes that take place within them and between them—it is a wider mind. Mind in the clinic is the sum of all of who we are, with our respective histories, thoughts, feelings, and body sensations, as well as the relationships and connections that are weaved between us. The two individuals share in a wider mind which creates their individuality, and at the same time these two individuals co-create the wider mind (to adopt object relations terminology, we might say that mind is the transference dynamics between our internalised models of the world).

The surrender into this shared co-creation strikes great similarities with Bion's reverie, particularly as it was conceptualised by Thomas Ogden (1997) as being an intensely personal and private event and, at the same time, an intersubjective event.

The theory of self in relational psychoanalysis developed independently from Bateson's philosophy (although both fields were influenced by dialogical philosophy), but there were many commonalities between the two. The two fields resembled one another in three main ways: first, the self was seen as a process (verb) rather than an object (noun), a principle of organisation instead of a concrete entity. Second, the self was de-centred. That is, the field of self expanded beyond the boundaries of skin to include connections with others (i.e., context was part of the self). Third, the relationship between the personal and relational was dialectic and cybernetic: they emerged from each other and interacted with one another. We co-created the wider mind and were created by it. The relational self was created by the tension between the continuous-and-individuated selves and the multiple-and-fragmented selves (S. Mitchell, 1993).

The concept of selfobject in self-psychology (Bacal, 1995; Kohut, 1959; Osterville, 1995) might be seen as parallel to the wider mind. This was the role that the (good enough) mother and father assumed by providing an expansive auxiliary self for the baby. The parents were part of the baby's self—they were not all of the self, but occupied part of it, therefore there was no clear-cut distinction between the object (mother/father) and the subject (baby).

We can consequently describe the mind (or self) in two fashions: as a personal object (belonging to me) and as an interpersonal organisational phenomenon. The two angels concurrently exist, and the tension between them creates intersubjectivity. These two ways of perceiving mind are similar to the two types of connection between body and mind, presented earlier in this chapter: one that emphasises their separated existence and complementary relationship (body–mind) and one that emphasises their unity (bodymind).

As psychotherapists, we sometimes work from a position of distinction and separation, focusing either on a psychological process or a somatic one, for instance by assisting the client to self-regulate or by increasing the client's self-awareness; at other times we work through and from the connection, while focusing on bodymind process, for instance by assisting mutual regulation or increasing awareness of the interactive relationship. We dance between the "either or" and the "both and". The therapeutic process and therapeutic act is no longer done *to the client* or *on the client*, but instead moves *through* the therapist and the therapeutic dyad (Aron, 1991). The therapeutic relationship then becomes a process of weaving mutual influence, mutual change, and shared creation of asymmetrical mutuality.

In the clinical setting, such a theory of self has many advantages as well as disadvantages. The psychotherapist is highly active in terms of her inner work and takes greater risks as a dynamic participant of the therapeutic journey (Maroda, 1998). The wider mind threatens to change us as therapists and people, demanding flexibility and growth from us; it does not permit us the privilege of being positioned as passive observers of the client, expert scientists in a lab, or doctors who are uninvolved with the curative processes, neither affecting their subjects and their recovery nor being affected by them.

Relational psychoanalysis uses the term *the intersubjective analytic third* (or *the analytic third*) which parallels Bateson's concept of *wider mind*. The term *intersubjective analytic third* was coined by psychoanalyst Thomas Ogden (1992, 1994a) to describe the third entity co-created in therapy between client and therapist, an entity which assumes certain autonomic characteristics. In the final account, Ogden—like Bateson—relates to the emergence process as having primacy over the individual selves of which it is made: "There is no analyst, no analysand, no analysis, aside from the process through which the analytic third is generated" (T. Ogden, 1995, p. 697). It is important to note that the intersubjective third is not unique to the psychotherapeutic relationship, of course, but could be found in many emotional-affective relationships. This is the deep and nonverbal connection "that permits us to say 'I know that you know that I know' or 'I feel that you feel that I feel'" (D. N. Stern, 2004, p. 75).

There is an immanent tension between the intersubjective third and the separated subjectivities that co-created it and are created by it. The family welfare, for example, could compromise and therefore be in tension with family members, even when these are the same members who created the family. Another familiar political example is the nationalistic ethos of "for the good of the country", where the collective takes precedence over the individuals (except for the selected few who dominate it, politically and financially). On the other hand, the consumerist and privatisation culture in the West can demonstrate both the advantages and the price we paid for abandoning *wider mind* values and almost exclusively praying to the god of the individual self.

The phenomenon of intersubjectivity—the existence of self that transcends our skin-boundaries, a wider mind in which we share, may provide one of the richest sources for therapeutic success and growth. Psychologist Edward Tronick and his colleagues (Tronick et al., 1998) differentiated between individual states of consciousness and dyadic states of consciousness, which are naturally shared by more than one person. This is a psychological view of the same phenomenon I described earlier in this chapter through the physiological explanation of mirror neurons. Thus, intersubjectivity challenges the myth of the mind as separated and isolated from others and its surroundings.

Influential relational psychoanalyst Jessica Benjamin (1995) depicted intersubjectivity as the paradoxical tension between our need to be identified and validated by the other and that of self-validation, between acknowledging the other and negating the other's existence. We yearn to belong to this wider mind, yet at the same time to maintain our separated identity and subordinate the other to us without surrendering to the shared creation. This particular translation of the tension may be the result of a patriarchal-dominated culture, where the masculine gender bias to possess and subordinate takes precedence over the willingness to partake and share. However, these movements exist in a gentler and more sublimated nature within us all. Our two bodies (or bodyminds) manifest complementary, yet sometimes contradictory needs too: to be different from the other and distinct from one another, yet to be part of the other at the same time.

But why am I discussing intersubjectivity and the relational context of mind in a chapter dedicated to body and mind? Aside from the structural resemblance in the questions both tensions pose (separation–integration), I believe that somatic processes are central for working with and doing therapy within the intersubjective field. That is, that body psychotherapeutic skills could assist also the non-body psychotherapist in encouraging the creation of shared space and working within it. By permitting affective and somatic dialogue in shared intersubjective levels, the psychotherapist can more easily cultivate the creation and sustenance of wider mind, of this therapeutic "us". Intersubjectivity, in my view, requires proficiency in nonverbal communication, which Wilma Bucci (2011) might regard as subsymbolic processes, and Thomas Ogden (1994b) might describe as *interpretive action*, which involves: "the analyst's communication of understanding of an aspect of the transference-countertransference to the analysand by means of activity other than that of verbal symbolization" (p. 108).

For example, relational psychoanalyst Steven Knoblauch (2012) related to the intuitive connection that helped bridge gaps both within and between subjectivities. These intuitive bridges were created, according to Knoblauch, by embodied cues such as gut feelings, muscular constricting or collapse, facial configurations, and other somatic expressions, both voluntary and involuntary. Another example is from Daniel Stern (1985), who touched on the limitation of verbal interaction in creating and working with intersubjectivity: "Language is a double-edged sword ... It drives a wedge between two simultaneous forms of interpersonal experience: as it is lived and as it is verbally represented ..." (p. 162). Stern (2004) further argued that attunement to the intersubjective field required the therapist to focus on the affective aspects of the experience.

Such focus on the here-and-now and the somatic self is more common in body psychotherapy than it is in therapeutic modalities, which work with conversation alone, and is facilitative to the expansion of self and surrender to the wider mind. Stephen Gilligan (2012) described the obstruction to flow as neuromuscular lock—a highly rigid organisation: "In such states of neuromuscular lock, consciousness is restricted to recreating the same experience over and over again" (p. 26). Gilligan continued: "Unfortunately, somatic intelligence is typically inhibited by the neurological lock of ego consciousness, reducing the body to an 'it' to be exploited, a machine to be programmed, or a dumb animal to be coerced into action" (pp. 89–90).

I believe that psychotherapists from different modalities would find that integrating elements and skills from body psychotherapy, such as attention to the body of the client and therapist, grounding, centring, embodiment, working with breath, and touch, will introduce a qualitative difference in their capacity to remain open to intersubjective fields and work with them. As a discipline, body psychotherapy is indebted to psychoanalysis for its depth and rigour. However, we can certainly return a favour; this book is also an invitation for psychodynamic and psychoanalytic practitioners to learn from body psychotherapy—without compromising their values and clinical position.

The relational approach enables us to adopt broader concepts of mind and self than those in frequent use in Western cultures. Such concepts are in fact common in shamanic cultures, by which Bateson's theory was influenced, as they emphasise connection, intimacy, shared creation, and love. In many Eastern spiritual practices and therapies we can find rituals for opening ourselves to shared fields of wider minds. In some shamanic practices, for instance, the Shaman specialises in mobilising the locus of identity from the personal to the communal (Keeney, 1994). Systemic psychotherapist and shaman Bradford Keeney (2005), who was a long-standing student of Gregory Bateson, illustrated: "When this relational, communal, ecological mind prays in harmonic resonance, the whole system reverberates with the pulse of life. Then it is life that heals" (p. 39).

Relational body psychotherapy, too, offers a multitude of therapeutic rituals, which allows the therapeutic dyad to better focus on shared affective fields: somatic attention, resonance, and touch all address the *us* that is created between us in immediate, concrete fashion. The clinical chapter on resonance (Chapter Eleven) demonstrates therapeutic work with the intersubjective body, which is illustrated as well at the end of this chapter with a ritual for opening into and strengthening the wider mind.

I find the idea that the self (and mind) is not just a personal object but also a part of a relationship very appealing. It allows me to think of self as a movement, streaming within fields, which are contained by wider fields still, and are maintained flexible and moving thanks to mutual tension. We are organised within larger frames, and the self we experience is forever changing, depending on context. Perhaps it eases my sense of fragmentation and appeals to my loneliness and insatiable need for the other. It comforts me to consider the self as partaking in varied wider minds, which change all the time: bodymind is therefore different when I sit with a client, work with a group, or write to you here. The resources available to the system, the attachment style of the system, the complexities of the bodymind, and the wounds and pathology of bodymind change all the time and are bound by context. For me, this is one of the most relieving thoughts I can hold—as a person, and as a psychotherapist.

Emergence phenomenon—between the mind and the brain

If we ask a biologist to tell us about the mind, what kind of explanation would we be given? The scientific Newtonian model holds a mechanistic understanding of the body, and a causal view of the interaction between body and mind. When seen through mechanistic eyes, the mind is but a complex expression of neural and biochemical activities. In this model's final analysis, the deepening of human knowledge will eventually equip us with understanding of the mind through biological explanations; in the last account, biology would suffice in explaining psychology. The causal aspect denotes a temporally linear connection between the two: we have thoughts *because* of neurological activities; we feel sad *due to* secretions of neurotransmitters and hormonal activity; we become who we are *because* our genetic code is translated into proteins and characterological traits. "It's all genetics," establishes Motti Shohat, the head of Raphael Recanati Genetic Institute in Israel, "Character traits, mathematical abilities, musicality and artistic tendencies, or alternatively attention deficit problems and learning difficulties—these are all genetic skills" (Lerner, 2011, p. 60).

The principle of emergence suggests a different order of an explanation. According to philosopher Donald Davidson (1970), when physiochemical processes achieve a certain level of complexity, novel characteristics which were not present before—such as mentality—appear as emergent qualities (Field, 1996). Physician Fritjof Capra (2002) further elaborates: "Emergence results in the creation of novelty, and this novelty is often qualitatively different from the phenomena out of which it emerged" (p. 36).

A few years back, preparing for a lecture, I asked my partner Tom (who is a biological scientist) (Rolef Ben-Shahar & Rolef Ben-Shahar, 2005) to help me with a metaphor for the mind-brain dilemma and the complexity of emergence phenomenon. She suggested the metaphor of a music box. Suppose we have a music box, which plays a lovely tune, whose source is unknown. Could we claim that the music is in the box?

Inspired by Motti Shohat's quote, we may argue that "everything is in the mechanisms", and explain the tune with terminology of gears and springs; according to this explanation, the music is *in the box*, weaved and structured in its mechanisms. First we had the box, and only then came the music. If the springs break, the music will no longer be in the box. Is this explanation sufficient when applied to human complexity? I am not asking whether this explanation is right or true; certainly, there is a deep connection between the music box's mechanisms and the music therein, but is it really a causal relationship? Does the music in the box exist *because* of the box? Furthermore, would such an explanation do justice to the complexity of the music and that of the music box? We might, for instance, argue that the music box expresses, through the music, its mechanistic richness, its functional aesthetics; that the music uses the box to express its harmony, to manifest itself—to embody.

Would it be more correct, then, to argue that the music is *not in the box*? Perhaps we can say that the music was created in the heart of a gifted (and mysterious) musician, who composed the music. Or that the music is in the mind of the music box builder (whose existence we do not know of, but we may—if we choose to—infer); or that the music does not exist without us listening to it. In each of these explanations, the music exists independently of the music box, and the box is but a mechanism for allowing the music to express itself in the world. While this is a lovely theory, we have neither the means of establishing it, nor ways of relating to the music-music box interaction. Moreover, such explanation ignores the obvious existence of the music box and the relationship between the music and the music box. Such a description leaves us with an ideal, yet without a possibility of manifesting this ideal in the world coherently.

But if the music is neither in the music box, nor not-in-the-box, then where is it? To properly examine the music-music box relationship we are called to assume a wider contextual perspective, while acknowledging both the complementary and the contradictory relationship between these two partial truths. The music is both in the box and not in the box. Both perspectives are partially true and partially relevant—at different times and contexts, and to different people. "Emergence phenomenon" could provide a broad contextual view which will allow the music (or the mind) to be deeply connected to the music box (or the brain/body) without us having to create a mechanistic causal relationship on the one hand, or adopt a lax spiritualist-idealist position on the other.

Emergence phenomenon relates to both Eastern and Western ideas. For example, the eminent theoretician Kurt Gödel (1931) presented his famous mathematical theorem, claiming that any sufficiently complex structure contained elements (propositions) which could not, even in principle, be proved true or false within the system itself. Gödel did not maintain that these arguments (mathematical sentences) could not be proved at all, but instead that they needed to be weighed from a larger mathematical structure, a different level of logic.

The ideas presented by Gödel and Davidson are relevant to psychotherapy both when looking at the relationship between mind and body, and when examining the I–thou relationship. Looking at these postulations as psychotherapists, we may come to consider that some changes cannot take place within a system, but require a broader system of which the original system is a part. Simply said—we cannot do it all by ourselves. Even if the mind did emerge from bodily structures (neurological, endocrinal, genetics, etc.), it would be incorrect to explain it in physiological terms. The mind requires a different language, one that takes social, cultural, and political aspects into account. To properly understand the pain of an individual within a family, we are called to examine and explore the familial, cultural, or social systems. Emergence theory claims that when a music box has reached certain levels of complexity, a new phenomenon might emerge from it—one that belongs to a completely different terminological world—music.

Despite the novelty inherent to the emergent self, it is very tempting to still use metaphors belonging to previous paradigms (older classes of logic), out of which the self was allegedly born and developed; using physiological metaphors to speak about the bodymind is seductive. There are some beautiful and poetic descriptions that provide such metaphors for the brain-mind interactions. The famous surgeon Leonard Shlain (1998), for example, describes the right hemisphere as "the realm of altered states of consciousness where faith and mystery rule over logic" (p. 19). Scientific and pseudo-scientific descriptions of body–mind interactions in general, and brain-mind connections in particular, are very common in therapeutic literature. Such descriptions are useful in bringing the readers closer to understanding the complex relationship between somatic, mental, and psychological processes—but such explanations do not come without a price.

In my view, describing mental and relational processes using metaphors of brain mechanics, physical localisation, and genetic sequencing is an epistemological and aesthetic mistake. It is a mistake not because the metaphor is untrue, since physical metaphors as well as systemic or relational ones are still just that—stories and metaphors, which present merely certain aspects of reality; it is a mistake because physiological metaphors continue to describe an emergence phenomenon in the terminology of its components. Such descriptions keep us glued to an inappropriate, old paradigm and further cultivate body–mind and I–thou splits, as well as confuse us by creating an illusion of causal connection. It makes us believe that the secretion of serotonin came before feeling good, and that we feel good *because* of this secretion; we lose our unfathomable nature to procedural and linear thinking.

Naturally, we can describe listening to the Rachmaninoff Piano Concerto No. 2 in terms of wavelengths, overtones, sound pitch, or auditory receptors and bioelectrical conduction, and this might be an illuminating and interesting description. However, such terminology misses the fact that the concerto creates a new language, essentially different—both in its aesthetics and in terms of emotional value to the components from which it emerged and developed. A much more contextually relevant metaphor might be one of joy (or suffering), of feelings and harmony, of images and sentiments. The physiological metaphor is unfaithful to the new phenomenon which was created by the notes and the technical skill of playing and conducting. Listening to music is an aesthetic, bodily, and emotional experience, requiring an emotional language. Similarly, good restaurant critics and talented wine critics write about food and drink in an affective language, one that is much broader and richer than merely describing the ingredients and methods of preparation.

Taking into account the historical context of psychotherapy, which was explored in Chapter One, and its efforts to be accepted by the Newtonian–Cartesian medical and scientific circles, it is no wonder that the medical-physical theory of mind was the predominant model for many decades. Some psychologists described the mind in cerebral terminology (or were looking forward to the day when such description would become possible), using causal connections to explain emotional experiences and relationships. Psychotherapy in general and body psychotherapy in particular used (and still does) similar terminology to strengthen its arguments and validate somatic interventions.

It is convenient and tempting to use neurological and biological data to forge erroneous causal connections between biochemical, genetic, or otherwise physical activities and the emergent phenomena. For example: "You are depressed *because* your brain-chemistry is imbalanced"; "You are only fat *because* you've got fat genes"; "Body psychotherapy works *because* of left-hemisphere inhibition and right-hemisphere predominance"; "You should do more physical activity *because* it would increase your serotonin secretion and then you'd be happier." In all these examples there are indeed important links between the two parts of the sentence, yet these are not linear and causal connections as the phraseology implies.

A mind that no longer resides in the brain

The influential physicist and system theorist Fritjof Capra (2002) wrote:

> The brain is a specific structure through which this process [cognition] operates. The relationship between the mind and the brain, therefore, is one between process and structure.

> Moreover, the brain is not the only structure through which the process of cognition operates. The entire structure of the organism participates in the process of cognition. (pp. 32–33)

Indeed, as a body psychotherapist, I am by no means attempting to dispute the mind-body or mind-brain connection. On the contrary, in my opinion our existence—and our mental processes—cannot be said to be anything but embodied. We cannot but be a body. We cannot think, feel, exist, or relate except as embodied organisms. However, I would like to wonder about the validity of a position which reduces the two fields into one language, and challenge the frequently presented linear causal connection between mind and body.

The bodymind is not similar to the mechanistic body or to the ethereal mind. The bodymind belongs to a different logical class of organisation than either body or mind, just like the *us-ness* (the wider mind) belongs to a different class of logic than you and me. A tension pulsates through and between the mind, the body, and the bodymind; contradictory pulls to integrate and separate complement one another. Gregory Bateson (1974) reiterated this position in writing: "An individual in a system is always part of that system and is therefore subject to all the constraints and necessities of the particular part-whole relationship in which he exists" (p. 27).

During change, the new organisation threatens the old paradigm, the old form. For example, when a baby is born, the two adults (traditionally) involved in its making become parents, and a family is created. This family now requires a new language, a new frame of contexts and relating. I say to my Zohar: "I'm ok with you eating this cookie, but let's ask mum how many you've already eaten." Tom became a mother, and we, as a family, are required to reorganise and find a new form—inventing ourselves as we go along.

Two weeks after the birth of Shuy Grace, our second daughter, I was sitting with Zohar who was sobbing loudly: "I love Shuy, but I hate the number four," she said. "I much prefer *three*, it is a much nicer number, so it was nicer being three." Just so that we are completely clear, she added: "I also hate five and six."

The bodymind in relationships—the intersubjective body

Up till now we have examined two types of splits and integrations: body and mind (and bodymind), I and thou (and the wider mind). Are these two processes connected? If the self is not simply a private entity but a process weaved within a relationship, then what happens to the body? Paraphrasing Winnicott's well-known quote "There is no such thing as a baby" [without a mother], psychoanalyst Susie Orbach (2003a) argued that: "There is also, I suggest, no such thing as a body, there is only a body in relationship with another body" (p. 10). If the mind indeed emerged from somatic processes, then the self (the bodymind of which I am a part) is an emergent phenomenon—I am created when I relate, and I can relate inasmuch as I have a body. This is a radical claim, and one that I find very exciting.

Looking at the body through the relational body psychotherapy lens, we no longer examine body and mind in hierarchical terminology (which is more superior, body or mind?) or causal language (which came first?). From this point of view, we examine a kaleidoscopic lattice of interactions and influence between body, mind, and environment. We are born thanks to a dialectic movement between somatic, linguistic, and relational processes, and our bodies receive meaning and blessing from our contact with another (Sella, 2011).

Should we choose to adopt this view, according to which the body belongs to the intersubjective field, which is sensory and somatic in its essence, then we are called to seriously reconsider the possibility of touch in the psychotherapeutic relationship (Asheri, 2009). Surrender to wider mind does not take place in a void, but occurs in our bodily, psychological, and relational organisation. The human context for such surrender is necessarily bodily. Our somatic experiences enable us to consider reorganisation, and embodied psychotherapeutic work can strengthen the psychotherapeutic relationship and the wider mind which develops therein.

Exercise: opening to a wider mind

(A therapeutic ritual or an exercise)

The following therapeutic process uses techniques from body psychotherapy and shamanism to encourage the creation of an intersubjective field, a wider mind. It also incorporates a mutual-validation ritual originated by NLP teacher and developer Robert Dilts.

1. Client and therapist face one another with both feet on the ground.
2. The therapist guides both sides internally, while emphasising some bodily relaxation: closing the eyes, focusing on the breathing and body sensations. The therapist encourages the client to loosen and unlock the jaw, to relax the eyelids, the feet and hands.
3. Both parties turn their attention inwardly, to sensations, feelings, images, and thoughts that emerge, without trying or making an effort to understand them, but instead allowing for a floating, witnessing observation.
4. The therapist guides both to softly open the eyes. The gaze is gentle, without attempting to focus on the other, but instead including the other within one's field of vision, with emphasis on peripheral vision. We aim to include the other, not trap the other.
5. Both therapist and client turn their attention inwardly—to thoughts, feelings, images, and sensations that emerge, without disconnecting from the other. How does this *togetherness* affect the flow of sensations (no need to verbally process now, there will be time at the end).
6. A possible verbal interaction to support the opening field: the client pays attention to her presence, and when she feels present—without losing contact with herself or the therapist, says: "I am here."
7. The therapist allows himself to receive the client's statement and replies: "I see you."
8. The last two stages (6 & 7) can be repeated three or four times, each time allowing for a deepening of the shared presence and its validation. If it is appropriate and acceptable to both sides, changing roles might be a powerful facilitative tool, so the therapist declares his presence and the client validates him.
9. Gently close and process together.

CHAPTER SIX

The bodymind character structure

My body was wiser than me
Its pain threshold lower than mine
It said enough
When I said more
My body
My body stopped
When I carried on (and oh, I carried on)
My body could not
It failed
And I got up and had to walk
And my body at my wake

—*Yona Wallach* (1992, p. 155), "My Body Was Wiser than Me"[1]

Introduction

One of the central notions in body psychotherapy is the understanding that developmental processes and developmental difficulties are both expressed in our body, particularly in our musculature. Learning about the development of character structure (and character armour) is central in the majority of body psychotherapy trainings. The term *character structure*, as it is used in this chapter, denotes three different facets: a developmental stage, a character rigidity, and character style.

Developmental stage: The first aspect of character structure relates to natural and organic developmental processes taking place during the first six years of our lives. Similar to early psychoanalytic models, body psychotherapy has a bodymind developmental model which characterises shared and parallel themes alongside the developmental axis. For example, all foetuses develop a startle reflex (where the arms are laterally jerked upon a sudden stimulus) and only later develop the Moro reflex, in which the arms jerk sideways and then, quickly, cling and grasp. The Moro reflex can be life-saving: it enables the baby to firmly hold on to the parent, thus to avoid falling if he is accidentally dropped. Another example is the move between horizontal posture (when the baby lies down or crawls) to vertical posture—when the toddler stands up and walks: during healthy and normal development, all babies transition from lying down and crawling, to standing and walking, a transition which carries great bodily and muscular consequences as well as psychological ones—a new bodymind organisation. The quality and rhythm of our bodily changes make sense, and could be relevant to understanding psychological processes in childhood and adulthood. As we shall later see, bodymind character structures indicate the natural progression of musculature and somatic organisation and development (and the erogenous zones identified with these developmental stages).

In its early days, body psychotherapy perceived those developmental stages as chronological, providing clear diagnostic criteria. Contemporary body psychotherapy, and particularly relational body psychotherapy, views these not as chronological stages but instead as themes or developmental issues, which may arise before or after the chronological stages which are offered here. The following developmental angles are central throughout our lives, and each person has one or two issues which had particular impact on her development, guiding her communication style and conduct with herself, with others, and with the world around her. These normal developmental stages allow us, as readers, to view those themes more clearly, but the themes in themselves are not limited to the developmental time span offered here.

Character structure rigidity: The second aspect of the bodymind character structure relates to disruptions in healthy development. Each developmental angle brings with it new bodily, psychological, and relational challenges. A marked difficulty or trauma, which is experienced during a specific developmental stage (or when a developmental angle is particularly active), may lead to bodymind rigidities at this stage and develop into pathologies connected with those rigidities. Character structure rigidities are, in fact, the typological system in body psychotherapy. We all express certain degrees of bodymind rigidities, and usually manifest one or two angles more than the others. For instance, when a toddler lacks the muscular maturity or emotional stability to walk for a long period of time, yet feels that she must not be small, she will have to inflate her chest and lock her lower back while walking. These two bodily movements might enable the toddler to walk with relative stability even in the absence of core muscles (spinal erectors and pelvic floor muscles) for strength. However, the price for such a posture will be weakened core muscles, a distorted sense of agency and capability, and restricted breathing patterns: to sustain this inflated position she would need to inhale a lot, while exhaling very little. This chronic holding, correlating with the "inflated" stage (or psychopathic), which will be further discussed, might result in issues of ego instability and an oscillatory sense of agency, both correlating with narcissism.

Most typological systems in body psychotherapy name the developmental stages after the rigidified state they might lead to (for example: schizoid, oral, psychopath, masochist, and rigid). Unlike the common categorisation and to remain faithful to my humanistic-generative therapeutic outlook, I chose to name those developmental angles after the main healthy developmental theme and not after the pathology.

Character structure style (or character style): A third aspect of character structure concerns lifespan developmental processes. The themes and issues every developmental angle emphasises are relevant to each of us throughout our lives. During the course of any interpersonal development we move through processes which resemble those early developmental processes: we arrive into the world—and into relationships, we attempt to have our needs met, we move between seeking support and wanting autonomy, we need to examine our own will against other people's wanting, and we oscillate between our capacity to tolerate sexual charge and pleasure—and repressing and contracting such charge.

Each time we come close to a relevant theme for us (where some developmental rigidity happened), we are faced with a challenge and a possibility for creating a novel movement. During the progression of therapy, the body psychotherapist expects that therapeutic processes might parallel the bodymind developmental stage. Each developmental style carries with it challenges, a potential for growth and healing, but also risks for suffering, regression, pain, and further developmental rigidities within the therapeutic relationship. Therefore, developmental styles are cyclical and repeating templates, which are bound to also be expressed in therapy on different levels: as an entire process (e.g., at the beginning of therapy, during therapy, and around termination of therapy), and in each session (e.g., at the beginning of a session, during the session, and at the end of each session). Understanding bodymind character structure will allow the therapist to foresee challenges during different stages of therapy and use stage-appropriate resources during those times.

Bodymind character structure typologies slightly vary between different body psychotherapy modalities. While there are great similarities in these methods, the names of stages vary, as do the exact division, the age of each stage, and more. In this chapter I chose to use Silke Ziehl's division (2000), but I was also assisted by other Reichian typologies (Keleman, 1985; Lowen, 1958; Reich, 1933a), and newer adaptations in body psychotherapy (S. Johnson, 1994; Totton & Jacobs, 2001). The work of Daniel Stern (1985, 2002) also influenced the structure of this chapter. I chose Ziehl's division both because of my affinity with her approach, and since it was based on psychoanalytic understanding and will therefore make sense to psychodynamic and psychoanalytic readers as well. Additionally, Ziehl holds a humanistic outlook, according to which each character structure (and character rigidity) is not just a developmental pathology—but also a manifestation of a victorious creative survival, bearing with it potential for growth and productivity.

The chapter examines the concept of character structure and character armour, and later explores the five main developmental angles and their respective developmental rigidities.

Atlas—the body as our biographical shadow[2]

> Indeed, the body is the shadow insofar as it contains the tragic history of how the spontaneous surging of life energy is murdered and rejected in a hundred ways until the body becomes a deadened object.
>
> —John Conger (1988, p. 108)

Atlas, the martyr, the hero, the beholder of skies. Another carrier of the primal sin, Atlas was punished by Zeus for his rebellion against the Olympian gods with the enormous task of standing at the edge of Gaia (earth) and holding the skies on his shoulders. The primordial Titan Atlas supported the sky on his shoulders, unable to let go for fear of the devastation that would occur if he did: Atlas, the one who oscillated between his omnipotent importance (the integrity of the world was dependent on him) and his helpless position and his inability to let go. As such, he was depicting the epitome of the narcissistic wound. So painful was his role, so intolerable, that he was driven to rigidity. Atlas requested the hero Perseus, who had just returned from slaying Medusa the gorgon, to allow him a glimpse of her face, which turned the onlooker to stone. Perseus obliged. Atlas committed suicide: he turned into stone, into the great chains of mount Atlas.

It is important to mention that while this hardening carried a grave price, it also expressed enormous gifts and value: the capacity to tolerate pain, to give meaning (narcissistic, but nonetheless meaning) to the holder of the sky, and, of course, the regal aesthetic value, the beauty and splendour of mount Atlas. Every rigid muscular organisation thus expresses both a tragedy and a victory at the same time.

Our body is our Atlas. In our bodies we assumed the forms which our developing organism perceived as necessary for our survival: "This body will make me more agreeable and acceptable, more loveable; this body will help me belong; this body will shelter me." Our muscular forms portrayed the unarticulated endeavour to balance the intrapsychic with the interpersonal: to shape ourselves so that we may survive and belong. "What a good boy you are," said the mother, "you never cry." The boy noticed his mother's distress in response to his crying. He was uncertain that she would survive his pain, yet helpless in his own need for her. For lack of choice he tensed his stomach, contracted his throat; he held his breath in. Gradually, rigidifying took place; a form with no movement; it may have no water: a tearless boy.

We develop an attitude to life, to others, and to ourselves. Throughout life, we assume bodily forms, which have muscular, emotional, mental, and relational components. Such an attitude may become rigidified if the experiences continue to occur—if the child is never welcomed in his tears, he will become a non-crying person; he will assume a somatic organisation that might have no space for grief. A somatic form is our self-image, our psychosomatic identity. Moshe Feldenkrais (1977), originator of the Feldenkrais method, expands on this: "In reality our self-image is never static. It changes from action to action, but these changes gradually become habits; that is, the actions take on a fixed, unchanging character" (p. 11). Those fixed habits, which we have created by regularly contracting our musculature and restricting our breath, were expressions of emotional attitudes, at the service of one of the most integral human needs: making love possible.

The character armour was created to support the character structure. Excess or deficiency in our emotional range could be expressed in muscular and respiratory chronic holding pattern: these coping strategies were not only emotional but also physiological—translated into posture and histology. Our somatic organisation attempted to protect us from harm and make us worthy recipients of love, to make the relationships with our caregivers feasible for them—and for ourselves.

Alexander Lowen (1958) explained: "The character is the medieval knight, his armour is his defence. Like all armour, the character armour creates a limitation of mobility and a decrease in sensitivity" (pp. 134–135). Therefore, emotional and physical stiffening resulted in limitation in movement, gradually rigidifying into habitual position. This might later lead to inflexible ego structures: like Atlas the Titan, we might find that our form has been set in stone.

This process is not merely a personal one—it is an organisational process of loosening and rigidifying. For example, a country that invests the majority of its resources in security and warfare limits its investments in education, culture, infrastructure development, and appropriate foreign affairs. There are, of course, circumstances where there are no other choices; when external threats require us to tighten our self-preservation instinct. Yet the near-exclusive investment in security also contributes to the creation of dangerous and threatening reality (among other ways, through social, cultural, and international binary projective identification, whereby we "deposit" badness with external agencies, thus cultivate them as such). The muscular character armour works similarly: it takes great energy to preserve it. Muscular holding requires physical and emotional effort, and is therefore limiting our lives. The more we invest in preserving our defence, the less access we have to resourceful cultivation of growth, development, and expression of our aliveness in the world. As a body psychotherapist, I assume that when the danger which necessitated the formation of muscular armour is gone, there might be value in loosening the rigid formation, allowing us to take new risks in our lives and invest our resources in building and cultivating life. The therapeutic relationship provides a safe space, where bodymind holding patterns might gradually become unnecessary and the clients would be able to examine the usefulness (or its lack) of their habitual muscular organisation.

"Life is a process of forming," writes body psychotherapist Stanley Keleman (Keleman & Adler, 2000). "There is a continual reshaping of our bodily-self, from the unformed infant to the formed adult. Either we live this forming unreflectively, or we volitionally participate in influencing our inherited responses" (pp. 50–51). By loosening rigid muscle structures while recognising their emotional sources and celebrating their original function, we reclaim the possibility for flow, and together with verbal and emotional therapeutic work, a reorganisation may be facilitated.

The boy who became a man still cannot cry; he cannot feel sadness. His neck and diaphragm are restricted; his breathing seems to have lost its joyous spontaneity and became controlled. His emotional range is now narrowed. Such armour leaves little space for flexibility: how can he surrender to his feelings when he is paralysed, when no mobility is possible? The body psychotherapist therefore aspires, among other therapeutic goals, to soften the psychosomatic organisation and encourage other, novel organisational choices.

We wish to melt the frozen history of our bodies, to awaken our kind Atlas and soften the illusive and elusive task of holding the sky, thus easing the guilt for our failure to hold the sky. We may soften the muscles, we may do breathwork, but more important, we shall contribute to the formation of a stronger and wider body: a shared dyadic body, a more stable wider mind. When muscles soften, breathing restrictions are removed, and we are better able to experience a containing relationship. When our breathing is freed, our musculature becomes softer and suppler. Our capacity to move freely and to choose is regained. Tears are permitted to flow now: the man who emerged here, becoming himself within and alongside the therapeutic dyad—and the therapist with him—can both support the boy that he used to be, as if reassuring him: "It's safe to cry now." A novel *us* was created, giving birth to a new Atlas, one that may not freeze into stone so quickly; an Atlas that may have more faith in his capacity to relate.

Bodymind developmental positions[3]

Every distinct psychotherapeutic modality holds a developmental theory. As I described in Part I (Historical), body psychotherapy developed out of a complex political context. Following Reich's eviction from the mainstream psychoanalytic milieu in the 1930s, body psychotherapy continued to develop primarily within humanistic psychology streams, and later as a part of the countercultural movements of the 1960s. Reichian bodymind developmental stages were based on psychoanalytic thinking and required a psychoanalytic framework to fully understand them; the developmental angles proposed here were influenced not only by Reich, but also by humanistic principles, which guided and informed body psychotherapy for many decades, hence these express integration between psychoanalytic and humanistic understanding (Wilkinson, 2000).

"The story of the growing child", writes Winnicott (1987), "is a story of absolute dependence moving steadily through lessening degrees of dependence, and groping towards independence" (p. 83). Each developmental position brings with it new challenges, as well as growing complexities of interactions between the baby, his attachment figures, and the external world. Character structure is created as a dialectic process between the baby and his environment, as an attempt to provide the necessary and sufficient conditions for meeting the organism's needs (and the needs of the baby's attachment figures too). This compromise between organismic needs and environmental pressures is inevitable. My understanding of organismic needs is different to the classical Freudian view of drive theory and id, but instead as seen under the lens of object relations and attachment theory, according to which the baby is attuned from birth to seek relationships (Hadar, 1997a, 1997b).

When the baby (or the child) attempts to express a spontaneous need and is confronted with limiting or oppressing reality (usually from attachment figures and other main carers), she may express difficulty (anger, sadness) towards the limitation, but with time will learn to internalise the negative message and subsequently limit the spontaneous manifestation of the need. According to Reichian theory, this emotional reduction is created primarily through constrictions of breathing patterns and muscular holding. These holding patterns become chronic with time, crystallising into the character structure, a psycho-somatic organisation parallel to Winnicott's (1960a) concept of the *false self*.

But character structure (and character armour) is not only pathological—it represents an existential necessity, telling us in the flesh of the main themes that accompanied the person since the earlier stages of his development, and about the creative resources and strengths that will characterise him throughout his life. Each theme portrays a pulsating and breathing dialogue between the desire for expressing oneself in the world, and the need for protecting the self in the world (Totton & Jacobs, 2001).

Character structure rigidities present us with a spectrum of many shades rather than a dichotomist division (oral/not oral), which characterised earlier Reichian theory. Perhaps we can adopt Otto Kernberg's (Caligor, Kernberg, & Clarkin, 2007; Kernberg, 1970) principle division and mark a gradient within rigid characterological styles: between normal (or adaptive) organisations, and the neurotic, borderline, and psychotic. Thus, a fragmented character structure (which will be discussed later in the chapter) could, for example, be expressed in a neurotic organisation (with adaptive perception of reality testing, that is, the ability to properly understand what is real and what is imagined and respond to these distinctions safely and appropriately): the clumsy waiter could be a good example for that, as he might be uncoordinated and awkward, but within a normative and functioning context. A borderline organisation of fragmented character structure might fit, for instance, a person with paranoid or schizoid personality disorder, struggling more significantly to connect the bridges between inside and outside, to function at work, or to form stable relationships. A psychotic organisation of the fragmented character structure could be found, for example, with a person suffering from schizophrenia.

In addition to the wide spectrum of severity in character organisation, the degree of the rigidity might certainly change. Even if therapy cannot change our character structure completely, it can certainly assist us in becoming more flexible and move on the spectrum towards a more adaptive organisation, just as secure attachment style could be earned with generative life experience and therapy (Roisman, Padrón, Sroufe, & Egeland, 2002).

It seems that the issues, which the developmental positions in this chapter present, actually develop much earlier than originally assumed (D. N. Stern, 1985), and that the astute chronological order offered by Reich, Lowen, and others is somewhat anachronistic. Therefore, the following developmental positions in this chapter suggest five angles of looking at life issues, and five main ways of positioning ourselves in relation to the world. Each angle is presented through its manifestation during child development, but it is also a way of looking at the character structure which is affected by those issues.

The five basic developmental stages relate to developmental challenges. They overlap in duration. In the *first stage*, the challenge is about existence, boundaries, and forming connection, and it lasts from intrauterine stages, through the birth, and until about three months old. During the *second stage*, the challenges concern nourishment and having our basic needs met. This stage lasts from birth or soon after until eighteen months. The developmental challenge of the *third stage* relates to balancing differentiation and support, between holding and autonomy, and it lasts from about eight months to two and a half years. In the *fourth stage*, the developmental challenges are about assertiveness: the child's capacity to express her will without losing validation and love, and it lasts from two years to three and a half years. During the last and *fifth stage*, the child's capacity to tolerate bodily and erotic charge is higher. In this stage the child's (bodily) sexuality reaches its first climactic peak, and the developmental challenges involve feeling erotic desire and expressing it in a secure and contained manner. This stage lasts between three and six years old. Many models in body psychotherapy divide this last stage into two separate stages or four substages (e.g., Kurtz, 2007; Totton & Edmondson, 2009).

The rest of the chapter reviews the three faces of character structure in light of five developmental angles. We shall explore the normative and adaptive developmental structures, their bodily organisations, and the consequences of developmental rigidities expressed during these stages. Each developmental style expresses the somatic and psychological strengths which emerge in this stage, the challenges faced by the individual and her environment during the stage, and the pathological risks and creative potential embedded in each stage.

First developmental position—arriving in the world: existence

Arriving in the world involves multiple and enormous challenges. The transition from a symbiotically regulated environment (mostly passive) to an environment which requires external dyadic regulation (active) is highly dramatic. Even in healthy and normal pregnancy and natural smooth birth, such transition is an extremely high-impact and possibly shaking experience. The first challenges the newborn faces are establishing his existence and ensuring his survival: to breathe, to sustain a life-enabling body temperature, to find his existence within the mother–baby dyad. From the latter stages of pregnancy, through labour and until the baby is about three months old, the newborn adjusts to the ex-uterine world through the necessary dyadic regulation provided by his primary attachment figure. Unlike the world of water, which he emerged from, gravity makes it difficult for the baby to carry his own weight and he loses much of his mobility and motor agency, which he had already acquired in the womb—he cannot even hold his own body weight. Faced with such deep and paralysing helplessness, the baby discovers his capacities and influential power over the parents.

Michel Odent (1994), one of the pioneers for advocating and promoting natural birth in Western civilisation, most beautifully described this first bodymind developmental stage. According to Odent, the huge adrenaline surge, which was later followed by activation of the parasympathetic nervous system, contributed to the alertness of mother and baby immediately after birth which allowed them to establish eye contact. This primary eye contact, validating the newborn existence, symbolised the main bodily segment of this stage: the ocular segment (relating to vision and eyes). Around birth and during the few weeks following birth, body psychotherapy described how much of the newborn baby's energetic investment was located around the eyes: in seeing, making eye contact with the mother (or primary carer), and perceiving the new world through the eyes and the ocular muscles. While the tactile senses were there from the beginning, eye contact secured connection in the absence of touch.

In fact, in a safe-enough environment the newborn baby should not exist. Her safety and security are not challenged, her existence is not challenged—there is continuity from the intrauterine containing to the maternal (or paternal) holding, thus the newborn is unaware of her existence. "In healthy development," writes Winnicott (1963) "the infant (theoretically) starts off (psychologically) without life and becomes lively simply because of being, in fact, alive" (p. 192). The infant, according to Winnicott, has a deep need for no self-consciousness (which Winnicott terms unselfconscious), since premature consciousness of her being alive presupposes an understanding (or consciousness of) her separateness, which is too intolerable during the first stages of life. If and when existence becomes a relevant issue during those first three months, the child might be predisposed to fragmented character structure dominance.

Throughout this chapter, when using the word *mother* I relate to the primary attachment figure, which could of course be someone else other than the mother (the father, or another parent, for example).

Character structure: When a baby experiences trauma at this early stage, the developmental style he expresses is frequently characterised by dissociative defence, since his very existence and being is threatened, thus this character structure is known as *fragmented*. It is also called *ocular, schizoid*, or *boundary* character structure. Schizoid fixation occurs as a result of injury to dyadic regulation functioning. The need for psychological non-existence (through dyadic regulation, the mother—or another primary attachment figure—enables the baby to be unselfconscious of his existence) is not properly met and the baby lives feeling there is nobody to support his liveliness, feeling unwelcomed into the world. Body psychotherapist Jack Lee Rosenberg (Rosenberg, Rand, & Asay, 1985) relates to the dissociative defence as protection from pain: indeed, we avoid sensations and feelings (pleasant as well as painful) but we also suffer a deadening of the self. Dissociation, for Rosenberg, is the high price we are willing to pay to protect ourselves from real death or psychic death.

In her endeavour to integrate psychoanalytic understanding of autism with body psychotherapy, body psychotherapist Renana Reis (2011) followed functional analyst Will Davis in proposing that the autistic encapsulation was not merely a psychological defence, but also involved physiological processes: more specifically, as Davis described, plasmatic contraction. There was, so Reis suggested, a concrete bodily shell protecting the autistic person from overwhelming (real or perceived) threat, and from avoiding a repetition of his early trauma.

The schizoid person was described by psychologist Yorai Sella (Aharon, 2013) as directly threatened by bodily sensations, which confront the schizoid with dread of death and annihilation, inherent to his bodily experiences. Therapy therefore involves an initial validation of the person's existence, and gradual expansion of the person's existence with his body and reality. In terms of attachment style, the fragmented defence therefore expresses disorganised attachment. Winnicott (1949) described the process of depersonalisation, inclusive of out of body experiences, as characteristic of the schizoid stage.

Main issues: Prenatal trauma, birth trauma, or mother's difficulty in establishing connection with the newborn, all position the baby in survival mode, between life and death. Existing becomes a central theme. The baby is forced to deal with dread of dying and find creative solutions to survive and exist in the world. The fragmented solution is a dissociative one (similar to the Kleinian paranoid-schizoid position (Klein, 1946)). Such a solution is a response to an extreme situation, requiring a deep emotional and physical split from the intolerable reality (Rolef Ben-Shahar, 2012b). In fact, the injury at this stage is at the heart of the baby's dyadic existence—the wholeness of the mother–baby dyad is severed, thus carrying with it severe abandonment anxiety and difficulty to trust the very existence of self, and of the world.

Bodily holding: The bodily holding characterising fragmented structure is *holding together*, as if the body is trying, with great effort, to hold itself together as one. This is the natural somatic response to the dominant feeling of fear and terror. We respond to threat by contracting our musculature. Such holding can sometimes be seen with very young babies, who seem to invest a great deal of energy in holding the body together, as if they would fall apart if they failed to make this effort. This is understandable, if we consider the transition from the intrauterine water world, operating as shock absorber, to the outside world, full of rich visual, auditory, and tactile stimulation. When fragmented character armour is created, the adult will seem as if he is trying to hold his body together. Functional analyst Will Davis (2008b), argued that: "The true schizoid character has a contracted plasmatic process, not a neuro-muscular armouring" (p. 4). He continued:

> The plasma is the internal sea within which we are swimming. Each and every part of our body is immersed in, totally surrounded by this semi-liquid. In fact, each and every cell is surrounded by this semi-liquid. In fact, each and every cell is filled with this semi-liquid. It is universally present and as a result, all of our psycho-somatic functions are directly dependent on it. And just as all life forms in the ocean will be negatively affected if the ocean becomes polluted, all of our life functions will be directly interfered with if our plasma becomes "polluted". For body psychotherapists, the most important form of plasmatic pollution is chronic contraction. And the earliest, strongest and deepest contraction is the schizoid state. (p. 6)

Nick Totton and Michael Jacobs (2001) offered the insecure and awkward character which Woody Allan often embodied as a good example for fragmented character structure.

Control issues: Issues of control are relevant and central to all developmental angles, yet they each have a different style of control. The controlling message (and illusion) of the fragmented character structure is mental: "I control my thoughts and ideas." In a chaotic world, where even my survival is at stake and I cannot trust another person, at least I can trust my thinking.

Breathing pattern: Faced with terror, breathing becomes strongly held (almost nonexistence) on the one hand, and chaotic on the other hand. The held and chaotic breathing pattern is not only characterising adults with fragmented structure; it is a generally common response to trauma: holding our breath is a normative response to extreme conditions.

Movement: The highly fragmented person is not completely embodied, as if he did not make up his mind yet whether to be a body or not, to exist or not. Body movements therefore frequently seem frozen, uncoordinated, or very small. To understand the fragmented characteristic movement we can call to mind a newborn baby, who recently transitioned from one gravitational world (water) to another, and the fragmented, jerky quality of its movements.

Bodily tension: Birth demands huge efforts from the baby. A lot of pressure is compressing the head, skull, and neck. The bodily tensions common to the fragmented structure express in ocular regions (around eyes), base of skull, and neck. These tensions also relate to the baby's efforts to make contact.

Eye contact: By and large, the fragmented character structure avoids eye contact or "grabs" eye contact fiercely and without letting go (as if life depends on maintaining it). When eye contact is established, the type of gaze tends to be staring, detached, and cold.

Touch: Touch is not just an intervention in body psychotherapy, but also an important diagnostic tool. Touch feels different with people whose issues, or character structures, are different. The quality of touch in people whose primary structure is fragmented is of "nobody's home". It is as if the person and his body are two separate entities, and it is difficult to sense the person by touching him. The skin might feel cold and the person may avoid physical contact, which might threaten him or feel invasive (Aharon, 2013). When touch does happen, it may feel awkward and disconnected from the relationship.

Fear: The fear when traumas occur around birth (or tap into these) is annihilation anxiety. Trauma during these developmental stages might create patterns of dread from extinction and emotional flooding, and indeed the person is easily flooded. It is difficult for the fragmented person to believe she could exist alongside another person. Terror of death envelopes relationships and life decisions—both big and small, hence decision-making is difficult.

Energetic phase: Energetically speaking, the fragmented character structure is dedicated to immense self-regulatory efforts and attempts for integration. The lack of necessary dyadic regulation (primary intersubjectivity, as advanced by Trevarthen (2004)) and the need to "grow up quickly" lead to fragmented and compensating self-regulation.

Strengths and resources: René Descartes, who embodies the fragmented character structure in his theoretical split between body and mind, arguably expressed in his philosophical ideas a dissociative defence against his early traumas (Withers, 2008). Yet Descartes's philosophy also demonstrated the strengths and resources of the fragmented character structure: flowing creativity and impressive intellectual abilities. Additionally, many people who experienced early traumas, and whose major character structure was fragmented, possess natural aptitude to spiritual qualities and often have a deep sense of belonging to spiritual realms.

Working therapeutically with fragmented character structure: The major therapeutic goal is allowing for safe and contained existence. The boundaries at this stage are unclear and amorphous—between the client and the world (or the therapist) as well as within the client, thus therapy needs to strengthen both dyadic and self-regulation. Body psychotherapy offers many tools for strengthening the somatic self, believing that connection to the boundaries of the body would gradually strengthen the ability to exist, enhance separation and connection, strengthen boundaries, and, hopefully, foster integration.

The fragmented character structure tends to deny anxiety and dissociate from it. When the fear is finally acknowledged, a paranoid anxiety might appear. Despite the dread that might overwhelm the clinic, it could be (when handled gently) a mark of therapeutic progress—when anxiety is made conscious, it becomes more possible to work with it.

Working with clients in the fragmented stage (or in fragmented stages of therapy) is slow, and is mainly trauma work: the therapist is relatively active, and emotional expression is limited to avoid flooding and retraumatisation; the therapeutic emphasis is on safety and security, containment, and gentle arrival into the world. The common defence here is escape into intellectualism, and so therapy aims at enabling, and gradually creating safe bodily-emotional experiences.

When the client arrives with deep spiritual connection, the body psychotherapist may also offer energetic touch, not working directly on skin but with the energetic field surrounding the client, with what Arnold Mindell (1982) called "the dreambody".

Extreme conditions: Schizophrenia, the autistic spectrum, and some forms of somatoform disorders, dissociative disorders, and borderline experiences could be understood as resulting from very early developmental traumas.

Clinical vignette

The following vignette integrates some parts of my work with Kate, who was diagnosed with dissociative identity disorder (DID) (Rolef Ben-Shahar & Wood, 2009).

During the first two years of psychotherapy with Kate, she would arrive in the clinic, lie down on the mattress, curl up into a ball, and rock—softly and gently. The majority of our work was nonverbal, through movement and gentle touch. Kate wrote: "I came to session after session and was unable to say more than a sentence or two" (p. 33). The following paragraph, written by one of Kate's parts, seven-year-old Karen, demonstrates a fragmented position:

> I was speaking in a whisper. He asked what my favourite colour was, but when I looked inside I couldn't tell. All the time I felt cold, but Asaf said the room was hot, and it was fear that was making me cold. Asaf asked, "Are you Karen?" and I nodded. [...] I told Asaf I was very sad. Asaf was shutting his eyes like he was sleepy. I asked why he was shutting his eyes, and he said so he could listen more carefully. "So you can listen with your tummy," I said, and Asaf said yes. I told Asaf the sadness was in my tummy, and I shut my eyes, and Asaf said, "Listen to your tummy." so I did and I said there was a lot of hurt there, as well as sadness, and as I felt it more strongly I said there was pain there too. I told Asaf about my cave which has little shelves with lights in and lots of cushions. (p. 44)

Kate herself relays: "I never felt that my feelings were acknowledged, that I didn't feel valued, so I was always trying hard, terrified of failure. I knew my parents loved me, but I didn't feel loved. They didn't show me or tell me that they loved me. I remembered the shock of going to a friend's house to a family that was much more openly affectionate than mine" (p. 36).

Exercise for working with the first developmental angle: breathwork for regulating anxiety

Different emotional states (or processes) are usually characterised by idiosyncratic breathing patterns. Stressful breathing is mostly flat, while the upper part of the lungs becomes more active (with the help of the diaphragm and intercostal muscles). This type of breathing is associated with activation of the sympathetic branch of the autonomic nervous system. Abdominal breath and lateral breath are mostly non-existent during stress situations and fear. Abdominal breathing tends to be more affective and emotional, while this basic lateral breathing exercise (inspired by Gay Hendricks, 1995) is excellent for down-regulating and calming anxiety.

1. The client is guided to lie on her back with bent knees and her feet resting on the ground. This posture loosens fascia (connective tissue) around the viscera and eases breathing.
2. The client places her hands on both sides of her rib cage. With each exhale she gently presses her ribs inwards (to assist the release of air), and with each inhale gently withdraws with the hands, to facilitate a regular breathing rhythm and "invite" the breath to the sides of the body. In fact, we move our hands as if we were supporting the organic work of an accordion, gently pressing it to direct the breathing to the sides of the body.
3. Repeat this conscious lateral breathing for a few moments.

Exercise for working with the first developmental angle: safe place

Working with terror requires the therapist to adopt a far more active role than in psychodynamic work. "Safe place" is a therapeutic process, which is valuable to establish, develop, and return to throughout therapy when working with very frightened clients. On the other hand, it can also be used ad hoc, when terror is present: an invitation to temporarily stop the therapeutic dialogue, reorient to the safe place and then continue.

This is a classic exercise for working with dread, which is used in one way or another in many approaches, certainly with trauma work, including EMDR (F. Shapiro, 2001), somatic experiencing (Levine & Frederick, 1997), and sensorimotor psychotherapy (P. Ogden, Minton, & Pain, 2006). I borrowed the following version from body psychotherapist Carolin Jakoby (personal communication).

1. The client is invited to sit in front of us and ensure he sits comfortably. Encourage and allow for natural breathing.
2. The client is asked to think of and imagine an external place in which he feels safe and secure (a real place, or if there are none—an imagined one). The therapist assists the client in doing so by asking him sensory-based questions and emphasising here-and-now: "What are you seeing there? What are the shades and colours? What kind of sounds are you aware of? Smells? What is the place's texture?" It is important to ensure the safe place is not ambivalent, and that there are no shades of fear or insecurity associated with the place. A good choice and creation of the place will allow for deeper and safer work later (even if this stage takes many sessions in itself).
3. Check with the client what kind of body sensations accompany the creation and tuning into the safe place. The therapist assists in amplifying and sharpening the experience of security, as well as in attending to the breath.
4. The therapist asks the client to scan his body, searching for a bodily place which has similar sensations to those of the external safe place. We are looking for an inner, bodily representation of the safe place.
5. The client is encouraged to place a hand over this place, connecting with his body sensations and breathing into this place. The sensation could be strengthened by calling upon an image or word that would anchor the safe place.
6. The therapist checks with the client what would help coming back to the safe place when needed, and encourages the client to practise (together with the therapist and on his own) coming and going.
7. During psychotherapy, whenever there is a threat of flooding (or when flooding occurs), the client is called to summon the safe place, before continuing with the narrative communication ("Let us return for a moment to your safe balcony: what did the flowers smell like there? What does it feel like to place your hand on this body part? And if you are feeling calmer, we can go back to what happened this week with your colleague"). The purpose of using the safe place is to create a less anxious space from which working and processing is possible, and to which it is possible to return when needed. Dance and movement psychotherapist Sharon Zack (personal communication) commented that the safe place could be drawn, and it might be the clinic (or parts of it): both additions may help clients who need a concrete image, or who have trouble imagining.

Second developmental position—dyadic regulation: neediness and nourishment

In one way or another, we have all arrived in this world; we have all discovered our first breath. Soon after breathing was activated, another bodily system begins to work in a very different manner to its intrauterine activity: the digestive system. During nine months in the womb we did not experience hunger; food streamed into our bodies through the bloodstream. Once the infant senses she is welcomed into the world, that she can breathe, suddenly her stomach contracts. Our first separated consciousness is not a cognitive or spiritual one, but a somatic consciousness. The stomach contracts—and the baby is hungry.

Hunger is one of the first experiences of lack: I want, I need, and it's not enough for me. With this lack also comes our first desire and passion, taking over our mouth and lips, our tongue, and our throat. If all is well, then shortly after this experience sweet warm milk flows in. In close proximity to the first intolerable separateness of the baby, as it manifests in the first lack and the first passion, appears the greatest satisfaction the baby has known since its conception. This is the void, which was described by psychoanalyst Christopher Bollas (1978), being transformed by the mother's milk to a feeling of fullness: pleasure is now spreading all over the infant's body, the lips are keenly tightening around the nipple (or bottle), craving more, and something inside can finally expand and surrender to the pleasure.

The pleasure requires the lack, and is conditioned by it; satisfaction is created by the need, and the entire world is now experienced through the lips and the digestive system, through the very same body-part that can give so much pleasure, satisfaction, and comfort. The mother, who is the main regulating agent of this dyad, places the baby next to her skin and her heartbeat is felt by the infant. And like any first experience of need, like any primal experience of lack being fully met, the first addictive pattern in our life is established: more ... more ... more ... An ocean of neediness opens inside us, through the lips it oozes out, through the lips it calls—in the only way a baby knows how to call—crying. And the good enough mother provides self-integration for her baby (Winnicott, 1962), and helps in establishing a transitional space where there is a place for the baby's need to need (to suffer, to tolerate the lack) and at the same time to have his needs met—quickly enough, but not too quickly.

Unending horizons of needs and wants characterise the second developmental stage. The parent–baby dyad hopefully recovers, as much as it is possible, the intrauterine environment and conditions. This is the first intersubjective stage (Trevarthen & Aitken, 2001), the primary dyadic state of consciousness (Tronick et al., 1998). This is also the last preverbal state. Here, too, like the first stage of arriving into the world, boundaries between inside and outside are not yet fully formed.

The world of nourishment and orality tends to be binary, oscillating between too much and not enough, and the transition between the two is sometimes sharp and abrupt. During this stage, the right for which the infant is fighting is the right to need, be fed, and nourished, and the main emotional hue is yearning and wanting. The developmental stage of neediness and nourishment lasts from around birth until about eighteen months, depending on how the baby is fed and weaned, and the fashion of meeting his needs in his relationship with the main attachment figures.

Character structure: When an infant experiences trauma during this stage, the injury is to his very permission to need and be regularly, consistently, and safely nourished. This injury, similar to the first stage, is in dyadic regulation, when the infant has yet to develop sufficient resources for self-regulation. To denote the active bodily centre during this stage, this character structure is called *oral*. It is also known as *collapsed* or *dependent* character structure. Difficulties in breast-feeding, reflux problems, malnourishment, strenuous external conditions, and hunger may all make their mark on the infant during this stage. Parental positioning towards the infant's neediness is also highly significant. Many parents struggle to tolerate such intense neediness and desire, particularly in Western culture, which idealises and idolises independence: "I can do it on my own." Oral injury may manifest in feelings of inner emptiness—or a void, lack of sense of agency, difficulty to care for self, or compensatory self-regulation (like the cartoon lover of Popeye the Sailor—Olive Oil, who forever needed saving). The oral position can also be expressed in a compensating manner—completely denying the need for another. One anorectic client prided herself, for example, that she could "survive on air alone". This compensatory position is related to the defence mechanism *reaction formation* (which can also be found in the inflated character structure, in the next developmental stage): if I do not get exactly what I want, then I need nothing whatsoever (from the relationship, from the therapist, etc.). The attachment style here is anxious (or preoccupied), that is, there is excessive preoccupation with feelings of abandonment and an experience of being unwanted as well as difficulty in forming genuine non-symbiotic connections.

Main themes: Nourishment and weaning, neediness, yearning and frustration, dependency and craving—these are the main issues during this developmental stage. When there is a major wounding during this stage, these themes might accompany the person throughout life. The unbridgeable gaps between too much and not enough, the righteous anger against injustice, and the frustrations concerning the need for others, all these become axes around which the person will revolve, and accordingly the psychotherapeutic process with predominantly oral character structure focuses on these themes. Addictions in general, and particularly oral addictions (food, cigarettes, alcohol) are frequent for people with oral character structure, who work diligently to attempt and quench the intolerable thirst, to fill the void in their belly.

Bodily holding: The bodily holding characteristic to this stage is holding on. Predominantly oral people struggle to let go, to complete, to say goodbye. This difficulty also manifests in the body. Endings are very difficult and emotional eating is common, serving as a clear substitute to needing the other (since "Food can never reject me," it can also fill the void, help me feel or not feel, hold me, and many other things).

Control issues: The control message of the oral character structure is about intake: "I am in control of what comes in and what does not come in to me."

Breathing patterns: Oral character structure is expressed in difficulty to take in. The neediness, dependency, and yearning might be obvious to those surrounding, but the person really is terrified of fully feeling and expressing these. Thus, inhaling is usually limited and exhaling is strong and long—it is hard to take in breath. The person will tend to breathe out much more than breathing in, being left feeling that "There's not enough air for me."

Movement: Imagine for a moment a breastfeeding baby, whose movements depend on the mother's degree of answering his needs. When needs are met, the movement is smooth; yet when needs are unmet, the infant gives up very quickly. The oral character structure has soft movement but is quick to give up, as if the movement lacks immanent energy. Body movements may be powerfully expressive, even mesmerising and seem promising at first, but lack impetus and last very briefly.

Bodily tension: During this developmental stage our world is largely experienced through our lips and mouth. The sugar in the mother's milk is our first drug, and sucking is a highly tiring—and very satisfying activity. When natural neediness is blocked, physical tension in the jaws and neck may become chronic. Wounding the infant's right to need does not only manifest in oral nourishment, but also in his needs for satisfying and pleasing intersubjective connection with the mother—being nourished in and by the transitional space (Winnicott, 1971a). Thus, oral character structure commonly holds muscular tensions in the hands and arms (mainly the wrist joints), the pectoral minor muscles, which are responsible for holding on and attaching, for cuddling, and for playing. Body tissues may feel as if they are inwardly collapsed. Body psychotherapist Ronen Levy (personal communication) offered the character of the "hanging-out junkie" as representative of the extreme oral character: loose, defeatist, wanting more and more hits, and inside the stomach lies an insatiable worm that knows not when to stop.

Eye contact: Oral characters might have a needing and "sucking" look, which is hard to ignore or refuse (sometimes may look like an abandoned kitten or a stray unwanted puppy).

Touch: The quality of touch in people with oral character structure is pleasant, safe, nourishing, and warm. It is pleasant to touch them and stroke their body; as if the skin is craving for touch. Touch is one of the most developed communication channels in oral people and they can be highly intuitive and astute with touch. The therapist who is comfortable working with touch could deeply enjoy the therapeutic relationship without falling into confusing erotic fields, common with later character structures. Predominantly oral people can also give nourishing, warm, and safe physical contact.

Fear: Fears during the neediness and nourishment developmental stage are from abandonment or being drowned and swallowed. Sometimes there is no nourishment at all and then the fear is of starvation and isolation; at other times the nourishment is toxic: the mother uses her baby to regulate her own narcissistic need to become the centre of her baby's world, and hence floods the baby with her love and milk without attentiveness to his own authentic needs. The dread of abandonment and wish for symbiosis on the one hand, and the fear of being enmeshed and swallowed on the other, both feed the terror of connection.

Energetic phase: The oral character is invested in building inner resources, needing to quickly take things in (because nothing will be left for later), or trying to survive without taking anything in (air, food, support). The energetic expression of these activities is *charge*—the effort to gather strength and energy, to accumulate just a little bit more, investing in continuous construction of a building which seems to collapse time and again. Together with the accumulation of energy and charge comes the collapse and defeatist despair: "If I cannot get what I want, then what's the point anyway?"

Strengths and resources: People who are predominantly oral can be very giving, nourishing, and empathetic. They tend to have a strong sense of righteous justice and will fight for what is fair. People who experienced oral trauma tend to be very sensitive—both to themselves and to others, and are able to introspect with astute intuition and attentiveness. Additionally, the infinite hunger for life is an important motivational force and they can "eat life to the full" and learn to enjoy a huge variety of activities and relationships.

Working therapeutically with oral character structure: Early psychoanalysis held the frustration of patients' oral needs as an important therapeutic value, a means of confronting the patient with the reality principle. The ability to tolerate frustration, and the therapeutic task of frustrating these needs at times has its place, but not necessarily during this stage. As Ferenczi

(1933) demonstrated, frustrating patients during the oral stage could create retraumatisation. The therapeutic goal when working with developmental orality concerns expanding the range between *not enough* and *too much*, and discovering the *good enough*—also through partial and boundaried satisfaction of the clients' needs.

Body psychotherapy with oral structures bares the quality of grace, since it might be non-verbal and has elements of reparative regression. It may nonetheless be highly uncomfortable, since the therapeutic dyad is very intuitive and it is difficult to find cognitive anchors for the clinical work. The therapy revolves around satisfying needs (or not). These are clients who tend to want more and the work is accompanied by discontentedness even if the needs are left unexpressed. With a predominantly oral client, the therapist might feel that the client misses the therapy but not the therapist. The therapist as a functional tool, an object (or part object), and as selfobject, is central here.

An important therapeutic question during these themes concerns therapeutic positioning with clients in early developmental stages (regression). Should we address the client at the development stage she is at, or aim at the stage we would have liked to challenge her with? Do we meet her as a child or call upon an adult? Should the therapist choose to meet the client at the earlier developmental stages, body psychotherapist skills and techniques might be of immense value, as orality primarily develops in preverbal fields, and therapy which is practised through talking alone might be limited in the extent of meeting oral and schizoid injuries.

Extreme conditions: Extreme oral conditions may manifest as depressive collapse, as well as bipolar disturbances. Eating disorders, which could be understood as disturbances in dyadic regulation and difficulty to take space (Bachar, 2001) can also express injuries during the oral developmental stage.

Clinical vignette

I worked with Gina, a forty-five-year-old single woman, for six months, until she successfully got pregnant with IVF treatments and decided to stop psychotherapy. When her son was three months old, Gina called, requesting an urgent meeting. On the phone she told me that her son was very fat and oedematous, severely suffering from reflux problems. The main problem, though, was that he was breastfeeding all the time. According to Gina, he was "... sucking me empty to death. I cannot sleep because he is feeding all the time. I hate him."

Gina arrived nervous to our meeting, and immediately began feeding Robert who was screaming already in the waiting room. His face was indeed swollen and his skin looked milk-white and oedematous. After about ten minutes of breastfeeding, I noticed that Gina was frowning and a moment later she withdrew backwards, in a very gentle and almost imperceptible motion. Robert stopped sucking and looked at his mum, and then barged on the nipple as if he was fighting for his life. Ten minutes later the process repeated itself—Gina's brow was beginning to frown, she withdrew, and Robert stopped and then resumed sucking even more forcefully. The third time, as soon as she began frowning, I asked Gina: "What's happening in you now?" "Nothing," she replied. "I'm feeding Robert." I insisted: "What were you thinking now?" Gina went pale. "I thought that he will never stop sucking." I shared my observation with Gina, and invited her to notice her stream of thoughts. We tried to remember times when she felt needy but also satisfied, and I asked her to call upon those moments when the dread of being sucked dry by Robert overwhelmed her.

After a few trials, Gina succeeded and within moments Robert stopped sucking, looked at Gina, and released the nipple. Within two weeks of shared work breastfeeding time was reduced to one hour at a time, with two hours between feedings. Gina embarrassingly shared how difficult it was not to despise Robert for needing so much. She later recognised her dread of needing—both Robert's needs towards her, and her needs for her baby. As for Robert, he gradually managed to breastfeed in a way that allowed his mother to breathe, live, and occasionally smile as well.

Exercise for working with the second developmental angle: exploring oral neediness

This is a very dramatic exercise, less befitting psychotherapy (particularly if the therapist is unfamiliar with bodily interventions) and more appropriate for experiential learning about oral development, with its challenges and resources.

1. Work in a couple, one is the sucking baby and the other is the breastfeeding person.
2. Position yourself appropriate to the developmental stage—the "baby" lies down, to allow for a horizontal centre of gravity.
3. The breastfeeding person gives the baby chocolate, or a lollipop (or, if you are feeling particularly brave, a bottle with sweetened milk).
4. The invitation here is dual: for the baby, allow your entire universe to be experienced through the mouth, the lips, the tongue, and the palate. You may oscillate between feeding like early stages of infancy, when there is little control over head and neck muscles and arms, or whether you prefer to be a slightly older, and more involved baby—take in when you want and push (or spit out) when you don't. For the breastfeeding person: allow the tips of your fingers to become the centre of your attention, the antennae through which you feel your way into the world. Check how you choose to feed the baby—how much autonomy you allow the baby, how much control? What happens inside you when confronted with this neediness and nourishment?

Consumerism, addiction, and orality: Oral injuries are not only highly common in our society, but also serve as a necessary aspect of consumerist culture and are therefore cultivated and perpetuated. Consumerist politics delude us with the possibility of satisfying the infinite void inside us. The oral illusion is that the void we experience is not an unavoidable and human condition, but a void *of something*, and that if we manage to find the right something to fill ourselves up, we could be contented. If I feel empty and hurting I can buy myself a watch (or eat, or look for a relationship, or go to the gym) and for a moment the emptiness eases. This is a classic addictive pattern and confusion between needing and needing *something*. As long as we are busy with the quest for the Holy Grail to fill our inner void, we cultivate and perpetuate the experience of lack, instead of looking at it or being with it. The ability to find satisfaction in "good enough-ness" while mourning the vast emptiness inside us is a healing movement that creates contentedness, which in reality is the ultimate dread of consumerist politics: a contented and full consumer does not buy. Since the goalpost of the promised land (the fifth generation iPhone, a more accepting partner, the new Botox treatment, the best therapy course) always changes, contentedness and the ability to be satisfied with what you have, while grieving for the needs that were not met, is an imperative therapeutic goal when working with oral themes. This therapeutic goal is very difficult to achieve since our culture preserves the ultimate satisfaction fantasy, forever seducing us to purchase, consume, fill ourselves up, and always change and return.

Third developmental position—standing up: between autonomy and support

And then one day, a toddler wakes up and looks at the world with new eyes, she gets up and starts walking. The months of crawling strengthened her back and buttock muscles, the pelvic and core muscles, the arms and legs. The body gradually ripens to take the next important and thrilling step. And then she stands up, unsupported, and starts walking. The world opens itself before us when we walk—our field of vision widens and our hands become free to explore. Suddenly we discover that we can influence our environment. We can take, we can grab. The source of the word manipulation is the Latin *manipulus* which means handful, and when we are free to stand and as our hands become free—we are at liberty to discover and shape our world with our own hands, to explore and experience our influence, and the limitations of this influence.

Alongside the transition from horizontal to vertical posture, our ability to sense our own body changes too. Gravity no longer acts on a wide surface, instead it presses against the joints, the back. Our spine stabilises and absorbs a lot of pressure. Our centre of gravity changes too, and from a widely spread impact it now moves to the abdomen and pelvis. Our capacity to tolerate the pressure of gravity is still limited, the bodily balance has not matured yet and the muscles supporting erect standing and walking are far from perfection. But we can explore and discover, try and fall. During this stage we are all explorers and discoverers, Vasco da Gamas, Christopher Colombuses, and Marco Polos. We stand and walk; fall and rise again, explore and come back home from our wondrous exploratory voyages.

The third developmental stage, most clearly expressed between eight months and two and a half years, is a time of exploring and discovery—and of coming home. It is not a coincidence that the attachment style test and the "strange situation" test are both done during this stage (Ainsworth, Blehar, Waters, & Wall, 1978; Bowlby, 1988). The strange situation is a psychological test devised to examine the quality of attachment between a toddler and his mother. While the tester is watching through a two-way mirror, the toddler stays with his mother in a room. A strange woman joins in, makes contact with the baby and leaves. Then the woman enters again and the mother leaves. For a very few moments the toddler is left on his own with the strange woman, and then the mother returns and a reunion takes place. The main importance of the strange situation test is in examining the quality of the reunion, looking at the toddler's capacity to express annoyance and anger, to be comforted by the mother, and return to normal and normative connection. During normal development, it is walking which distinguishes babies from toddlers, as it allows the toddler a new and increased degree of somatic autonomy. During this stage object-constancy (perceiving objects as existing regardless of our sensing them) strengthens, language begins to develop, symbolic thinking develops too, and relationship with attachment figures becomes more distinct as well.

The standing toddler holds his head high, and the body therefore loses its simian curvature which maintained a supple and flexible spine. From this stage onwards, the head is held by the neck muscles and by inflating the chest muscles. In order to remain erect we need to reorganise our balance. The sense of self in space—proprioceptive sense—changes here. The feet change too: they become our main source of contact with the ground and the three arches of the feet develop and strengthen—they become the main support of the entire body-weight. We have all paid a heavy price for standing up—we carry a huge burden on our back and spine and the spinal vertebrae pushed into one another. Gradually the erector muscles strengthen and mature to support this new and weird posture. Additionally, the most vulnerable and protected body part is now publicly presented—we exhibit our bare belly to the world. Despite this heavy toll, most of us choose to pay this price for the privilege of moving on two feet, being able to see wider and into the distance, and freeing two limbs, hands which are completely at liberty to explore and play.

During this stage we indeed explore, play, and practise manipulation and influence: hence, narcissistic issues are central here. We discover our impact on the world. The rectal muscles begin their maturation process, which is usually completed between the age of eighteen months and thirty months, and with them they bring great pleasure at making things concrete in the world: our own consciously conceived creative artefact (this is why this stage used to be called early anal). Alongside our exploration and monitored separation from the primary attachment figure, object relations deepen and relationships become more complex and possible: the parents are revealed and the toddler enjoys examining and exploring his parents and their differently looking bodies. Dance and movement therapist Yona Shahar-Levy (2005) described the changes during this stage as transitioning from the "cradle envelope" position where the body of the baby is enveloped by the bodies of the parents (dyadic regulation) to the "facing relationship" position, where the body of the toddler is facing the parents (the other) as an individual (self-regulation). The egocentric body positioning is challenged here, and the desire to return and be a cradled child might be distinct and powerful, if sometimes repressed.

Character structure: Let us observe this character structure style through developmental eyes. When a toddler starts walking, he requires two types of support. On the one hand, the wish to explore the world and discover its impact is prevalent, and therefore the wish for autonomy is central. The toddler needs his separateness and going-out into the world validated and encouraged (support in developing self-regulation). On the other hand, the toddler is not yet ready for complete differentiation, and still needs to return to his attachment figures, be small and supported (and rely on dyadic regulation). Home needs to be a safe place for us to explore the world.

The toddler begins to move things around, examining her impact on the world and on others; she wishes to enjoy her impact and therefore continuously challenges boundaries. This stage involves manipulation of discovering the influence over others: the child as an agent in the world. Developmental arrests and rigidities during this stage consequently concern distorted sense of agency, and inappropriate balance between autonomy and support. The injury is narcissistic: when the child needs to choose between autonomy and support, her sense of agency is harmed and she might later, as an adult, struggle to believe it is possible to be in connection without full control. She tends to pendulate between a deep sense of impotence and omnipotent illusions. This character structure is therefore known as *inflated, anal (early), control, narcissistic*, or *psychopath*.

Main themes: There are two possible injuries during this stage: to the right for autonomy, or to the right for support. When the wish for autonomy is not validated, the child needs to choose whether to remain small (sacrificing the wish to individuate and separate) or grow up and leave (sacrificing love and support). For example, a highly narcissistic mother may take great delight from her oral baby: the baby needs her indefinitely, and she can experience herself as the centre of his universe and delight in dyadic regulation. The wish for autonomy may threaten her, and she might experience great discomfort when the baby suddenly grows and moves away: "Why are you leaving? How can you do this to me?" The second injury concerns the return to safety and security, and the wish for receiving support. The need to be little again is not validated or rejected and the parent conveys the message of "You are such a big boy, you are too big for that, let go of my leg." For instance, the father might have suffered from the oral stage—he felt that he had lost both the mother and the baby and was unable to penetrate their tight dyadic connection. When the toddler starts walking, the father takes pleasure in their newly formed relationship and is worried that the child's need for support will retrieve the earlier condition, hence he shames the child's wish for support: "You don't need it anymore, come on, go back to play." The parents (as well as the therapist who works with inflated character style) are called to open a transitional stage, whereby both orality and the wish for independence and autonomy are concurrently validated and celebrated.

The narcissistic child fears that he will only receive support by recruitment: "I cannot be big (or little) unless I manipulate." Extreme conditions are seen as psychopathy and sociopathy. The true heart's desire is that "someone will allow me to be big and small, that someone will see me with both my bigness and smallness".

Bodily holding: During the inflated stage holding is high and up: "Look at me! Look how big I am!" Like an animal inflating itself with air to look bigger, so does the inflated character structure makes itself big by puffing up the chest and locking the lumbar back.

Control issues: The message of control of the inflated character structure is external: "I control my environment. I can control others and make them do as I will."

Breathing patterns: To maintain the mask of bigness and capability, and faced with the dread of having its helplessness discovered and shamed, the inflated character structure mainly breathes in and exhales very little. The body is held, with breath, like a tight balloon—and there is a strong holding and control in the diaphragm.

Movement: Imagine a toddler taking her first steps in the world, bigger than life, holding her body with great effort to make this feeling of agency, bigness, and strength last as long as possible, and then collapsing and falling, only to quickly rise again. The movement of predominantly inflated character structure is similar—big and quick, dramatic with extensive arm movements and larger-than-life gestures, full of energy yet short lasting.

Bodily tension: The toddler who just started walking is not ready yet for long distances. When a child needs to hold herself erect before the core muscles have sufficiently developed to provide systemic support, a gap is created between the outer built tension (and charge) and the inner collapse. Like Popeye the Sailor Man, the inflated character maintains a polarity between highly developed and strong upper body to a nearly non-existent lower body. The bodily holding of this stage manifests in locking the shoulder and pelvic girdles, which allows an inflated erect posture at the expense of flexibility and supple movement. The chest, shoulders, and pelvis are highly tense. The stereotypical macho figure expresses the bodily tension of this character structure. Other classical inflated figures are the father of body psychotherapy Wilhelm Reich, who was discussed in Chapter Two, Jean Martin Charcot, who was discussed in Chapter One, Buzz Lightyear (from *Toy Story* films) and, as mentioned, Popeye.

Eye contact: Inflated characters actively seek confrontations and tend to establish competitive, challenging, and confrontational eye contact (who would last longer?). Eye contact may seem competitive and is part of a constant power struggle—the world is a battlefield, and eye contact is an opportunity to establish a hierarchy of power.

Touch: People with predominantly inflated character structure may have very thin skin which can sometimes feel oedematous. Touch can be very charismatic (both to receive and to give) and has seductive qualities. Unlike the warm touch of the oral character, the quality of touch here is more sweeping and more manipulative.

Fear: The main repressed feeling in the inflated character is helplessness against the difficulty to hold the tension between wanting separateness and wanting support: the narcissistic helplessness. There is a great fear of losing connection. Manipulations stem from the dread of severed connection.

Energetic phase: The body is charged and energetic, and there is a constant discharge of energy. These are the clients who burst with anger (yet quickly calm), who cry a lot (and quickly recompose). There seem to be endless ideas, energy, enterprises, and possibilities. Yet the energy does not last long and collapses; toing and froing between quick inflation and quick deflation of air. Inflated characters are very creative and excellent entrepreneurs, for example, but they struggle to maintain a sufficient level of excitement and functioning over a long period of time to follow through with their ideas. Accordingly, they tend to seek energetically charged thrills (extreme experience, extreme sports, etc.)—an addiction to adrenalin.

Strengths and resources: The world-exploring toddler is an excellent example of the strength of this character structure: the capacity to express the joy of creativity and play. These are people with amazing ideas, who can sweep everybody off their feet, lead, and convince—they know how to impact and charm others, and they have deep capacity to influence, possessing charisma and charm, ability and willingness to be challenged and challenge others, and have good leadership skills. Good lecturers, politicians, and leaders require some inflated developmental style (healthy narcissism) to believe that their influence is possible and important—and to translate it into action.

Working therapeutically with inflated character structure: Narcissistic clients need therapists who are willing to challenge them (who are able and willing to work with negative transference, for example) and be challenged without shaming. Therapy ought to validate the power and autonomy of the clients, but also insist and see the neediness and the importance in support. Therapeutic positioning is of utmost importance, since the client may experience the potential humiliation in the inflated stage as threatening. These clients find it difficult to perceive the other person's reality as different to theirs (see the other as a subject), thus struggle to show trust. The therapist should cultivate his presence, be mindful of manipulations, and set clear boundaries—yet at the same time remain attentive to the softer aspects of the client. The psychotherapist is required to insist on his own truth, and his own subjective experience, all the while respecting his client's reality.

The main themes of autonomy and support are challenging in psychotherapy, since this character structure may easily challenge the therapeutic framework itself. Being sucked into power struggles may feel inevitable, yet it is an assured therapeutic loss; but how can we allow the client to come and go without harming the therapeutic relationship? The invitation here is to remain in contact: to be able to communicate and maintain dialogue even when the client wishes to leave; acknowledging that we are willing and able to negotiate around issues of control without having to assume a controlling language. The therapeutic gift is validating and blessing both needs, along the lines of: "Blessed be your coming in and leaving."

In terms of bodywork (but also relevant for psychoanalysis), working with the client always lying down might be a mistake here, since it might preserve and shame the desire for autonomy. It might deliver a castrating message, conveying to the client that she will only be supported if she remained little. Since the inflated structure has not fully matured its capacity for self-regulation, lying down may easily enable and encourage regression to oral positioning, with the shame and associated dread of helplessness. When clients express a need for individuation, bodywork could also be done sitting up or standing up, and when they tire and wish to lie down, then working with oral fields could be done without the ominous risk of shaming.

Extreme conditions: Psychopathy, sociopathy, and some cases of borderline personality disorder. While there is very little literature concerning body psychotherapeutic work with psychopathy or sociopathy, body psychotherapy offers interesting and innovative approaches to working with clients with borderline personality disorder: the therapist, for example, may frequently reflect her somatic resonance to her client. The experience of spending time with a therapist, "who genuinely discovers who I really am and still loves me (even if she hates me too)", is a transformative and potentially reparative experience. Body psychotherapist Tom Warnecke (2008, 2009), who specialises in working with borderline personality, offers a myriad of fascinating approaches to working with borderline experiences, which include interventions with movement, touch, and use of somatic transference.

Clinical vignette

Chris has been in therapy with me for three years. He shares his utter frustration with the gap between his huge sense of agency and capability, and his shame and helplessness. Chris gives me an example, yet the speed of his speech confuses me. I feel flooded. I ask him to show me, as well as tell me, what he means. Chris demonstrates an inflated body position and marches into the room as a proud rooster, while making very loud sounds and stomping his feet in the ground, then he immediately hides under the table. I find myself actively looking for physical exercises to do with Chris, but feel increasingly distant from him and fearful of being with him. My inner dialogue becomes very alert; I am frightened of his explosive anger and try to be nice. Chris senses something and immediately yells at me: "I'm doing your silly exercises and you can't even bother to be with me. What's the point?" He sits down.

I feel my own desire to puff up, to retract, and to offer Chris a wounding transferential interpretation regarding his anger. I genuinely have interesting things to say to him, yet I can sense my defensiveness and desire to attack him. I notice that for a long while I haven't exhaled, that all the air is held up. Slowly, I breathe out and come closer to Chris. "You are right," I say. "I am busy being scared of your shouting, and it's unfair. I want to be with you but sometimes I am too frightened of the volume of your power." Chris is taken back with surprise: "How can you be scared of my power? I am so little." I smile, "You are also little, but you are not only little. And also, sometimes I am little too." We both exhale together, with a big sigh. Chris comes closer, "I didn't know you sometimes feel little too."

Exercise for working with the third developmental angle: walking

In Feldenkrais (1977), walking is seen as a series of controlled fallings—we lose our balance and retrieve it, fall forwards, and block the fall with yet another step. This simple exercise can experientially demonstrate the fascinating developmental processes involved in walking together with the advantages and disadvantages of the narcissistic inflation. The exercise is better done outdoors and in a large space, and is appropriate to teaching, supervising, and therapeutic purposes.

1. Client starts walking with the therapist behind her.
2. The therapist guides the client to gradually slow her pace, until reaching a "slow motion" speed. The slower the walk is, the easier it is to notice the multitude of muscles involved in walking. The client is invited to note which muscles she uses, and the therapist takes care that the client does not fall by supporting her back (if needed).
3. The therapist invites the client to inflate her chest forwards and high, lock her lower back, and experiment again with walking and slowing down. Walking slowly becomes much easier, yet the bodily prices are heavy. Together, client and therapists can examine the differences and process them.

Fourth developmental position—assertiveness: between needing and wanting

Many important developmental processes take place between the ages of two and three and a half years. Vertical posture and walking have completely matured, the core muscles hold the body with supple mobility, and the child can walk and run while remaining balanced. Language too becomes more complex and the child usually has more command over his verbal communication. The toddler begins to discover his will, and wishes to explore this against his parents' will: to exist alongside them.

During this period, the rectal muscles completed their maturity and most parents begin potty training. The toddler, who earlier learned to take pleasure in letting go of faeces, now enjoys his ability to hold and not let go, taking pleasure in frustrating his parents and exploring the impact of his will on theirs. The significance of relationship increases and the child, whose linguistic and expressive abilities have broadened, can now be in a relationship with his parents, a relationship with growing complexity. Potty training asks of the toddler self-control, and is much more convenient to the parents, who no longer need to deal with messy changing of nappies. But the same longed-for self-control also brings with it new developments of willpower and the need to exercise it against his attachment figures. Not only is it important for the toddler to want—it is important for him to want differently to mum or dad, and for them to be strong and stable enough to tolerate his separate and different will—not necessarily satisfy his wanting, but validate it as legitimate.

The first two developmental angles, of existence and nourishment, explored issues of dyadic regulation; the third angle, between support and autonomy, was on the threshold between dyadic and self-regulation. This developmental stage concerns the emergence of clear, separated, and distinct qualities of self-regulation (for this reason, body psychotherapist Cäsar Schwieger (1998) claimed that the inflated character structure was not a real characterological position, but an intermediate stage between orality and masochism).

The journey to individuality moves through distinction—between me and the other-than-me, and the "terrible twos" characterises this distinction and differentiation. The parents become holders of will, and it is against their will that the child yearns to discover his own—and he requires a stable yet non-defeating counter position.

For the toddler to become a child he needs to be distinguished and allowed his separateness; for his wanting and differentness to be validated (even if not always accepted), while remaining in connection. If during the earlier stage the toddler moved from separation (self-regulation, autonomy) to symbiosis (dyadic regulation, support), then here the separateness is actualised, and it is from this separateness that the toddler wishes to connect: "Accept me as I am, allow me to be who I am, and still remain connected with me and love me as I am."

The capacity for independent and assertive expression is the central theme during this stage. The developmental challenge is no longer personal, but familial—surviving the battle of wills peacefully and without using love as a bargaining chip for negotiation. An injury to the child's right for assertiveness and expression of his wanting (and not wanting) oppresses the child's crucial separation rebellion, defeating his wish for self-regulation. In such cases the child understands that in order to maintain love and connection he needs to sacrifice his desires, his will, and his independence, and the *dense* or *masochist* character structure is created. Every psychotherapist carries an emphasised masochistic aspect: the mere willingness to tolerate long hours of other people's suffering, drawing our worth and sense of self from being needed and from listening (providing a service) has a certain masochistic quality.

Character structure: The military service in Israel is mandatory (after high school, men are required to serve three years, women two). I remember the first day of my induction, in the south of Israel. We had left the military buses, which stood idle in a huge parking space, and were instructed to stand in a big U shaped structure. It was dark and Sergeant Michael arrived, walking among us and yelling at the top of his voice: "You are pathetic and whining little girls." I was holding my breath and trying to take as little space as I possibly could. Michael continued: "We're going to get these little girls out of you, we're going to change those mummy's boys. We'll take every drop of humanity out of you and make you into soldiers." I will never forget this horrid experience, which marked the terror that accompanied me throughout my military service. The dense character structure is the internalisation of Sergeant Michael and the subsequent becoming of "a soldier".

While the fragmented character structure was insensitive to self and her body because of the body–mind split, the dense character structure gave up sensitivity to herself in favour of attunement to her environment, particularly to others. In her famed book *The Drama of the Gifted Child,* Alice Miller (1981) described the child who developed skills of attunement to others and recognising the others' needs. The right for independence and assertiveness was blocked here later than the inflated structure. The child has already experienced love and acceptance, and these are both too precious to lose. Wishing not to risk the loss of love and validation, the child sacrifices herself, sacrifices her will, and becomes highly sensitive to others (her parents) and their will. This role reversal between the parent and the child, which Wilfred Bion (1963) related to as reversed dynamics in the container–contained relationship, is also common in the dense character structure (as well as in the inflated character structure, who also had to prematurely grow).

The dense character's ethos is making herself worthy of love and approval—and she does so by internalising her parents' critical voices (highly active superego) and shaming herself accordingly. Her own will becomes associated with pain, and the deep association between pain and pleasure, accompanied by self-sacrifice, gives this character structure the name masochist. This character structure is also called *endurer, dense, anal (later), self-defeating personality* (Daum & Hartman, 2010), or *held*.

Notwithstanding the defeated self-sacrifice, this character structure already had ample love and connection, and is thus full of resources—she might have experienced secure attachment. The dense child (and adult) is responsible and dependable, has endless energy and is very hardworking, loyal and rarely complaining, generous and loving, caring and investing in connection. On the other hand, her self-sacrifice is accompanied by resentment—a very violent inner dialogue and self-hate which can consume every cell inside her body. The dense personality is like a pressure cooker: anger and inner charge are always growing, full of guilt and fear of disappointing another. The dense character easily placates, yet is bitter about it; helps the other and is loyal—yet full of judgment towards the other and herself, supportive—yet self-abandoning, very stubborn and yearns for intimacy—yet struggles to be present since she believes that in order to receive love she must suffer. She finds it difficult to express herself and her own will, it is far easier to satisfy others and be frustrated and bitter about it.

A dense character structure is created when the child is defeated by her parents; the parents are unable to tolerate their child's separateness and her need for independent expression of her will. It may manifest in controlling potty training, pressure to "Behave yourself" and "Do not mess." It might be the mother who proudly exclaims "I know you better than you know yourself, and I know better than you what you need and want." The parent uses love as a trading currency to secure obedience, and the child, feeling guilty for having her own separate needs or anger, eventually placates and obeys. The classic "Jewish mother" who says "If you truly loved me you would have at least tasted it," is a caricature example for the making of the masochistic/dense character structure. Self-sacrifice could therefore be a response to a manipulative parent, a highly needy parent, or a (perceived) weak parent who cannot withstand the child's strong will. The main feeling the parents are striving (consciously or unconsciously) to evoke in the child, as a means to control her behaviour, is guilt, and these guilt feelings are at the heart of being of the dense character structure.

Main themes: The rights of freedom and of assertiveness are central here. The dense personality requires a long time to listen to his own wishes, and is easily confusing his own will with others'. Issues of responsibility and will, the ability to say yes—and no—are of great importance. The dense character structure tends to develop difficult and complex relationships with authority figures, which are perceived as threatening and castrating. The most repressed and accumulated feeling is anger, and the capacity to express anger is central for healing and balancing here. The masochist would struggle to initiate an angry rebellion, but could stoke anger in another person and then join in, or express anger in other indirect ways (passive aggressive). One common fashion of discharging anger here is through projective identification: he will infuriate the other, who will respond on his behalf ("Stop it; I'm fed up with you always being so nice, say no already!"). Thus, he can outsource his true anger, depositing it in the hands of others. The belief that love needs to be paid for with self-sacrifice attracts to the masochist people who need infinite support (for example, oral characters) and he senses his self-worth through providing services, being "a soldier". Patterns of placating and self-punishment are very common here. Due to the developmental connection with potty training (and mess) the dense character tends to need—sometimes compulsively and obsessively—order and structure as well as strict time management (which he expects from himself, not from others).

Bodily holding: The dense character structure holds it all in. The image of a pressure cooker is very appropriate to understanding masochistic quality, and indeed there are occasional (mostly unconscious) steam emissions—the masochist will support and love, but would accidentally spill a glass of hot tea on the other; anger will find its way to be expressed, even if indirectly. The inner sense is of someone who might burst with holding, even if it is not always visible to the observing other. This body holding provides the dense person with reasons to complain and hold grudges. This muscular holding allows an expression (even if distortedly) of the real difficulty of asserting his will and anger. The body structure is appropriately dense and firm, yet accessible and warm.

Control issues: The main control of the dense character is self-control: "I control what I take out and what I don't, what I express and what I hold in (mainly anger), and the degree which I allow the other to see what is really happening inside me." The control issue is central to the dense character but differently from the inflated structure. While the inflated character will attempt to control (via influence and manipulation) the environment and the other, the dense character will try to control himself and shape himself accordingly.

Breathing patterns: The need for control is expressed here too. The message which the dense personality internalised is: "I must not be who I really am, I have to control the way I am seen and perceived, in my actions, and in my words." Hence, breathing is controlled. It is as if the breath lost its spontaneous organic quality. There is great fear of "letting go" of breath—for fear of bursting, destroying the other with my fury, or messing up.

Movement: Imagine a disciplined soldier, who lost the joyous spontaneity of movement. Her entire demeanour is goal oriented. The movement of the dense structure is slow, scarce, and extremely measured. The movement lacks initiative, and is instead answering a call to duty.

Bodily tension: The dense character structure is very held, with overall high muscular charge. The upper back is large, strong, and stretched, and shoulders are broad, carrying high muscular tension. The buttock muscles too are held (not letting go for fear of messing up). The mythological Atlas, whom I mentioned at the beginning of the chapter, is an excellent example of masochism. The neck is often very thick and the eyes tend to be sunken in the head (part of the holding-in pattern). The character of Ben Grimm (The Thing) in the *Fantastic Four*, played by Michael Chiklis wonderfully illustrates masochistic body structure.

Eye contact: Warm and suffering. The dense character structure is forever self-sacrificing and enduring, and her eyes express the warmth and connection she offers, together with her defeat and her suffering. It is hard for her …

Touch: A predominantly dense person knows how to give. Her touch (and touching her) is pleasant and warm, with a sense of genuine connection. Tissues and muscles feel full, contracted, and dense. Unlike the oral touch, which is also very pleasant, touch in the dense character is not as magnetic—there is a sense of real presence and willingness to connect.

Fear: More than everything, the masochist fears loss of approval and love. The fear is within relationships—particularly with authority figures (or authority transference dynamics in friendships and romantic relationships). A dense person is hard to get to really know, because she is so frightened of showing herself fully and risking losing connection; she is highly attentive to how the other person needs her and wants her to be and will quickly change to meet those needs, often without even realising it.

Energetic phase: The dense character structure is, as mentioned, a pressure cooker. There is amplification of energetic charge with a lot of holding. While outside the movements are small and gentle, inside volcanos threaten to erupt.

Strengths and resources: If you want a job to be done from beginning to end, without giving up or getting discouraged, the dense character is your person. The masochist is attuned to others, can give, and impeccably functions under any circumstance for long periods of time. She is dependable, trustworthy, and could be leaned against, knowing she will be there. Her ability to tolerate is also accompanied by very strong will (and she can be very stubborn)—and when she learns to listen to herself and her needs, there is a rewarding and loving work with willingness to go through processes and changes. The dense is highly organised and keeps time, is able to be independent and self-regulatory.

Working therapeutically with dense character structure: The dense client is tricky to work with. On the one hand, he is an ideal client: always on time, respectful of the therapeutic setting, loyal and unchallenging, able to participate and support the therapist (positive transference), progresses gradually if slowly and keeps on showing up to therapy. On the other hand, he really struggles to find his own will—and may become lost and swallowed with a strong-willed therapist. He gives no space for his urges, needs, and their spontaneous expressions. Sometimes he "slips"—forgetting a session, forgetting money, and mainly rebelling against the therapist by remaining suffering—he does not get better. The difficulty bares the promise for love. The real therapeutic challenge is in not resting too comfortably in his placating gifts, but insisting on his true self, his true desires and wants.

Therapy with dense character structure is slow. It is important to encourage the client to listen to himself and his needs, to develop self-awareness and express it—to say his yeses and nos. Working with negative transference is imperative, particularly expressing anger, but this work takes time as it threatens the client who fears he would lose the therapist's love and approval. Reich believed (1933a) that the masochist's needs are predominantly held in the body, and that he required deep bodywork to liberate these natural impulses and discharge them. The client struggles to feel himself and would therefore often ask for deep and penetrative bodywork, but if this request is met without attentiveness it might only strengthen the muscular armour (as the therapeutic vignette below will demonstrate). One of the therapeutic goals is to assist the client internalise an authority figure (superego), which can accept him as he is, with his differentness, without having to bend his will against the therapist's—to extract the "want" from the "need", thus allow a kinder internal dialogue.

Extreme conditions: Masochism, obsessive-compulsive disorder (OCD), depression. The masochistic depression is different from the oral one. While in the earlier, oral depression there is genuine scarcity of energy, thus there is charge with quick collapse, as if the person needs to be charged all the time (hypotonic), the masochistic depression is an active (inner) oppression of energy. There is great investment in making sure the vital energy does not manifest itself (hypertonic). Hence, clinical work with these two types of depression greatly differs.

Clinical vignette

Jef volunteered to work with me in the centre during a workshop. We have all sat on cushions on the ground, and Jef shared how he had always been a carer: as a child he took care of his sick parents, doing whatever was needed, and also taking care of his younger siblings. "It was too much for a child," he said. "I know it but I don't feel it." Jef is short and firm; his neck is very thick. Even today, as a male nurse, he knows that he carries far too heavy a burden both at home and at work, but he cannot feel the burden. Instead, he holds. I ask Jef to locate the sense of burden in his body and Jef answers, "It's like carrying sacks of potatoes on my shoulders."

With Jef's permission, I leaned against his shoulder with my elbows. The elbows dug deep into the flesh. "It hurts," said Jef, taking a deep breath, "but I can take it." I leaned deeper, giving him more weight, leaning against his shoulders with my entire body weight and Jef breathed: "I can take it, give me more." Asking another participant to join in, a heavily built man, who now further leaned on me and we were both digging into Jef's body.

Ten minutes later, four people were standing and leaning into Jef's shoulders. His breathing was constricted, yet he seemed in a meditative state: breathing with utter concentration and impressive control. "I can take it, give me more weight," he smiled triumphantly. "I have a feeling that even if every participant leaned against your shoulders you would still be able to take the weight," I said. Jef nodded with a smile. I asked everybody to let go and we released the pressure. "And what is the price for being able to take it, Jef?" Jef was quiet. Following was a few long minutes of silence in the group; a tense and nervous silence. Finally Jef responded: "I abandon myself and what I want, I cannot even feel what I want, I lose myself in internal dialogue and lose connection with myself and with you."

Exercise for working with the fourth developmental angle: yes and no

This is a simple and valuable exercise for encouraging assertiveness and shifting positions in relationships. I learned it from Silke Ziehl and have used it since in many of my trainings and sometimes (if less frequently) in therapy.

1. Client and therapist decide on time frame (I propose to begin with four minutes, two minutes each direction). Time frame helps in containing the emotional and energetic charge of the process.

2. The therapist presents the exercise to the client: the client chooses one word, either *yes* or *no*, and the therapist gets the other word. For the agreed time, the only conversation is done with these two words—having a yes-and-no dialogue. This is an opportunity to play, move around in the room, and use the body to speak: change tonality, and experiment in as many ways and patterns of saying yes and no as possible. For example, yeses could be begging, seductive, playful, unafraid, placating, authoritarian, or stubborn. This is not a ping-pong game, there is no need to await the other's yes before you say no (and vice versa). The therapist can role-model flexibility.
3. After two minutes therapist and client swap roles (the person who said yes will now say no and vice versa).
4. Process together. What did it feel like to say *no*? To say *yes*? What was easier? What was difficult or challenging? How did it affect the therapeutic relationship?

Fifth developmental position—"I am here!": sexuality and passion

Donald Winnicott (1960b) suggested that good enough parenting took place in three different stages, each of which carried different challenges and demands: (1) holding, (2) mother and infant living together, and (3) father, mother, and infant—all three living together. During the first two stages, the role of the father (or the secondary attachment figure, when the organisation of the family was different or in single sex relationships) was less significant to the infant. The third stage of triangular position of father-mother–infant (or parent-parent–infant) is the one relevant to the fifth developmental position, a shift from a dyad to a familial field.

Two highly significant processes are interwoven between the ages of three and six years: an amplification of energetic and somatic sexual charge, and a familial process climaxing in the oedipal process. While all the previous developmental stages took place in pre-oedipal spaces, this developmental angle marks the emerging sexuality of the child (and the person) in all its might. The first process concerns the falling in love with one parent (classically speaking, even if culturally biased, the parent from the other sex) and our wish to possess the parent to ourselves, while removing any obstacle in the way (i.e., the other parent, traditionally the one from the same sex). To avoid the traditional gendered bias which gave the oedipal complex a bad name, we can relate to it as a desire for shifting from a linear dyadic position to a spatial position (from couple to a family). The shift from dyad to field makes space for the world. The heightened charge involves a desire to have one parent and to be like another, to identify and possess. Once more, if we zoom out from the masculine-conditioned language of possession, we can relate to two movements in the world, "wanting to be" and "wanting to have". The second process is the discovery of genital pleasure and the capacity (increasing yet still limited) to tolerate the volume of sexual and sensual pleasure brought by genital arousal.

Before expanding our dialogue on these two processes and their connection, let us return to consider the second developmental angle, of neediness and nourishment. As I have illustrated and argued earlier, during the first stages of his life the infant is not a completely separate entity from his main attachment figure—and the first lack is followed by the first desire, which are experienced as seeking symbiotic reunion with the mother. This search still belongs to what the researcher Colwyn Trevarthen (1974, 1993) termed "primary intersubjectivity", as mentioned in Chapter Four. This is a symbiotic connection, a wider mind which is still missing its separate awareness, its informed consent to submit. Not so during the oedipal stage. The child's separateness has been sufficiently established, and the yearning for union and connection with the parent is now mindful—it is a yearning for secondary intersubjectivity—for surrender to a wider mind, which would not come at the expense of individuality and subjectivity but instead complement it. The essence of the oedipal wish, as I understand it, is to unite with the parent without losing subjectivity, to concurrently be apart from and a part of this dyadic wider mind.

As Ferenczi wisely noted in *Confusion of Tongues between the Adult and the Child* (1933), the language of the child is essentially different to that of the adult. While the child exists and functions in a field of tenderness and delicate being, the adult also occupies life with passion. The child's sexual awakening, which is also expressed in masturbation and greater capacity to tolerate the bodymind arousal and sexual charge involved in genital stimulation, is first and foremost a process of self-regulation. The child learns to build up charge and delights in her ability to tolerate it—but this charge is unlike the adult's which can reach its orgasmic climax. The child takes pleasure in body sensations, the ability to create these, and experience these. This emergent sexuality is hugely different from adult sexuality; it is not "goal oriented" or directed at intercourse, which require an entirely different maturation (tolerating the other's arousal as well as my own, withstanding sexual amplification, and remaining connected with self and other through this arousal). The child's sexuality is not yet mature enough to engage with this secondary sexual intersubjectivity; it will take many years before she can withstand such deep connection and maintain both the connection and her separateness amid the sexual charge.

Alongside this bodily development, of being able to tolerate higher sexual and energetic charge, the child uses the parent as an object for this huge surge of feelings—and frequently falls in love with the parent. The awoken sexual desires bring ambition and depth to the heart's yearning for unison, and at the same time the soft feelings of the heart mobilise the sexually charged desire towards connecting with the other. This is the child's first attempt at creating secondary intersubjectivity, to unite without losing her differentiated self. The child, who successfully moved through the earlier developmental challenges, now dares to attempt and challenge the triangular structure and return to a dyadic formation (Rolef Ben-Shahar, 2010d). The parents are now assuming an unpleasant role of breaking the child's heart without shattering it to pieces. When the child can grasp the realistic boundaries of her agency, the parents will narcissistically wound the child in a consolable manner, which she stands a chance to recover from, without terminally wounding her.

As psychoanalyst Harold Searles (1959) explained, during the oedipal stage the child needs her parents to validate her sexuality and appropriately admire her without transgressing or meeting those needs. Two terminal narcissistic injuries could therefore be inflicted here: the first is concerned with colluding with the child's sexual wishes, and the second with rejection of her sexuality. The extreme example of colluding with the child's call for love and her attempt to break the family triangle is sexual abuse: the parent confuses the child's sexuality with adult passion, and is seduced into romantic and sexual relations with the child (I am not implying in any way that the parent is passive in the seduction, but instead that it is imperative that the child could safely seduce the parent—that this is developmentally OK, if not necessary). Sexual abuse is not merely a sexual act, but has wider consequences—breaching and collapsing the transitional space between desires and realising them, between fantasy and reality, and shattering the familial space. The child who has been abused might grow dreading her immanent destructive powers ("If I managed to separate mum and dad, I am dangerous"). In a paper on body psychotherapy with oedipal injuries, I have termed this omnipotent injury "narcissistic anxiety".

At the other end of the spectrum from collusion we can find the injury of rejection—the parent (or parents) shame the child's attempt for getting close and her falling in love, condemn it, and despise the behaviour. The child's heart is shattered to pieces, and she moves into the world with a deep sense of incompetence and helplessness ("I couldn't even impact or influence mum or dad, what chance do I have of impacting anyone"). I have termed this impotent injury "narcissistic depression". This child might grow with a poor sense of agency, perceiving herself as having little impact on the world.

A good enough heartbreak might allow the child to trust the relational transitional space as a supportive field and amplifying platform for her inner feelings—even ones as strong as passion, love, and sexual desire. The child will learn to surrender to her heart and to her passion, and gradually allow her heart and genitals to integrate within relationships—to create a wider mind inclusive of love and passion, storm and comfort. A coarse heartbreak, resulting from confusion of tongues, might contribute to the creation of the rigid character structure and an oedipal complex awaiting resolution.

Character structure: A developmental trauma during the sexual-oedipal stage could break the organic connection between the heart and the genitals—love and passion. Love and sex might become separated, sometimes even opposite forces to each other. The bodymind solution is expressed in splitting the pelvis from the chest and avoiding surrender: rigidifying the capacity to fully be in connection. The character structure is correspondingly called *rigid*, and sometimes *phallic*, *oedipal* or *hysteric*.

Injury during the oedipal stage may be of a collusive nature (abuse) or rejection (humiliation). Full sexual abuse is deeply traumatising to the child, making it difficult to later trust in fantasy spaces and holding safe boundaries. Since this developmental stage involves a familial space and not a dyadic one, the reactions of both parents might change, appropriately creating four subcategories of the rigid character structures. While there are many other possibilities for injuries during this stage, these four subcategories are considered classic in body psychotherapy. It is important to emphasise that while both sexual orientation and gender orientation may seem clear-cut here, we all move on a gender spectrum (we are all masculine and feminine, anima and animus), and sexual orientation spectrum (between homosexuality and heterosexuality) (Freud, 1905d).

In fact, the rigid character structure is the one most suffering from gendered bias in the history of body psychotherapy and, in my opinion, requires significant revisions to better accommodate modern understanding of sexuality. The reader is invited to look at any injury presented here as feminine as potentially taking place in the boy's/man's feminine parts and vice versa. We may think of these conceptualisations as relating to the archetypes of anima and animus. The use herewith of the traditional heterosexual family is only for simplifications and the oedipal stage does not demand, in my opinion, such a structure—but a triangular structure (a spatial rather than dyadic organisation). Single parent families pose a great challenge to this limited view of character structure, but exploring this properly is beyond the scope of this section.

The four subcategories of the rigid character structure typify earlier forms of body psychotherapy which I am less identified with. These are the *hysterical* and *masculine aggressive* (in women) and the *phallic* and *passive feminine* (in men). It is sad to note, that none of these traditional subcategories include abuse by the mother, or—from a very different angle, a child that chose to identify with the parent from the same sex out of preference and not pathology. Perhaps it is important to remind ourselves that this typology, when looked at from a relational point of view, is contextual and partial—and should be used as a means of developing sensitivity to body–mind manifestations, rather than guidelines for labelling clients. Or, in the words attributed to American humorist Robert Benchley: "There are two kinds of people in the world: those who divide the world into two kinds of people, and those who don't."

After great deliberation, and despite the valuable information these may carry, I decided to omit the description of these subcategories from this book to remain more truthful to my current theoretical and clinical orientation. Readers who wish to learn about these categories could find them elsewhere.

Main themes: Love and sex are the main issues here, alongside the deep desire to live in a connected place between the rejected and broken passion and the heart. Common rigid defences are perfectionism ("Perhaps, if I'll be the best, the most perfect of all—I can get love"), seduction, romanticism, and conquering. The yearning to be all of who I am without leaving rejected parts of me behind, and the real readiness for connection (when the person manages to overcome the dread of contact) characterise the rigid structure.

Bodily holding: Withholding, holding back. The rigid character structure oscillates between deep desire to bring all of himself into connection—with all of his love and passion, and the fear of being shamed and humiliated. The body holding is therefore one of avoidance and withdrawal—holding back of bodily and emotional energy. The rigid personality holds himself like a wild bull in a small rodeo pen, still prevented from barging out with its full force. Unlike the dense holding, the bodily holding here is more directional—not like a pressure cooker, but like a reined-in bull—where the direction would have been towards surrender. Furthermore, while the dense holding is primarily of anger, the rigid holds back from surrendering to connection, to love, and to passion.

Control issues: The controlling message of the rigid character structure is about surrender: "I control the degree of giving in (or not) to connection and surrendering all of me to another person."

Breathing patterns: The bodily holding creates a split between genital sensations of passion and the softness and loving emotions of the heart. Accordingly, there is a sharp division between the chest and abdomen, and between chest breathing and abdominal breathing.

Movement: This is a tango-like character structure—wanting to move forwards, but fearing rejection, wishing to come close and allowing for connection, but withdrawing to the back and holding back from surrender. The movement characterising this stage is, therefore, backwards and forwards movement. Rigid characters can be very expressive in their movements, but it would not be an exaggerated movement. There is ample movement, full of vitality and contact.

Bodily tension: The muscular armour of the rigid character structure principally expresses the split between the heart and the genitals. Coming back to Charcot's experimental work with curing hysteria, which was described in Chapter One: the Victorian culture humiliated the oedipal process and the organic place of sexual desire and emphasised, particularly in women, the disgust from sexual expression. We could better understand the very frequent hysterical passing-out episodes as a result of chronic abdominal holding (which splits the heart and genitals). The tight corsets provided an extra layer of bodily armour, retaining and strengthening the split between the (sexual) prostitute Mary Magdalene and the (lovable and virgin) sacred Mother Mary (Freud, 1912d). In this character structure there is a tension between permission to be a sexual man or woman and the risk of losing connection, and the validated and loved childlike quality, which lacks sexual charge. Rigid characters often have muscular tension in the extensor muscles, responsible for holding back, primarily those supporting the spine (erector muscles). There is hard muscular armour throughout the body with strong charge, strung muscles, and tense tendons: a quality of a highly tight string.

Eye contact: While the rigid character structure does not surrender easily, it is certainly present. Eye contact tends to be present yet distant.

Touch: The rigid character structure is very soft inside, yet somewhat hard and string-like outside (highly tense tendons). Touch can be deep, loving, connecting, and sometimes seductive, but is inconsistent—like the movement and holding, touch also moves in rhythms of towards and away from, coming and going. Being in physical contact with someone predominantly rigid we may feel completely seen and connected in rare moments of intimacy, only to feel lonely and abandoned a moment later.

Fear: The rigid character structure fears rejection of different aspects of herself—either having her heart and broken-heartedness rejected, or having her passion rejected, shamed, and castrated (or both), thus there is fear of surrender to connection.

Energetic phase: There is a lot of charge in the outer parts of the body (including the extremities, the physical organs responsible for reaching out for connection), yet inside the body there is relatively low charge (looser holding). The energetic movement is allowing the other person in—the capacity to cross the divide between inside and outside, and mainly loving connection, a meaningful relationship.

Strengths and resources: Predominant rigid character structure presumes a successful and not-too-painful transition of previous developmental angles, and therefore there are many resources here including capabilities, ambition, grounding (the next chapter will expand the notion of grounding), capacity to engage in relationships, and connecting to self and others. The rigid person can be charming and possess considerable social qualities, "the life of the party", very loving and idealistic, and has the making of a leader. The body structure can be very beautiful, well-proportioned both externally and internally. The need to be "the best of the best", as a compensation for the parental rejection of aspects of the self and an attempt to regain their love, is a tremendous ambitious resource, and can drive many people with rigid character structure to succeed in their field and sweep others along with them.

Working therapeutically with rigid character structure: The British poet Alfred, Lord Tennyson is perhaps best known for his writing: "'tis better to have loved and lost than never to have loved at all" (1849, p. 31), and this is the therapeutic motto of working with rigid character structure. Therapy with the rigid character involves surrender and heartache. It is likely that transference love will take place, that the client will fall in love with the therapist (and often the therapist will fall in love as well) and will go through a heartbreak that ideally does not shatter the heart—a love that is neither castrating nor abusive, neither rejecting nor seductive. The therapist strives to encourage the client to challenge the love and sex divide and find inner integration between the two, as well as bringing them together into relationships with others (including the therapeutic relationship) by remaining connected to both heart qualities and to fire and passion.

Closeness, intimacy, and surrender may be experienced as humiliating and the therapist might quickly become an enemy against which the client has to protect. Through the language of tenderness, the therapist might provide a more human model of connection, integrating softness with fierceness. It is easy to be seduced into a power struggle, which ends the very moment it begins, as it amplifies the rigid defence. The client will struggle to remain in contact and the therapist would be required to be present and transparent, allow for genuine connection to take place, and reflect both the wish for, and the fear of connection to the client.

How can we allow space for passion and surrender to passion without losing safe therapeutic boundaries? How safe is it to feel sexuality and love in general and within therapy in particular? Is it better to feel or to disconnect? The therapeutic process needs to encourage issues of love and sexuality to surface, and the therapeutic emphasis is—more than any other character structure—the therapeutic relationship between client and therapist as a dyad, in the here-and-now (while still working through the there-and-then).

Relational body psychotherapist Shoshi Asheri (2004) suggested that therapeutic work with erotic material in the oedipal stage invited the therapist to validate the client's emergent sexuality, celebrate it, and welcome it. At the same time, the therapist ought to be "dealing with the disappointment that this cannot be consummated with you, the parent/therapist".

Extreme conditions: Sadism, paranoia, hysteria, phobias, and hypochondria. Some types of dissociation, including dissociative disorders, could result from splits during this developmental stage (primarily due to sexual abuse).

Clinical vignette

Rosie came to therapy wanting to experience body-oriented psychotherapy, which included Reichian bodywork, and was less interested in pursuing a psychotherapeutic exploration. She was beautiful with luxurious red hair, full of vitality and depth, intellectual and creative. With her I felt electrically animated and threatened from the storm; I was mentally, emotionally, and bodily awake and excited. Just like her hair, therapy felt like dancing around the fire—and the fire element was always present.

Rosie could not understand why her boyfriend was so possessive of her, and why she needed to limit her sexual exploration to her partner. Equally, she mocked me for "your funny boundaries" and for my refusing her explicit requests for a sexual relationship between us.

Rosie's father left shortly after she was five, and Rosie remembered his dread of her sexuality as a child (I believe a part of her thought she sent him away with her sexuality).

Inside me I moved through stormy weathers while working with Rosie; between my omnipotent saving fantasies (from Rosie's unspoken loneliness) and my diverse sexual fantasies, I made great use of supervision, which allowed me to see both the loving and sexually powerful woman as well as the young girl begging to be seen, without reducing Rosie to one or the other.

After eighteen months of therapy, Rosie asked one day to work on the muscles along her spine (erector spinae), which were hurting. A few months previously she had left her boyfriend, who was able to meet her emotionally but unable to meet her forcefully, to rejoice in her passion; she wanted more. Rosie lay on the mattress on her stomach, and I sat beside her. After some deep Reichian bodywork with the erector muscles, I gently placed my hand on her back and Rosie immediately reported feeling sexually aroused. I felt my body awakening too, and alongside the excitement and dread I could recognise another feeling, one of deep love towards her and wanting to protect her. Hesitant and apprehensive, Rosie asked what I felt, and I shared these three sensations with her—the excitement, the dread, and the protective love. I felt very exposed and fearful and Rosie started crying—"You are not leaving me," she said.

In the following year our therapeutic relationship changed dramatically, moving to and fro between erotic transference dynamics and deep oedipal love. With great trepidations and with the invaluable support of my supervisor and psychotherapist, I did not stop to touch Rosie, but we also avoided working with the same affect-laden manner which characterised our early relationship. Together we mourned our decision to not consummate our passion—and alongside the grief, our love deepened. Rosie began dating a man who was attentive to both her heart and her sexuality and moved to live with him and shortly afterwards stopped therapy. While she later updated me that the heart and sex divide was a recurring theme in her new relationship too, Rosie was committed not to give up aspects of herself—or of her relationship.

Exercise: opening to a wider mind

This is a very simple and non-threatening exercise, combining movement and breath and providing an emotional and bodily experience to the love-passion connection. It is done in pairs, and if the therapist is comfortable enough with this positioning it could be exercised in therapy or the therapist be guided how to practise it with another person. I often use it when working with couples. I learned this exercise from Silke Ziehl.

1. Stand about two meters apart, unlock knees and close your eyes to allow for inward attention. Both parties note their breathing. Open your eyes and look at one another with an open gaze and soft focus. Synchronise the rhythm of breathing.
2. One of the partners breathes while exercising the following movement: the hands are positioned by the side of the body facing upwards. With the inhale the hands move upwards towards the heart and then extend towards the other person while exhaling. The movement and breath carry the message: "I allow my heart to fill with passion and from there I open to you"—the movement is from me to you, through the heart connection.

3. The other partner breathes while exercising the following movement: the hands begin where the movement of the partner stopped: they face upwards and outwards. With the inhale, the hands move inwardly towards the heart and then down towards the pelvis. With the exhale, the movement continues outside towards the partner (now the hands face downwards). The movement and breath carry the message: "I allow the fire of my passion to fill with the softness of my heart and from there I open to you"—the movement is from me to you, through the genital connection.
4. Continue breathing together for a few breathing cycles and change over. In fact, the synchronised movements create the sign of infinity (∞) between the pair: connecting with another person who moves inside me, connecting to myself which is enabled through the other.

Bodymind character structure—summarising table (based on this chapter as well as on Ziehl, 2000)

Developmental angle	**Existence**	**Neediness & nourishment**	**Autonomy & support**	**Between need & want**	**Sexuality & passion**
Character structure	Fragmented	Oral	Inflated	Dense	Rigid
Other names	Ocular, schizoid, boundary	Collapsed, dependent	Anal (early), control, narcissistic, psychopath	Masochist, anal (late), endurer, self-defeating, held	Phallic, oedipal, hysteric
Age (classic)	Prenatal, birth up to three months	Birth to eighteen months	Eight months to thirty months	Two years to three and a half years	Three to six years
Main themes	Early trauma, annihilation anxiety and abandonment anxiety, the right to exist	Food and nourishment, weaning, yearning, frustration, the right to need and depend	The right for autonomy and support, exploration and playfulness, manipulation	The right for freedom and expression, assertiveness, anger and expressing anger	Love, sex, relationship, surrender, and perfectionism. The right to be fully accepted
Bodily holding	Contraction and holding together	Holding on	Holding up	Holding in	Holding back
Control	Thoughts and ideas	What comes in and what does not	The environment and others	What comes out and what does not	The degree of surrender to connection
Attachment style	Disorganised	Preoccupied	Avoidant	Secure with hues of preoccupied	Secure with hues of avoidant

(*Continued*)

Table. (*Continued*)

Developmental angle	Existence	Neediness & nourishment	Autonomy & support	Between need & want	Sexuality & passion
Breathing pattern	Held and chaotic	Difficulty to take in and inhale	A lot of inhale, little exhale	Controlled and not spontaneous	Division between chest and abdomen
Movement	Frozen, non-coordinated, little	Soft but quick to collapse	Big, quick and short lived—inflated and deflated	Slow and measured, "like a soldier"	"Tango" like, backwards and forwards—a lot of movement, vital
Bodily tension	Head, skull, neck, around eyes	Hands, pectoral minor, jaws and neck	Shoulder girdle and pelvic girdle	Upper back, buttocks, shoulders—a lot of bodily tension	Back extensors, diaphragm
Eye contact	Avoidant, staring, disconnected or grabbing	Needing and sucking (like a kitten)	Confronting—looking for eye contact, competitive and challenging	Warm and suffering	Present yet distant
Touch	Avoidant, disconnected from context	Pleasant and safe, craving touch	Thin skinned, seductive, sweeping	Pleasant and warm, connected	Present and deep yet inconsistent
Fear	Annihilation anxiety	Abandonment or being swallowed	Loss of connection	Loss of approval and love	Rejection of love or rejection of passion, castration
Energetic phase	Self-regulation and integration	Charge—building inner resources	Quick move between charge and discharge	High charge and holding in	High charge outside, low inside
Resources and strengths	Creativity, clear thinking, spirituality	Capacity to nourish and give, empathy, sensitivity and intuition	Charisma and charm, influence and ability to challenge and change	Reliability, generosity, attention to other, endurance, strong will, discipline	High capabilities, ambitions, groundedness, connection with self and other, beauty

(*Continued*)

Table. (*Continued*)

Developmental angle	Existence	Neediness & nourishment	Autonomy & support	Between need & want	Sexuality & passion
Therapy	Trauma work: slow work, focus on boundaries, regulation and connection to self and to body	Reparative regression, satisfaction and frustration of needs, therapist as selfobject	Work with negative transference and challenge without shaming. Establishment of trust and boundaries	Slow work. Inner listening and self-awareness. Work with negative transference, mainly anger	Work with surrender and heartbreak, intimacy, risk and security; oedipal work
Extreme conditions	Schizophrenia, autistic spectrum, dissociative disorders	Depression, bipolar disorders, eating disorders, addictions	Psychopathy, sociopathy, borderline personality disorder	Masochism, depression, obsessive compulsive disorder	Sadism, paranoia, hysteria, phobias and hypochondria, dissociation (following sexual abuse)

Notes

1. The poem is reprinted here with permission of Hakibbutz Hameuchad—Sifriat Poalim.
2. This section is an expansion of a paper previously published in *Attachment* journal (Rolef Ben-Shahar, 2012e). I would like to thank Karnac for its kind permission to use this material here.
3. Body psychotherapist Ronen Levy greatly assisted me in organising character structure material.

CHAPTER SEVEN

The language of the body: further concepts in body psychotherapy

Story Water
A story is like water
that you heat for your bath.
It takes messages between the fire
and your skin. It lets them meet,
and it cleans you!
Very few can sit down
in the middle of the fire itself
like a salamander or Abraham.
We need intermediaries.
A feeling of fullness comes,
but usually it takes some bread
to bring it.
Beauty surrounds us,
but usually we need to be walking
in a garden to know it.
The Body itself is a screen
to shield and partially reveal
the light that's blazing inside your presence.
Water, stories, the body,
all the things we do, are mediums
that hide and show what's hidden.

> Study them,
> and enjoy this being washed with a secret we sometimes know,
> and then not.
>
> —*Rumi* (1995)[1]

Despite the differences between modalities in body psychotherapy, there is nonetheless a terminological common ground and shared conceptual understanding. This chapter will present some of the basic concepts in body psychotherapy, in addition to those touched upon by the last three chapters. Many of these concepts, which are presented here from a relational body psychotherapy perspective, overlap and interact with one another.

Energy

> Man has no body distinct from his soul, for that called body is a portion of soul discerned by five senses, the chief inlets of soul in this age. [...]
>
> Energy is eternal delight.
>
> —William Blake (1790, p. 75), "The Marriage of Heaven and Hell"

Whatever name we give it—be it libido or orgone, chi, animal magnetism, or life force, energy is here, demanding our attention. Many therapeutic modalities, including psychoanalysis in its early days, have made use of the concept of *energy* as a basic facet in their theoretical and clinical foundation. As Harry Stack Sullivan (1953) bravely wrote: "The ultimate reality in the universe is energy" (p. 102).

Reich's energetic understanding, which was discussed in Chapter Two, was essentially biological. Focusing his research on biological conductivity (primarily of the autonomic nervous system and skin conductivity), Reich believed he had discovered life energy, which flowed throughout the universe—the orgone. This energy, as Reich postulated, was not only responsible for our human health or ill health, but moreover affected all organic matter, the weather, and the planets and stars (Reich, 1942).

Alexander Lowen (1975) abandoned the concept of orgone, and instead extensively spoke about bioenergy—the bodily metabolic energy which affected bodymind organisations.

As noted by Nick Totton (2003), most body psychotherapists today used the term energy more vaguely and loosely than Reich's bio-electric or Lowen's biological energy. However, energy is still a central concept in the work of many body psychotherapists, who observe their clients (and themselves) and evaluate their energetic organisation. These observations in turn shape their clinical interventions. Totton expands: "Therapists decide how to approach a client by their assessment of the state of the client's 'energy', and the perceived movement and variation in body 'energy' gives them crucial feedback on the effect of their interventions" (ibid., p. 63).

Totton (ibid.) suggests that body psychotherapists frequently use the term energy to describe "an emotional hue", which manifests in the client's bodymind and could be sensed by the therapist. Indeed, some research supports the idea of bodily energy, which allows for body-to-body communication and creates interactive connections. Researcher James Oschman

(2000), for instance, offers some explanations for this body-to-body communication, including inter-organismic electromagnetic communication, peripheral nervous system, and his "entrainment" model, according to which energetic patterns in one organism tend to resonate and replicate in organisms who are in close physical proximity (for example brainwave frequency).

According to some spiritual understandings and Eastern philosophies, our bodies are surrounded by an egg-shaped energetic field, broader than our skin, and we are all sensitive to what takes place in that energetic field, which is forever interacting with our environment (Myss, 1996). To examine the concept of energy through therapeutic eyes, let us first direct our attention to modern physics. The influential physicist David Bohm (1957) writes: "There is a universal flux that cannot be defined explicitly but which can be known only implicitly. [...] In this flow, mind and matter are not separate substances. Rather, they are different aspects of one whole and unbroken movement" (p. 11).

But what is this "implicit knowing" of the universal flux which Bohm refers to? Could this energy only be described through physical language? In Chapters Four and Five I shared ideas regarding body–mind organisation and the concept of bodymind. One of the arguments I wish to propose here (suggested by writers like Daniel Stern (2004)) is that intersubjectivity cannot be perceived cognitively but requires somatic attention; that the main way to feel into the intersubjective space (and intersubjective body) is through body sensations. We feel our wider bodymind through our six senses (the familiar five senses and proprioception), through our own body. To simplify the argument: when we are attentive to our own bodies we can feel "the other" alive and moving through us. This implicit knowing Bohm speaks about and many body psychotherapists relate to is, so I believe, *resonance*—our connection to the other through the interface of our own body.

Whether we search for a physical, biological, psychological, or spiritual explanation for the concept of energy, the clinical applications of energetic evaluation of the client, the therapist, and the therapeutic process are central tenets in the work of many body psychotherapists. Chapter Eleven will exemplify the body psychotherapeutic skill of working with resonance.

Embodiment

I have mentioned and discussed embodiment in Chapter Five, while exploring the bodymind understanding in body psychotherapy. Embodiment relates both to the inevitable unity of our bodymind experiences (being) as well as to the skill of strengthening and cultivating the connection between somatic and psychic dimensions of our experience (doing). The body psychotherapist aspires to assist her client (and herself) to fully embody her experiences—to experience the world through the body, as a body: to be at home in her body. Family therapist Andrew Roffman (2003) elaborated: "Embodiment as a concept specifies that we are, as human beings, living organisms whose experience in the world is embodied experience, that there is no contradiction between being a mind and being a body, and that neither mind nor body is reducible to the other" (p. 58).

The therapist uses her own bodily presence and her practice of embodiment to provide a role model for her client, and to nonverbally (or subsymbolically, to use Bucci's, 2011, terminology) invite the client to experience her world through her body. The body psychotherapist assumes that embodiment allows for a more comprehensive processing of her life experiences, and that it could encourage fuller surrender to her own vitality (Totton, 2003).

Many body psychotherapeutic skills are reliant on embodiment as a basic skill. Observing another person's body or the shared body (the intersubjective body), working with somatic countertransference (elaborated later in this chapter), or offering active somatic interventions, all demand that the therapist is attentive to her sensory channels, and therefore invests in her own embodiment. When "being at home in my body" becomes a practised and cultivated skill, then difficulty in feeling our body and embodying provides highly valuable information to the therapist. In my work with dissociative clients, for instance, my lack of embodiment and losing the sense of my body become an important compass for indicating early signs of traumatic flooding (Rolef Ben-Shahar, 2009; Rolef Ben-Shahar & Wood, 2009).

Body psychotherapist Jack Lee Rosenberg (Rosenberg, Rand, & Asay, 1985) added: "Our success has come from recognising that our being, our Essential Self, is grounded in the body; that ignoring the body is to have very limited lasting success in the treatment of psychological pain" (p. 14). Similarly, body psychotherapist Stanley Keleman (1985) exclaimed even more conclusively that: "Without anatomy, emotions do not exist. Feelings have somatic architecture" (p. xii).

Traditional body psychotherapy supposes embodiment as a prerequisite for relationships. For a relationship to exist, we need at least two bodies (two bodyminds). Relational body psychotherapy adds a dialectic tension to this claim: we need bodies to relate, and at the same time we need to relate to have bodies. Relationality requires a dance between two feeling bodies and two embodied psyches, which create and condition one another.

To conclude the discussion of embodiment, I would like to offer Will Davis's (2012) call for reconsideration of the place of the body in psychotherapy, which nicely places the quality of embodiment within a larger frame of bringing the body back into therapy. Davis writes:

> It seems that the question of including the body in psychotherapy should be rephrased. It should instead be: why not include the body in psychotherapy? It is a necessary part of developmental themes, emotions, beliefs and the therapeutic process. The body and mind are deeply interwoven. As a result the best approach is a body/mind unity within psychotherapy. (p. 72)

Somatic awareness and levels of consciousness

> "I can't explain myself, I'm afraid, sir," said Alice, "because I'm not myself, you see." "I don't see," said the Caterpillar.
>
> "I'm afraid I can't put it more clearly," Alice replied very politely, "for I can't understand it myself to begin with; and being so many different sizes in one day is very confusing."
>
> "It isn't," said the Caterpillar.
>
> —Lewis Carroll (1865, p. 54), *Alice's Adventures in Wonderland*

Stanley Keleman (1981) refers to awareness as the process of life itself: "The continuum of our self-forming is what we are conscious of" (p. 19). According to this understanding, the awake and living body *is* consciousness and awareness.

Awareness has many facets: we may speak of the mind which can observe itself, that is—the ability to develop an inner witness, mindful of the mental and cognitive processes taking place inside us. This is a goal in itself in some forms of meditation, as well as therapeutic processes. We may also describe a person who is aware of her feelings and the manner in which she is activated by her own biography and history (someone who is "in touch" with herself). Another facet is sensory: awareness of the information we receive from our six senses (the capacity to discern, differentiate, and report): visual, auditory, olfactory, gustatory, tactile, and proprioceptive (the sense of self as it is organised in space).

The *levels of consciousness* describe the degree of complexity of information we are exposed to, within which we may develop conscious awareness. Freudian understanding of the body considered sensations as non-organised *primary processes*—the therapeutic task was therefore to support the patient in gradually developing these into *secondary processes*, cognitive and linguistic ones. I adopt a different outlook, of psychoanalyst Wilma Bucci (1994, 1998, 2001, 2011) who described parallel ways of encoding information (inclusive of somatic information) which were still organised and structured, even when they lacked words. Forerunner of relational psychoanalysis, Hans Loewald (1977), similarly offered an interesting take on awareness. Loewald suggested that mental activity involved both primary and secondary processes interweaving with one another, and that analysis (by encouraging free association) was an endeavour to move the patient closer to primary processes.

Thus, both Loewald and Bucci offer us a fresh perspective on levels of awareness, where nonverbal processes are no longer seen as inferior; on the contrary—these are essential entry points into change. The levels of awareness offered herewith are therefore not hierarchical but instead mark developmental degrees of complexity.

The first level of processing information (according to Reich, 1933a) was sensory and motoric: the baby was primarily a somatic entity. He was flooded with sensory and motoric information and gradually learned to discern different types of sensations (cold and hot, contracted and relaxed, light and dark). According to Daniel Stern (1985), this primary and primitive sense of self began already in the womb, and developed prior to any other type of self-awareness. Some of these sensations were organised into nonverbal language (which Bucci termed subsymbolic). Like Bucci, Eugene Gendlin (1962), subsequently the originator of *Focusing* (1978), claimed that not only did body awareness exist before language, but that it often did not require language to express itself. To successfully communicate with subsymbolic organisations, the therapist needed to speak with the body in its own language, and body psychotherapy provided a highly valuable therapeutic direction in offering ways not only to speak about the body (or about the pain), but also to *speak the body* and *to speak with the body* in its own language (body-to-body conversation). "The possibility of offering direct body contact, body observation, or touch," wrote relational body psychotherapist Liron Lipkies, "creates a connection between symbolic language and subsymbolic processes" (2012, p. 7). The psychologist and bodyworker Alan Fogel (2009) added: "Language is neither necessary nor sufficient to describe embodied self-awareness. […] Language is also not necessary as a means of communicating my embodied self-awareness to others. Body movements, facial expressions, and gestures are often sufficient" (p. 31).

The next level of complexity involves clusters of sensations which are organised and grouped into emotions and feelings (e.g., contracted stomach, dried lips, and pressure in the forehead create frustrated hunger); parental naming assists in organising a bridge between sensations, movements, and emotions ("Oh, so you were just hungry, here's the breast. All is OK now"). The formation of images and shapes is a later phenomenon still, more complex than emotion ("What's happening inside you?" I ask a client; "I'm like a concrete wall," he replies. The anger and helplessness form into an image of a concrete wall). Finally—symbolic thinking (linguistic) represents an even later organisation. Awareness could therefore be cultivated and developed in any of those levels: sensation, movement, emotion, imagery, and thought.

Body awareness (or somatic awareness) includes both sensory and motor awareness, as well as the ability to communicate this awareness to another person through symbolic means (verbally), or via subsymbolic conversation. For example, when I am asked "How are you?" I may respond with a verbal "I'm OK, thanks," while presenting another, subsymbolic answer: I could smile widely, gesture a very small nod, pull my shoulders up, or heavily sigh. The meaning of my answer will be deduced from the combination of these two levels: the symbolic and subsymbolic; my communication need not be verbal to be understood. The body psychotherapist will relate to the variety of body sensations as crucial sources of information regarding the person's state, and hence she might be curious about (and ask questions regarding) details such as: skin sensations, gut feelings, breathing patterns, bodily locus of the current experience, gestures, temperature, texture, bodily tensions, pulsations, and bodily streams and rhythms. All these provide the psychotherapist with diagnostic data and substance for intervention. This knowledge forms a deserving field to be learned by other modalities of psychotherapy.

But body psychotherapists understand somatic awareness not only as a valuable therapeutic skill, but also as being valuable in its own right and worthy of cultivating with clients, as a basis for self-awareness. We believe that our clients will benefit by becoming more aware of their body. Movement is the basis of awareness, argues Moshe Feldenkrais (1977), the originator of the Feldenkrais method: "Most of what goes on within us remains dulled and hidden from us until it reaches the muscles. We know what is happening within us as soon as the muscles of our face, heart, or breathing apparatus organize themselves into patterns, known to us as fear, anxiety, laughter, or any other feeling" (p. 36).

Therefore, the body psychotherapist encourages his client to familiarise himself with his somatic self, to listen to his body, and to cultivate clear and sympathetic communication with body sensations. Body psychotherapist Adi Kashi-Kark (2011) describes this as moving from the pain that shouts to speaking the pain. She writes: "Body psychotherapy offers a connection through the body into feelings, which provide a bridge to deep knowledge of our emotions and sensations. Thus, the body no longer needs to scream the psyche, as legitimate expression is given to the inner psychological world" (p. 88).

Faced with pain and suffering (emotional or physical) we tend to objectify our hurting part, often turning our body to an *it*—the nonself object. Somatic awareness assists us to reinhabit our bodies, to reclaim our embodied nature—gradually making the body ours (I have a body), and later repossessing the selfhood immanent in our bodily self, as part of me (I am a body). To reiterate, we move from "there is a body" through "this is my body" to "I am a body".

Body psychotherapy assumes a functional identity between body and mind (please see the psychosomatics section below) and therefore somatic awareness is a crucial facet in personal, as well as therapeutic, development. The Feldenkrais method, for instance, is almost entirely based on developing awareness through movement and somatic observation. According to Moshe Feldenkrais (1977), somatic awareness necessitates movement. Feldenkrais maintained that we operated in the world in accordance with our perception of self, which was in turn based on our body image. Yet this body image was not necessarily accurate to our bodily reality, and instead was influenced by our character structure, our history, and the defensive organisations we have adopted over the years (a similar conceptualisation to the one proposed in Chapter Five). The Feldenkrais method is a systemic effort to correct body image distortions by increasing our somatic awareness. Part III (Clinical) will exemplify how increasing somatic awareness could be used as a therapeutic skill.

Psychosomatics

> Pain is a language of sorts, with its uniquely encoded messages. It is a language written in the person's flesh, psyche, and spirit. The client learns this language. The quality of immediacy in encountering the pain in body psychotherapy forms a new experience, and a fresh point of view, which may lead to the source, the origins of the pain.
>
> —Adi Kashi-Kark (2011, p. 65)

In her book *The Body Speaks* (*הגוף מדבר*), Israeli psychoanalyst Nitza Yarom (2001) examined some fascinating bodily and psychological aspects of hysteria, through analysing the character of Saint Francis. What was it that made (and still makes) hysteria such a focal point for curiosity in the field of psychotherapy? As Chapter One showed, psychoanalysis emerged from studies in hysteria, from the deep quest to find connections between somatic and psychological phenomena. It is no wonder that extreme conditions, where body and mind took turns speaking of the person's suffering, formed the meeting point for the exploration of both. After all, it was much easier to realise the interaction between body and mind when pain is prevalent. Alexander Lowen (1965) protested this injustice: "For too long, Western thought has regarded the body as a mechanism, an instrument of the will, or a repository of the spirit. Modern medicine, for all its advances, still holds to this view. We do not take our bodies seriously except when something goes wrong" (p. 316).

The term psychosomatics (or psychosomatic illness) has sadly become a shaming label, a condemnation describing an illness with no organic (bodily) findings: "It's all in your head," "It's only psychological," and so forth. Psychosomatic illness is commonly understood as a psychological condition *creating* unreal bodily symptoms. Chronic pain sufferers are often confronted with demands to prove the reality of their pain via biochemical tests. The subjective experience of pain is frequently met with explicit or implicit professional denunciation.

But pain is neither somatic nor psychic, but always carries both dimensions. The psychotherapeutic difficulty to relate to somatic pain as having its own (somatic) meaning and not solely psychological meaning, parallels the medical difficulty in relating to emotional suffering as having important meaning in its own right, not only as a result of an organic experience (hormonal imbalance, serotonin deficiency, etc.). When faced with pain, the psychotherapist will be predisposed to looking for emotional meaning, the medical practitioner—for organic sources.

Body psychotherapy has a unique way of relating to psychosomatic pain, categorically different to both classic psychoanalysis and medicine. Body psychotherapy understands people to a priori be psychosomatic systems. The somatic and the emotional aspects operate both as functionally identical systems (bodymind), and as two systems, which influence, condition, and complement one another (body–mind) (Reich, 1942). Therefore, every somatic phenomenon will also have a psychological expression and vice versa—every emotional event will manifest in our physiology. It goes without saying that any illness and pain are also psychosomatic. While the hierarchical and causal search is tempting (regardless of whether we see the psychological trauma as causing the physical pain or the physical pain contributing to a chronic victim-positioning which attracts abusers), but the relationship between emotional and somatic aspects is not causal but complementary (two phenomena that parallel one another) and dialectic (two phenomena, which create one another).

In his regular column, "The Body's Voice" (קולו של הגוף), relational body psychotherapist Ronen Levy (2012) traced psychosomatic contexts in psychotherapy, illustrating the complex relationship between emotional and somatic expressions. Levy wrote: "Verbal language, with all the depth it can offer, is sometimes found wanting when embodied and nonverbal processes are presented. We are requested to develop new channels of communication, until we can extract the wordless story told by the body" (p. 62).

Psychoanalyst Norman Doidge (2008) related to pain not only as a reflexive response to injury (organic pain), but also as a compass, providing an inner review of the person's health. To heal pain, we are consequently asked to reorganise our bodymind. Body psychotherapy is unique in its ability to communicate directly with the pain—to speak with the hurting person through the soma—the body. Bodily interventions communicate with the client exactly where she expresses pain. By looking at the pain, the body psychotherapist will be curious to discover the physiological expressions of any emotional difficulty, while also examining the emotional expressions of physical pains and difficulties. Body psychotherapy offers therapeutic interventions which could serve as novel and varied "entry doors"—both through the emotional and the bodily channels.

I would like to return to Kashi-Kark's (2011) discussion on psychosomatics, which illuminates some of the major aspects of working with pain in body psychotherapy:

> During the therapeutic process, verbal dialogue is created alongside a somatic-motoric dialogue. The bodily fields of client and therapist touch one another and communicate with each other, creating a secure therapeutic space. Body psychotherapy provides the client with a direct and unmediated dialogue with the body and the emotions expressed through the body, in a unique way which a solely verbal treatment cannot provide. (p. 68)

Another concept worth mentioning when discussing psychosomatics is "functional identity". The concept of functional identity is close to the concept of bodymind (which was mainly expanded on in Chapter Five), describing the functional identity between our body (physiology) and our mind (psychology). The main difference between the two concepts is their historical context: bodymind is a modern conceptualisation, a concept which developed in and from body psychotherapy, while functional identity is a concept coined by Wilhelm Reich (1933a) and is earlier than bodymind.

To conclude, let us return to Reich's basic argument: "It would be wrong to speak of the 'transfer' of physiological concepts to the psychic sphere, for what we have in mind is not an analogy but a real identity: the unity of psychic and somatic function" (ibid., p. 340). The body psychotherapeutic understanding of psychosomatic phenomena is directly connected with Reich's functional identity (or with the bodymind). To this extent, all psychotherapy—and all physical illness—is psychosomatic.

Charge and discharge

Reichian tradition perceives a cyclical energetic and organic rhythm, which is expressed in the body and involves energetic charge and discharge. Many problems are seen as a result of obstructions to this energetic motion—either due to lack of sufficient charge (as in certain depressive states), or due to hypercharge with insufficient discharge (for instance, held anger or unexpressed crying). The therapist would respectively assist in building charge or finding legitimate and healthy ways to discharge the repressed bodily energy. The concept of discharge is close to the Freudian *catharsis*, but is a part of a broader energetic cycle. In presenting the charge-discharge cycle, Reich was ahead of his time in understanding autonomic nervous system functioning. Vegetotherapy (Reich's therapy, presented in Chapter Two), focused on regulating the autonomic (vegetative) nervous system.

In a way, the charge-discharge cycle integrates Western therapeutic and medical knowledge with Eastern philosophies and outlook on energy and life. One of the basic principles in traditional Chinese medicine (TCM), for example, is the cyclical rhythm of life, which is very different from the Western understanding of life as advancing in a linear fashion (Connelly, 1994). The healthy person in TCM is not necessarily the person who always moves forward, but instead one who can move smoothly through the seasons of life, which keep repeating and inviting us to surrender. Likewise, the charge-discharge cycle has a wavelike quality—it begins with excitation and energetic tension, continues with the building up of charge until it reaches a climax, where discharge begins. The climax is characterised by surrender to body rhythms and letting go of (or losing) voluntary control of the process. After discharge there is a period of relaxation and rest. In body psychotherapy philosophy, this cycle is expressed in most psychosomatic (bodily and emotional) patterns, but is most significantly pronounced in the sexual-arousal cycle (Painter, 1984; Rosenberg, Rand, & Asay, 1985). Reich believed that only through full orgasm was an ultimate completion of discharge possible (Klisic, 1992; Lowen, 1965; Reich, 1942). However, modern body psychotherapy is less dogmatic and extreme in its energetic work. Some of the earlier cathartic interventions offered by Reich involved very strong emotional, bodily, and affective activation, which most contemporary body psychotherapists will hesitate to use in the same fashion.

Charge and discharge interventions may include encouragement to express sounds (from yawns, through sighs, to shouting and swearing), uncensored emotional expression (crying, shaking, or laughing, for example), bodywork, breathwork, and movement and dance. The body psychotherapist may use cushions and other props for expressing feelings (for example, kicking and hitting a cushion with a baseball bat). These interventions aim to release obstacles to the energetic charge-discharge cycle, which may have disturbed the natural flow and ability to surrender to pleasure, to the body, and to relationships. The 1960s counter-cultural movements (as well as some spiritual and pseudo-spiritual disciplines, among them followed by Osho's disciples, who developed famous methods of active meditation), were profoundly influenced by Reichian discharge techniques (Osho, 1976), but often implemented these outside a safe and containing therapeutic framework.

Jack Lee Rosenberg (Rosenberg, Rand, & Asay, 1985) argued that the early methods of body psychotherapy used powerful cathartic techniques (discharge) without minding the complex relationship dynamics between client and therapist. He proposed that the value of energetic discharge was severely limited when it took place outside an emotionally attuned therapeutic relationship, which gave it meaning, containment, processing—and more than anything—context.

Despite the criticism, the ability to assist a client in being more proactive in regulating his charge and discharge cycles and his energetic management (emotional, mental, somatic, and sexual) is one of the significant contributions of body psychotherapy. Breathing exercises, for example, can provide immediate and important assistance to panic attacks. Familiarity with charge and discharge techniques could help the therapist in accelerating recovery processes from depression or helplessness as well as to connect (alongside the grief) to the client's bodymind resources and the organic patterns of healing immanent to the organism, which have become disconnected due to body–mind dissociation (see "Self-regulation and dyadic regulation" later this chapter).

Somatic experiencing (SE), which was reviewed in Chapter Three, is an excellent example of contemporary adaptation of charge-discharge cycle. SE practitioners are particularly attentive to autonomic nervous system arousal (the sympathetic branch, which is associated with the bodily rhythms of alertness, the trauma vortex), and assisting their clients in developing a relaxation response (the parasympathetic branch—associated with the healing vortex) (Levine & Frederick, 1997).

The orgasm reflex

Reich associated the ultimate surrender with submitting to the involuntary rhythms of the orgasm, which he considered the clearest indicator of psychological and physical health. The healthy person, for Reich, was able to function and take pleasure in her work, and surrender to loving sexual relationships without inhibitions. Reich (1942) considered the "orgastic potency" as a measure for health—this potency was not the mechanical sexual release, but the ability to let go of defence mechanisms and control, giving into the rhythms of the body—surrendering to the energetic stream and flow, letting it take us without losing contact with ourselves or the other. Reich identified four stages in the orgasm: tension, charge, discharge, and relaxation, which he considered characteristic not only of the sexual orgasm but also of any other affective bodymind process (see "Charge and discharge" in this chapter).

According to Reich, we could not consistently surrender to the forces of orgasm and the orgasm reflex as long as we had neurotic defences. Not only did he consider sexual blockages as obstructing the orgastic streaming, but he moreover believed that full orgasm was a sign of liberation from neuroses: that the ability to surrender sexually was a testament of the person's health.

Reich examined the extent of his patients' orgastic potency by observing the orgasm reflex: a gentle and non-sexual reflex that occurred when both the neck and the pelvis were relaxed and loose with every exhale, allowing free streaming between the two. This flow of energy had an open wave-like quality of motion (Reich, 1933a). The degree of surrender to the orgasm reflex informed the therapist about the patient's capacity to surrender to his life (not just sex), as well as marked areas of bodily and emotional blockages requiring therapeutic intervention (Lowen, 1965).

When we watch an infant breathing, we can see how its entire body moves with each breathing cycle in a wave-like motion—the flow of energy in the body is concrete and visible. Similarly, after a deep emotional and physical discharge (for example, after an orgasm with a loving partner—but not just after an orgasm), this wave-like movement is clearly visible.

Most body psychotherapists today, including neo-Reichian, believe that Reich exaggerated the importance of orgasm to human life (Totton, 1998). While the ability to surrender—to pleasure, to connection, to being, and to sex is still central to the work of many body psychotherapists, the exclusive focus on the orgasm became more refined. Nevertheless, some body psychotherapists are still curious about the nature of orgasm and use the subtleties of orgasm as a diagnostic tool and therapeutic compass. Body psychotherapist Ljiljana Klisic (1992), for example, characterised five types of orgasm, each representing a different developmental level and capacity for bodily, emotional, relational, and spiritual surrender.

Body psychotherapists with Reichian training might take explicit interest in their clients' sexual lifestyle, asking direct and open questions about sexual experiences in general, and particularly about the nature of orgasm, the bodily experience of surrender, and the nature of relationship that was created during the orgasm. For example, the therapist might enquire if the client "had" to close his eyes during the orgasm, whether there was an emotional connection with the partner in those moments, what happened immediately after climaxing, and whether the sexual release was experienced only in the genital area or in other parts of the body too.

Body segments

The concept of body segments is deduced from the body psychotherapeutic developmental theory presented in Chapter Six. Reich divided the body into horizontal bands (segments), which corresponded to different developmental stages and manifested correlating bodymind qualities (Keleman, 1985; Totton & Edmondson, 1988). When contracted regularly, the following seven bands tend to accumulate tension, thus creating the muscular armour. Most training in body psychotherapy included organised methodology for working with these segments energetically, by paying attention to them, with voice, movement, touch, and breath. Furthermore, when a certain developmental angle was pronounced in a client, the body psychotherapist might pay particular attention to the body segments commonly active during the particular developmental stage, and be mindful of these parts alongside the idiosyncratic psychotherapeutic dialogue. For example, a language rich in tastes and textures might emotionally activate a client with predominantly oral character, while using authoritative language could trigger clients with inflated or dense characters (although they would respond differently).

There is an important theoretical and clinical connection between the bodymind character structure and the body segments. The theory of bodymind development provides a theoretical grounding for clinical interventions with body segments. Dividing the body into segments is an applicable practice, which translates character structure and developmental processes into therapeutic interventions. These are complementary bodies of knowledge, mutually informing one another. The psychotherapist who possesses developmental knowledge but lacks the skill of working with the segments might miss opportunities of softening bodymind organisations and offering somatic changes, while the bodyworker who is well able to clinically work with the segments but lacks developmental understanding will be missing the appropriate context (and therefore timing) for interventions.

The body segments are:

The ocular segment: Eyes, brows and forehead. Muscular armour around this area could express in chronically contracted muscles and limited mobility around the skull, the forehead, the eyes, and tear glands. Sometimes there is an empty-looking facemask, with a vague and expressionless gaze (especially related to terror and fear—first developmental angle).

The oral segment: Mouth, jaw, and chin. In this area we tend to muscularly hold repressed desire to bite, suck, and yell.

The cervical segment: The neck, throat, and upper shoulders. This is where we tend to hold anger and "swallowed" feelings.

The thoracic segment: Chest and back. This area could be held back as part of controlling feelings and avoiding surrender (fifth developmental stage) or be chronically collapsed from exhaustion, sadness, and shame.

The diaphragmatic segment: Lower chest and diaphragm. Holding here might separate the upper from the lower body—between the head and the heart, and the pelvis.

The abdominal segment: The belly and viscera: intestines, stomach, kidneys, liver, and pancreas. Common holding here relates to repression of deep gut feelings such as disgust, shame, or fear of death.

The pelvic segment: Pelvis and legs. Pelvic holding could repress deep sexual feelings of yearning and longing. Holding in the legs might express insecurity and lack of grounding (Painter, 1984; Totton & Edmondson, 2009).

The body segments correspond to the body psychotherapy developmental theory, and they also correspond to the energetic centres in yoga philosophy and psychology (chakras). According to yoga philosophy, different energetic centres are activated during corresponding developmental stages as well as life challenges and body challenges. Working specifically with certain energetic-somatic bands might therefore surface their relevant and corresponding developmental issues, allowing us to process these and work through them (Judith, 1996).

For further elaborated reading on body segments please see:

Marcher, L., & Fich, S. (2010). *Body Encyclopedia: A Guide to the Psychological Functions of the Muscular System*. Berkeley, CA: North Atlantic.

Painter, J. W. (1984). *Deep Bodywork and Personal Development*. Mill Valley, CA: Bodymind.
Totton, N., & Edmondson, E. (2009). *Reichian Growth Work: Melting the Blocks to Life and Love* (*2nd ed.*). Ross-on-Wye, UK: PCCS.

Pulsation, streaming, vibration

> Movement is the unifying bond between the mind and the body, and sensations are the substance of that bond.
>
> —Deane Juhan (1998, p. xxv)

Petals open and close; muscles contract and relax: life pulsates and vibrates through us. To be more precise: we partake in life's pulsation. We breathe: opening our chest, we let the world flow in with every inhale. For a fraction of a second all seems possible, if not yet realised, and a second later we choose: the air is no longer outside us, quickly it organises inside us adopting shapes and spaces within our cells. The digestive system follows a similar route: we begin a dialogue with an apple; we look at it, reach out with our hand to grasp it, to connect with it—while it still has a quality of apple-ness that is different to us. We chew the apple, speedily absorbing it within us, turning the apple into us. Within a short while, the apple-ness is no longer separate from who we are.

As Chapter Four demonstrated, we constantly move from form to flow, from adopting organisations to deconstructing these, to readopting newer shapes and forms. These forms begin their life in the body—in the manner we hold our muscles, our connective tissues—contraction and relaxation, even sooner they do so on cellular and histological levels. As organic and living beings we continuously organise ourselves—we actively partake in the dialogue between form and flow; we share in the organisations we adopt, yet we are also influenced and organised by external agents.

More than any other therapeutic modality, body psychotherapy takes an interest in bodily rhythms, in the music of our somatic reality, in bodily streaming and bodily organisations which call for a direct and unmediated language, one that can be conveyed and celebrated with somatic attunement and touch; we seek ways of feeling into the pulse of these rhythms, of life pulsation. Stanley Keleman (1981) suggested that when we were able to freely flow between organisations, the pulsation of life was renewed and our vital aliveness could then flow more freely. In fact, he described individuality as our "personal rhythm of pulsating" (p. 39).

Keleman indicates three states of aliveness: pulsating, streaming, and vibration: "I feel the world as continuum of vibration, a shimmering field of excitation. This vibrating field gives rise to an increase in excitation, which tends toward expansion" (ibid., p. 35). When Keleman speaks of excitation, he describes a movement wishing to transcend its boundaries—the yearning to express the inner vitality, as early as from the cellular level. Keleman illustrates how, when our skin is deeply cut, our first response is shaking and vibrating, and then we begin to sense the pulsation—the world flows inwardly and outwardly: "When pulsations occur rapidly and in series, you have streaming. Streaming is a continuity of pulsation, a stream of rhythmic excitation that maintains itself in a particular direction and in a particularly organized form" (ibid., p. 35). Keleman exemplifies this: when we hold our breath, we can sense the movement of bodily excitation. If we make a tight fist for long enough, we can sense gentle pulsation throughout our body. In Western civilisation, Keleman continues, we have accelerated the organic processes of individuation and self-regulation: the child was separated from its mother far too early following labour. Both weaning and potty training frequently preceded the child's organismic readiness for it. Therefore, the child developed compensatory mechanisms of self-regulations without having developed the abilities to be attentive to its own rhythms and the rhythms of life around.

When the process of individuation is hastened and does not follow the organic pace of individuation, it may result in a premature organisation of separate self, before it was safely established within a dyadic-self. In such conditions we may lose our ability to naturally listen to our pulsating life rhythms. In such cases, when we are exposed to deep feelings of pulsation, streaming, and vibration, which are at the heart of our organismic vitality, we might view these as threatening or dangerous and attempt to stop this natural and organismic process in its tracks.

By accepting the body psychotherapeutic assumption that bodymind energy could be felt and interacted with, a new world of diagnosis and intervention could open before us. The quality of energy and its conduction become a focal point of reference to the body psychotherapist, who, like the Chinese medicine practitioner, learns to recognise different types of energy flow—pulsation, vibration, streaming—towards the centre or from the centre to the periphery, downwards or upwards through the body, and more (Totton, 2003).

"Energetically speaking," writes Alexander Lowen (1975), "the whole body can be viewed as a single cell with the skin as its membrane. Within this cell excitation can spread in all directions or flow in specific directions depending on the nature of our response to a stimulus. [...] One can experience the flow of excitation as a feeling or sensation which often defies anatomical boundaries" (pp. 51–52). Reich (1942), however, was less determined regarding the biological nature of the streaming feeling, which he saw as bioelectric, an expression of the cosmic energy—the orgone.

This energetic pulsation is the movement flowing from the centre of the body outwards and from outside in. Pulsation has many emotional and bodily manifestations, including breath, pulse, heartbeat, shivers of excitement, and other emotional expressions. Crying, for instance, has a rhythm, which tends to bring with it involuntary rhythmical pulsatory movements (Keleman, 1981). The body psychotherapist might be curious about the client's bodily rhythms and attempt to engage with them, sometimes incorporating bodily interventions around somatic pulsation, streaming, or vibration.

The following vignette demonstrates therapeutic use of bodily rhythms:

Beverly came to therapy following a traumatic car accident, in which she was seriously injured and the driver who hit her died. She was only able to speak of the accident by completely dissociating from the sensations of her body. One day, Beverly arrived twenty minutes late to our session; she was angry and irritable, and complained about the traffic jam that held her back. Her lips were shaky as she spoke about being late and the traffic jam. Beverly quickly moved to another subject, which she wanted to discuss in therapy.

I stopped her and asked her to tell me about the traffic jam again: "Do you notice that your lips are shaking when you talk?" "Now, once you've drawn my attention to it, yes, I do," she replied. "Let the gentle shaking do what it needs to do, give it space," I asked. Beverly reached out with her hand, and asked that I held her hand. She sat, our hands held together, and the vibration spread out—from the lips to the neck, to her arms, her chest, to her stomach and legs. It was as if a wave of vibration moved through her. While she shook, Beverly reported having images but I asked her to keep focusing on the sensations. After about ten minutes of shaking the vibration stopped. Beverly lay down on the mattress, her hand still holding mine. Her breathing was full and calm; and she told me—tearful yet calmly, the story of her accident. Her body moved gently, still following waves that became rhythmic and gentle but were no longer a flooding tsunami.

Boundaries

Within the psychotherapeutic world, the concept of boundaries denotes several different levels, each of them concerning questions of liberty and safety, of in and out. Nick Totton (2003) poetically elucidates this:

> Just as a cell needs a surrounding membrane to define it, human beings need "edges," psychological boundaries which resist change—in order to delineate where they are; in order to exist at all. One can think of these edges as our grip on embodiment. While it may be helpful to relax any particular edge, we cannot do without edges altogether. (p. 59)

In this section I shall relate to four facets of boundaries: three dimensions of therapeutic boundaries and how they communicate with body psychotherapy and a fourth dimension where body psychotherapy has an important contribution to make to the general field of psychotherapy.

Frame boundaries

A central goal in most psychotherapeutic systems is the establishment of trust and safety within the therapeutic space—for both the client and therapist. This is also one of the first challenges in therapy. Frame boundaries mark the bounds of the clinical work within time, place, and a clear contract of value and exchange. These are the necessary conditions for the existence of therapy. Different therapeutic disciplines hold different positions regarding the rigidity or flexibility of frame boundaries.

Some body psychotherapists adopt frame boundaries from psychodynamic psychotherapy, which are considered relatively fixed; but the majority of contemporary body psychotherapy modalities have adopted boundaries, which are closer to those common to the humanistic practice of psychotherapy than to psychoanalytic boundaries. It means that while frame boundaries are seen as central and crucial to the therapeutic work, the therapist might show a degree of flexibility regarding frequency of meetings, session duration, and the possibility for making contact between sessions. These boundaries, different as they might be from the psychodynamic ones, would still be contracted, that is—they form part of the therapeutic dialogue and are transparently and clearly discussed.

A special note regarding the duration of sessions should be made here. Attention to body requires time, and body rhythms are often slower than the rhythm of thought. Often, and particularly when therapy incorporates bodily interventions of breathwork, movement, or bodywork, a clinical hour of fifty minutes simply does not suffice to create a safe and contained therapeutic encounter. Many body psychotherapists may therefore offer longer sessions—of ninety minutes or two hours. Sometimes longer sessions are planned specifically ("Next week we could work with the tension at the base of your skull, so I would like to suggest that we meet for ninety minutes"), and at other times in accordance with the client and the client's needs. Contracting for longer sessions could be ongoing: there are, for instance, clients with whom I meet regularly for weekly (contracted) ninety minutes or two hour sessions.

Conduct boundaries

Conduct boundaries relate to the psychotherapeutic act, or more specifically to therapeutic interventions, and include the therapist's position regarding her ability and competence, her therapeutic style, the relevance and appropriateness of her interventions, and her ethical standing and beliefs about psychotherapy. If we take, for example, a classic intervention of dream interpretation, the manner of interpretation will depend on a few factors:

- **The therapist's ability and competence**: Ability relates to the measure of skill and knowledge the therapist possesses; how much she understands the dream, how knowledgeable she is in the theoretical thinking and different approaches to dream interpretation. By *competence* I refer to the translation of her abilities into practice—how comfortable the therapist feels in exercising her understanding in the here-and-now of the therapeutic situation, and how available and retrievable the knowledge is to her when needed. These factors are connected to the type of clinical training she had and its quality, as well as to the fabric of the therapist's personality and to the nature and quality of the therapeutic relationship.
- **Therapeutic style**: Does the therapist take a waiting or an active stance? Would the interpretation be Freudian or Jungian, or perhaps Gestalt style dream interpretation (where each part of the dream represents part of the dreamer)? Body psychotherapy, for example, offers a number of ways of embodying dreams (such as psychodramatic methods, which invite the client to "show the dream" rather than speak about it as an observer). This factor is influenced by the type of therapeutic training as well as by her personal style of clinical work.
- **Relevance and appropriateness**: How important is it to present this interpretation to the client? Would it advance therapy? Is the timing right? Is this interpretation (or any interpretation) the appropriate therapeutic act right now, at the therapeutic stage we are at, and to this particular client? This boundary relates to contextual examination of our interventions.
- **Ethical standing**: What is allowed and what is forbidden in therapy? What is right and what is wrong? Does the psychotherapist believe that disturbing the flow of associations to propose an interpretation is an important therapeutic intervention? Perhaps she sees such interruption as a crude and inappropriate act? What is the ethical standing the therapist holds regarding the type of intervention and its timing?

Some conduct boundaries are shared by all psychotherapeutic modalities. For example, the framing of the psychotherapeutic relationship as a professional and transferential relationship, and the resulting taboo against sexual relations between client and therapist is a consensual conduct boundary. Like psychotherapists from other modalities, body psychotherapists continuously deal with questions and challenges of conduct boundaries. One of the common criticisms against body psychotherapy regards the "lack of boundaries" in body psychotherapy because of the possibility and reality of working with touch. Chapter Ten in Part III (Clinical) further explores issues of touch in body psychotherapy; but I would like to reiterate here that although body psychotherapists adopt *different* boundaries to those of the psychodynamic psychotherapist, it does not make their work (or them) lacking in boundaries. I believe that there is a common confusion in the field between issues of competence (and ability) and ethical issues.

Body psychotherapeutic interventions are a result of appropriate and thorough training. Most body psychotherapists are comprehensively trained in anatomy and physiology; they acquire clinical tools for intervening with touch, movement, and breath, and are able to justify and explain their intervention both clinically and theoretically. Body psychotherapist Arnt Halsen (1995) argued, for example, that knowing when to touch or not touch, how to touch and not to touch, required training and depth no less than knowing when to offer an interpretation and how to offer it. And indeed, therapeutic interventions exercised incompetently or without sufficient training are certainly problematic—both ethically and professionally.

Even within body psychotherapy, different approaches (and certainly different psychotherapists) hold varied conduct boundaries. For example, there are some modalities which refrain from using touch—Babette Rothschild's trauma work (2000) and Stanley Keleman's formative psychology (1981) are examples for such modalities. However, most body psychotherapists have trained in touch interventions and are competent and able enough to use these while holding to clear, safe, and appropriate boundaries (Totton, 2003). One of the conduct boundaries shared by all therapeutic modalities is avoiding touch when it is directly exercised to create sexual arousal (of either client or therapist).

Transitional space boundaries

Darren, a recently trained body psychotherapist, has been seeing me for supervision for the last two years. For a few consecutive sessions, Darren brought to supervision a client who kept asking for bodywork, but Darren blatantly refused: "I find her too attractive," he explained. I asked Darren to imagine what would have happened if he were to gratify her wish ... "Let your imagination go wild," I encouraged him. Darren froze, "I can't even go there in my mind; it's too dangerous."

Psychoanalyst Donald Winnicott (1958b) beautifully phrased what I call transitional space boundaries:

> There is a constant struggle in the individual throughout life, distinguishing fact from fantasy, external from psychic reality, the world from the dream. The Transitional Phenomena belong to an intermediate area which I am calling a resting place because living in this area the individual is at rest from the task of distinguishing fact from fantasy. (p. 123)

Transitional space boundaries—of both client and therapist—directly relate to the boundary (or the horizons) of fantasy, to the ability to challenge inner boundaries and dare to stay open to uncertainties, to flow, to undecidables, while remaining safe and protected. The degree of liberty the therapist, client, and the therapeutic dyad allow themselves would largely set the therapeutic volume and landscape—how threatening or safe, exciting or boring the clinical exploration would be. In the spirit of Winnicott, psychoanalyst Ofra Eshel (2005) boldly related to this context: "An analyst cannot expect a patient to make a breakthrough into previously unbearable, threatening, dissociated territory, unless the analyst is willing and able to risk entering and being in there, and survive" (p. 722).

Body sensations and bodily charge are immensely powerful experiences, and a significant part of the body psychotherapist's task is in assisting the client to learn and contain the challenging task of being a human being in a human body; to expand the client's capacity to trust in and work with transitional space between experience and action, to open to fantasy spaces *while still holding safe and firm boundaries*: kicking the cushion representing the boss without kicking the boss. To succeed in constructing safe yet expansive transitional space boundaries, body psychotherapists (like any therapist, really) need to have undergone a thorough psychotherapeutic process themselves, and have regular, consistent, and ongoing support for their personal and clinical anxieties and hopes (in forms of supervision or peervision, ongoing training, psychotherapy, and self-care).

Self-boundaries

The muscular armour, which was discussed in Chapter Six as part of exploring character structure, is in itself a boundary: a self-boundary created to shape the space between inside and outside in a way which supports the organism when faced with pressures and demands (both external and internal). Psychologist and bodyworker Yorai Sella (2005b) relates to the muscular armour as "a second skin" (p. 97). Self-boundaries are formed through behaviour and personality, in our conversation, in how we organise our relationship, and in our bodies.

Self-boundaries concern the way our organism perceives and creates both its separateness from the world (being apart from) and its connectedness to the world (being a part of), the dynamics between inside and outside, between "mine" and "not mine". In his book *The Skin Ego*, the French psychoanalyst Didier Anzieu examined some somatic aspects of self-boundaries, and particularly those concerning the surface of the body (Anzieu, 1989; Sella, 2011).

Different body systems contribute to developing a sense of boundary and definition to the organising self. Bones may help us in perceiving boundaries, groundedness, and positioning in relation to the world, the connective tissue in strengthening connection between different systems, and the lymph system may provide us with a sense of protection and security (Hartley, 2005).

Self-boundaries define the construction of self (like Totton's quote at the beginning of this section, which compares boundaries with the cell membrane). In this context, we might speak of the bodily and energetic perception of boundaries (Rosenberg, Rand, & Asay, 1985): How much space do I occupy? How much space do I need to feel safe? Does my body feel as my own, and can I accurately appraise my body's impact on my environment and the environmental impact on my body? To what extent am I able to embody my experiences? Do I need rigid boundaries to feel safe? Are my boundaries clear to me and to others?

These questions might be explored in the psychotherapeutic process in bodily ways as well as verbally, and the body psychotherapist will attempt to be mindful of such expressions, and particularly of the somatic aspects of boundaries, the use of external boundaries, the use of gestures and postures, and finally—of the boundaries of the body. Following are certain aspects of self-boundaries which may be explored and worked with therapeutically:

- **Relational body boundaries**: The capacity for eye contact or lack of it, the physical relationship between client and therapist (for example, a client who needs physical proximity and dissociates when there is distance), the quality of breath (held, free, etc.) and its location (diaphragmatic, thoracic, lateral), when the therapist comes closer or moves back—all these tell the body psychotherapist about the client's safe space and the intimate space needed to establish safe boundaries. Thus, body psychotherapists would not keep a rigid proximity distance (one size fits all) with all clients, but be mindful of those boundaries and be willing to play with them to best suit the therapeutic process.
- **Use of external boundaries and buffers**: How many layers of clothes does the client wear? How visible is the body beyond the clothes? How distinct is the body? Is the client wrapped in a thick layer of fat, and if so—is it uniformly held or are certain areas of the body fat and others not? How long is the hair—how much does it reveal and how much does it cover? Make-up, perfume, jewellery, tattoos, piercing—all these could at times be used as strengthening body boundaries and are therefore worthy of checking by the psychotherapist.
- **Gestures and postures**: The manner in which clients are sitting, standing, moving, and physically conducting themselves could indicate their boundaries. The body psychotherapist will develop sensitivity and curiosity towards these messages.
- **Boundaries of the body**: The skin, the sense organs, the hair, the face, smells, and breathing: all these express boundaries in unmediated and direct ways—the boundaries between inside and outside. Body parts on the border between inside and out are of immense importance to the boundaries of self. Repetitive skin conditions, short- and long-sightedness, unpleasant mouth odour—such information (and more) could, for example, provide the therapist and client with crucial data regarding the boundaries between inside and outside, and the body psychotherapist might relate to these directly, as part of the material which is shown and handled in the clinic.

This bodily observation, which is grounded in anatomic and physiological knowledge, on top of the psychological understanding, provides the body psychotherapist with an invaluable set of tools for examining the boundaries of the client, and the boundaries of the therapeutic relationship. This observation serves as a compass for navigating within the stages of therapy and to better gauge the degrees of interventions offered by the therapist, as well as supporting the therapist in either flexing the self-boundaries of the client, or strengthening them—depending on what is called for. I believe that acquiring training and experience in such somatic elements of self-boundaries could profoundly enrich psychotherapists from other modalities.

Grounding: three levels of leaning

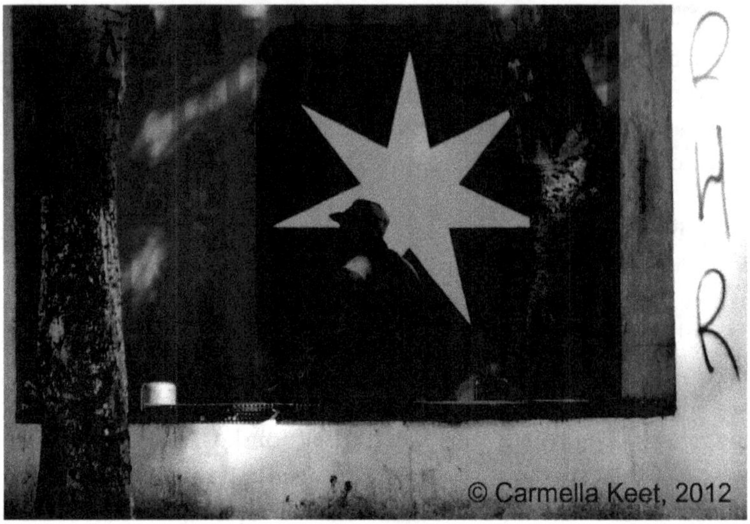

Rene Magritte's window opens to eternity
it only seems to be of this world
In reality: it is a sacred dense portal;
angels move through it
And insects of infinity creak from both ends
happiness and love can move through
And suffering, it too can cross the divide of Magritte's window

—Asaf Rolef Ben-Shahar

Grounding is a central concept in body psychotherapy, describing the bodymind interaction with its environment. To illustrate the meaning of grounding, I would like to turn our attention to the shamanic worldview. Shamanism emphasises the interconnectedness of all levels of being, a unity which manifests in actual connection between us and the world around us. In the shamanic worldview, we are connected with energetic strings emerging from our bodies upwards (to the sky), downwards (to the ground) and horizontally—connecting us to others (Keeney, 2005). These strings affect us by vibrating, and we similarly impact our environment. Thus, the healthy person can directly lean against and connect with the resources of the land (connecting to earth, to the ground, surrendering into gravity), the resources of spirit (connecting with levels of meaning, providence, and faith; surrendering to a force bigger than us), and interpersonal resources.

Grounding therefore portrays the quality of our connection with these support systems: our ability to be supported, to lean against and surrender to gravity (*earth grounding*), to resources of the spirit and to faith (*spiritual grounding*), and to the wider mind opening between us and our fellow persons (*intersubjective grounding*). Body psychotherapy commonly uses the term grounding to indicate earth grounding, but I have chosen to look at these three levels of leaning here and relate to all three as different aspects of grounding.

Earth grounding

> Grounding is an expression of our planetary life. Grounding connects our processes of excitation with the earth, forming us both. Just as the groundedness of a tree routes the flow of sap from earth to leaves and from leaves to earth, so does our groundedness channel the flow of excitement from ourselves to the environment and from the environment to ourselves.
>
> —Stanley Keleman (1981, p. 27)

Gravity is a continuous reminder for both the possibility of bodily life and its limitations. As early as in the womb, gravity is used as an organisational principle—a point of reference against which the tissues can organise—up and down, right and left, in and out. To be aware of our bodily, as well as our emotional, boundaries, we need ground, the capacity to lean against our physical existence: how much force do I need to exercise in order to lift my leg and take a step? How much energy do I need to invest to reach out and touch the other person's shoulder in a way that attracts his attention but does not hurt him?

The concept of grounding relates both to the psychological and the physiological aspects of our relationship with support and the degree of our bodily presence. Alexander Lowen writes: "Not to know how one stands is equivalent to not knowing where one stands or to have no standing as a person" (in Totton, 2003, p. 68). Earth grounding manifests in our connection with our legs; in the ability to remain anchored in our emotional-bodily experience without disconnecting from one aspect or another of our being.

David Boadella, founder of "biosynthesis", describes grounding like this: "The therapeutic work of grounding is concerned with establishing a good relationship between the voluntary, semi-voluntary and involuntary modes of movement and with recreating a more appropriate muscle tone" (1987, p. 15).

As illustrated in the last chapter, moving from lying down (the first two developmental stages) to standing up (the last three developmental stages) involved significant paradigm shifts in our relationship with the ground. When we lay down, surrender to gravity equally spreads over the entire body surface. Practising grounding exercises lying down could cultivate our ability to surrender to support by the ground and to lean into earth more fully. In contrast, vertical posture is much more focused, since gravity then operates mainly on our joints and spine; accordingly the body psychotherapist will apply different practices for increasing awareness to the relationship with earth and strengthening it, both lying down, and sitting or standing up.

The following exercise, inspired by Anodea Judith's (1996) "splitting the earth", will demonstrate earth grounding:

This is an excellent practice to assist us (or our clients) in coming back to our bodies, strengthening our sense of bodily self and connecting to the ground. It is best done barefoot, to directly feel the contact of the body with the ground and to amplify sensory awareness.

1. Begin standing up straight, with the feet spread shoulder-width apart. The feet are slightly inwardly turned and knees are gently bent to avoid locking.
2. With the exhale, apply pressure on the feet downwards and outwards, as if trying to split the earth into two. Let go with the inhale and repeat a few times.
3. Add to this a gentle bending and straightening of the knees: with every inhale bend the knees, and straighten them (together with pressing down and out with the feet) with each exhale. Repeat a few times.
4. When there is greater energy flow to the legs, and the connection to earth is amplified, you might notice changes in body sensations, like pins and needles, streaming, vibration, or temperature changes—or even emotional shifts. Allow each of them its space with as little intervention as possible.
5. The last stage includes adding some sound. Repeat the process: breathing in while bending the knees, breathing out while straightening the knees and applying pressure on the earth down and out. With each exhale allow some sound to come out, ideally lower tonal registers. Repeat it for a minute or two.
6. Notice sensations, feelings, images, and thoughts. Notice your breathing. You may wish to walk about for a while and notice the quality of your contact with earth. Can you note differences from the beginning of the exercise? Has something in your relationship with the ground changed?

Spiritual grounding

Nick Totton and Em Edmondson (1988) coined the term "skying" to describe our capacity to achieve contact with the cosmic and spiritual aspects of our being, which I refer to here as spiritual grounding. Totton (2003) wrote: "Like a tree, human beings function best with their roots in the ground and their branches reaching for the heavens" (p. 69).

As I have suggested before (Rolef Ben-Shahar, 2012b), spiritual practices which lack grounding might be dangerous and indicate escapism, both from connection and from embodiment. Nonetheless, without our capacity to trust, to lean, and to attribute meaning which is not only material we may lose our flexibility and vitality: "Without the sky connection," writes Totton (2003), "grounding will tend to become over-grounding, a heavy, stodgy practicality" (p. 69).

Spiritual grounding does not require a particular religious faith, but instead a willingness to surrender and lean, trusting in the organising principles, trusting in life itself. Nineteenth-century philosopher Franz Rosenzweig wrote: "Just as we are—and no less than that—we are obligated to maintain the boundaries of not-knowing. Indeed, God is beyond all our knowing. Yet even preceding your not-knowing, God gives himself to you, to your call, to your ascending attunement, to strengthening you, to your life—God gives himself to you" (in Bergmann, 1974, p. 219). Spiritual grounding therefore expresses our willingness to open to the unknown and surrender to it, as a leap of faith.

Body psychotherapist Oshrat Kartin-Korman (2011) explored the impact of spiritual grounding on the therapist's positioning:

> Directly linked to the understanding that every belief impacts the person's life, and understanding the person's feeling faced with God's love, which provides him with purpose and meaning, one might say that when a person can sense the love of God, he positions himself differently in himself, in his world, and with his fellow others. A person who believes that God loves him and that he is loved, is differently organised. This inner organisation is expressed in reality through sense of purpose and connection. (pp. 43–44)

Intersubjective grounding

By using the term "intersubjective grounding", I relate to our capacity to lean against another and use another for support, regulation, and growth; to our wiliness to open to a co-created shared self, a wider mind. In biosynthesis, the concept of "facing" (Boadella, 1987) denotes a similar practice of balancing hypersensitivity to the surrounding with hyposensitivity: an emotional-mental-bodily connection to the other through the eyes and the voice, the perception, emotion, and language.

As I suggested in Chapter Five, the willingness to surrender to connection and consciously submit to intersubjective connectedness requires a steady-enough ego structure, since the wider mind threatens the separated and individual subject; the independent self. Notwithstanding the fact that such wider mind could deepen and strengthen the individual, relaxing ourselves into it involves great fear. Surrender, claimed psychoanalyst and musician Emmanuel Ghent (1990), was not a voluntary activity: "One cannot choose to surrender, though one can choose to submit. One can provide facilitative conditions for surrender but cannot make it happen" (p. 215).

In clinical terms, the body psychotherapist is attuned to the client's capacity to surrender to the therapeutic relationship, as well as to her ability to allow for the relationship—and the therapist—to become meaningful in her life. The body psychotherapist may offer interventions for strengthening earth grounding or (according to her worldview) spiritual grounding, thus providing a supportive platform for the client to surrender to the therapeutic relationship. Falling backwards into somebody's arms is an excellent example for such an exercise. Indeed, this exercise has become a cliché due to its wide overuse in workshops and business settings; nevertheless it does cultivate and exercise our willingness to lean and surrender. Sometimes the body psychotherapist might use intersubjective grounding to strengthen the client's connection to earth or meaning. To a great extent, these three levels of grounding condition one another and enable each other.

The creative and innovative psychiatrist and psychotherapist Milton Erickson (Erickson & Rossi, 1989) astutely portrayed the spirit of surrender into therapeutic relationship: "But somehow or another you will realize that you are safe, that you are secure, that there is somebody you know and can trust, and whom you can recognize who will be with you, with whom you can talk, with whom you can shake hands" (p. 31).

My friend and colleague, relational body psychotherapist Elad Hadad (personal communication) drew my attention to the fact that grounding (of any kind), like centring, can either be defensive and reactive, or a cultivated conscious act. Therapists and clients alike may withdraw from connection or from life when threatened, quickly cultivating the "coming home" practices of grounding to actually avoid surrender. To reiterate: despite the fact that grounding is a practice of surrender, it could be used for the exact opposite—to escape surrender and avoid the threat of loss of self within contact. This reactive aspect of grounding is often a defence mechanism preserving the fear of intersubjectivity.

Centring

Centring is first and foremost a stance, a way of being within oneself and in relation to the world. In *The Teachings of Don Juan*, Don Juan explains to Carlos Castaneda the essence of centring:

> *Does* this path have a heart? If it does, the path is good; if it doesn't, it is of no use. Both paths lead nowhere; but one has a heart, the other doesn't. One makes for a joyful journey; as long as you follow it, you are one with it. The other will make you curse your life. One makes you strong; the other weakens you. (Castaneda, 1968, p. 106)

Influenced by Eugene Gendlin's (developer of focusing) concept of *felt*-sense (Gendlin, 1978), psychologist Stephen Gilligan (1997) outlined the first premise of his "self-relations psychotherapy": "An indestructible 'tender soft spot' exists at the core of each person" (p. 4), he posited. Many clients arrived into therapy having tried, time and again without succeeding, to find the same solutions to the same problems: "This suggests that they have lost connection to their center, to their own ways of knowing, to the place where they can feel renewed, resourceful, and confident" (ibid., p. 5). For Gilligan, not only our strengths and resources have a centre; moreover—every emotional-affective experience, including symptoms (bodily or emotional) has a somatic centre and our ability to track it and identify it supports the therapeutic work. Gilligan's work may provide a somatic platform for working with multiple self-states (Bromberg, 1996).

Gilligan's description of our dynamic centre, identifying it as the connection to the river of life, to the potential for flow, was highly influenced by Carl Jung (1934). At the core of this centre, our bodymind defences are inactive, and from there our bodily energy expands and spreads into the body. But life moving and flowing through us is not always pleasant, as it sometimes may even pose threats to our organism: "As life flows through you, it brings difficult and overwhelming experiences at times. So we have the capacity to shut down around the 'tender soft spot,' protecting it from damage" (S. Gilligan, 1997, p. 10). The price we pay for such protection, though, is disconnecting from the flow of life.

Centre is therefore both real and a metaphoric concept, relating to the centre of self as well as our bodily centre (Totton, 2003). Most people intuitively sense their centre around their heart or stomach regions (viscera/gut); the concept of *gut feeling* might be worn, but we can mostly identify gut feelings even if these are sometimes hard to conceptualise and verbalise.

Centring is also a skill, allowing us to rekindle the connection between mind and body functioning, repossessing ourselves as bodyminds. Gilligan (1997) illustrates:

> When a person is feeling stuck or isolated, attention is often concentrated in the head or projected away from the body. One simple principle to restore balance is to center and drop attention lower into the body, its different centers of consciousness, and the earth supporting the body. This principle is central to all martial arts. (pp. 80–81)

Centring skills—the active cultivation of minding our centre and investing in the skill to return to it, cultivating the skill of coming home, are at the heart of most body psychotherapy modalities. We use centring as a way of establishing somatic awareness, of familiarising with our felt sense, and to strengthen our embodiment. Different therapeutic methods offer a variety of ways to sharpen our somatic awareness of our centre, and subsequently use this awareness as a compass (or auxiliary compass), guiding us in life—as well as guiding the therapeutic process.

The body psychotherapist endeavours to assist his client in feeling his centre: to centre himself and relate to his centre. Furthermore, the body psychotherapist cultivates his own practices of centring, using these skills to help him in making clinical decisions—our ability to sense ourselves from the inside can help turn unexplainable intuitions into deep skills of inner consultation, of connecting with the wisdom of our organism.

Two centring exercises are offered here: the first assists us in finding our centre and cultivating it, the second in finding symptomatic centres and working with these.

Centring exercise: coming home

This simple process is appropriate both for therapy and for the therapist who wishes to centre himself before therapy. I wish to encourage the therapists among the readers to dedicate a few moments to centring before a session and notice the impact of centred positioning on their work.

1. Sit comfortably, ensure your clothes are loose, take your shoes off and make sure your feet touch the ground.
2. Place one hand on your chest and the other on your belly, breathing effortlessly to these two regions. Stay there for a minute or two.
3. When breathing is as full as it can be right now, think of a time—in the distant past or recently, where you felt at home in yourself; when it was OK to be who you were just as you were; where you could stay with yourself at ease. Allow yourself to assume the posture and breathing pattern of that time, and check where you sense this inner home in your body. Let the feeling amplify.
4. Imagine that each breathing cycle begins in this very centre, flowing and spreading to the rest of the body, both from within to outside and from outside inwardly. Allow the breath to become a channel through which inner and outer can meet and interact.
5. Is there a voice that could accompany the feeling? An image? A movement? A word?
6. For some people, this sense could be amplified by saying sentences (either aloud or quietly) such as: "I am here, I am present, I am centred, this is me."

Exercise: touching the centre of disturbance

This is a therapeutic exercise (more appropriate for training or workshop setting), based on an exercise by Stephen Gilligan (1997). The process demonstrates working with centres of disturbances—the symptomatic centre of the client, and retrieving connection with the generative and resourced centre.

1. The client shares an emotionally meaningful experience/event/process, which requires processing.
2. Therapist centres himself and listens—less to the narrative and more to his own body. Where does he sense the centre of disturbance in his own body when the client speaks? Where does he experience the difficulty in his own body?
3. The therapist invites the client to check where he experiences the centre of disturbance in his body as he speaks of the experience/difficulty.
4. The therapist asks for permission to touch the centre of disturbance identified by the client. The attention of touch is a declaration of presence: "I am here, with you." In self-relations psychotherapy terminology—we bless the place with human presence.
5. Client and therapist both pay attention to sensations, thoughts, and feelings: share and process. If the exercise is done in a workshop setting than swap roles.

Self-regulation and dyadic regulation

> The best way to heal a forest is to leave it alone. It has its own self-corrective processes that restore the ecosystem. People are the same.
>
> —Gregory Bateson (in B. A. Erickson, 2006, p. 79)[2]

Self-regulation

In the field of psychotherapy, the term self-regulation relates to the person's capacity to maintain systemic balance and retrieve systemic balance. We understand self-regulation as a dynamic and homeostatic phenomenon, an ongoing process of correction and adaptation: an attempt to support the forest in its self-corrective capacities, to leave the forest alone.

But what does it mean to leave the forest alone when we talk about psychotherapy? Does it make the therapist redundant in the process of therapy? Are we simply asked to provide the client with tools for removing the obstacles for healing and regulation and then step back? If so, what about the therapeutic relationship? Does it mean that Bateson understood the therapeutic relationship as only important as a functional means to removing obstacles for flow?

While this model might be appropriate to the early thinking of body psychotherapy, it does not sit well with relational thinking. Moreover, this is a strange statement coming from one of the most significant contributors to systemic thinking and to cybernetics, from the developer of the double-bind theory of schizophrenia (Bateson, 1972), who viewed schizophrenia as a familial rather than a personal disturbance. By deepening our understanding of what Bateson meant when talking about self (or in this instance, the forest), we would discover an almost opposite meaning to the first reading of this beautiful quote, one which is much closer to contemporary therapeutic and relational worldviews than to the earlier organismic understandings of the self. We would see that expanding the notion of self to include the other-than-myself and the environment within it presents a different notion of "leaving things be".

Wilhelm Reich (1942) believed that a person capable of somatic self-regulation will also be emotionally regulated: autonomous, ambitious, motivated, and adaptive. He continued the Freudian perception of moving between the reality principle (environmental pressures) and the pleasure principles (seeking physical discharge for urges and drives, the pressure of the id). As a Marxist, Reich believed that the healthy person should not surrender to environmental pressures without thoroughly examining these, and insisted on maintaining his rights. A man or woman capable of self-regulation could therefore accept other people's beliefs and values without forcing themselves on the other.

Indeed, one of the greatest contributions of body psychotherapy to the general field of psychotherapy concerns somatic self-regulation. Following from Reich's orientation, traditional body psychotherapy placed great emphasis on somatic self-regulation: learning how to better manage and monitor our feelings through attention to our body. Applications of somatic self-regulation have a psycho-educational component: we teach our clients how to down-regulate and up-regulate, how to calm and how to build charge (often by modelling, at other times through active engagement). In a way, traditional body psychotherapy involved practices and exercises for helping the forest to remember its self-healing capacities, helping the person to remember his or her organismic self-organising principles.

The somatic aspects of regulation have been incredibly valuable for the entire field of psychotherapy and particularly to trauma work. Today, many mainstream trauma systems of therapy include, involve, and incorporate aspects from body psychotherapy (including EMDR); this goes as far back as Reich with vegetative therapy and regulating the autonomic nervous systems.

Today, most contemporary body psychotherapists adopt a more relative view regarding bodily self-regulation. Even though somatic regulation is still understood as important, even central to our well-being, other factors might be as crucial, such as emotional regulation, or the therapeutic relationship. Fritz Perls (Perls, Goodman, & Hefferline, 1951), for instance used the term "organismic self-regulation" to describe a person who is able to know, by listening to his body, what he needed. Nick Totton (2005) portrays two main self-regulatory directions: the need for full self-expression, and the need for self-protection.

The character armour (which was extensively discussed in the second and sixth chapters), is of course one way of self-regulating. It is an emotional and muscular holding which allows flow (not ideal, but the best under the circumstances) between self-expression and self-protection, between needs and wants and environmental pressures. Bodywork directed at softening and flexing the muscular armour (or with classic Reichian therapists, at breaking the armour), represents a search for a more adaptive regulation.

Early body psychotherapy related to regulation primarily in intrapsychic (or intra-psychosomatic) terms, which did not include the environment—the therapist and transference dynamics, the quality of relationship, and the dynamic nature of self. The body psychotherapist used skills to support clients in strengthening their bodily regulation. For example, the breathing exercise I offered in Chapter Two, and the breathing exercise for anxiety reduction in Chapter Six can both help clients in developing greater control against anxiety-provoking events. Learning and practising skills of grounding, centring, embodiment, and streaming—all these were at the core of praxis of early body psychotherapy, and are still important skills even for body psychotherapists who are more dynamic, analytic, or relationally oriented.

Relational body psychotherapist Roz Carroll (2009) creatively pointed at the shift in understanding self-regulation in body psychotherapy. According to Carroll, when body psychotherapy opened to analytic influences, particularly those of object relations and attachment theory, "'self-regulation' started to become a more complex, qualified notion. There was a focus on understanding and getting a bodily sense of internalised relationships and the way in which unconscious structures are perpetuated" (p. 92).

In some body psychotherapy modalities, self-regulation still forms the central clinical axis: such as somatic experiencing (Levine & Frederick, 1997) or Babette Rothschild's somatic trauma therapy (2000). It is no coincidence that these methods are focused on trauma work. Strengthening the vertical axis (the intrapsychic) allows for a relatively quick process in helping sufferers reclaim the course of their lives. In many cases, trauma work calls for more focused intervention and is less process-oriented, requiring particular emphases and an appropriate toolbox for "quick retrieval" of life skills. Opening and surrendering to the therapeutic relationship and the therapeutic process is mostly a later process. First we make the world safe.

One of the central questions behind regulation concerns the way we understand the self, and what constitutes the *self*. We can conceptualise the question slightly differently, in light of Bateson's opening quote, and ask what is the forest? Perhaps, in simpler words still, the question is *who is doing what and to whom*? Gregory Bateson (1974) had a very interesting answer. For him, "An individual in a system is always part of that system and is therefore subject to all the constraints and necessities of the particular part-whole relationship in which he exists" (p. 27). Bateson's answer reveals his systemic approach. His self is always understood as part of a larger context. In fact, for Bateson (1979) (as we have observed in Chapters Four and Five) mind is a cybernetic system—including both the intrapsychic qualities (the separate trees, the relationship between the trees in the forest) and the interpersonal connection (the relationship between the forest and its changing environment—including me, when I walk inside the forest). He therefore describes mind as a relational process, "the patterns which connect" (p. 10).

When we allow the other to be understood as part of our system; when we understand the mind as a dynamic process of becoming in the field—as Bateson did, then the psychotherapist can no longer remain a technician of somatic skills applied on the patient. The therapeutic relationship emerges as an impactful central axis and with it, the invitation to dance to and fro between self and mutual regulation. For me, this is a true application of what Reich referred to as the functional identity between body and mind: me, my body, and my mind; you, your body, and your mind; and us, our shared-body, and our shared-mind—all constitute a cybernetic system whose primary characteristic is mental activity (what Bateson considers as *mind*): self-organisation and self-healing.

Dyadic regulation

Chapter Five discussed the wider mind, this intersubjective entity which emerged from, and was co-created by a meeting between two persons, and subsequently created them. I have already mentioned Tronick's notion of dyadic states of consciousness (Tronick et al., 1998) and Stolorow and Atwood's claim (1992) that intersubjectivity challenged the myth of the isolated mind. Wider mind rests on a primordial bodymind experience—on our being born into a dyad. There are many parameters which the newborn baby cannot regulate by himself: bodily (e.g., digestion, immune system, body temperature) as well as emotional. During these stages, the mother (or primary attachment figure) is required to serve as a selfobject (Lichtenberg, 1991), helping her baby regulate himself by partaking in a broader self.

To fully experience our subjectivity, our individual agency in the world, we need an other to relate to, to recognise us and validate us. We also need an other to regulate and validate the other. Relational psychoanalyst Jessica Benjamin (1990) proposes that: "The psychoanalytic process should be understood as occurring between subjects rather than within the individual" (p. 184). The psychotherapeutic process therefore oscillates between the two poles—recognising the other and surrendering into connection with the other (wider mind) and separating and distinguishing ourselves from the other. Each of these movements requires different therapeutic skills: the psychotherapist may assist the client in discovering herself as separate, strengthening her body and mind and her distinguished consciousness through *self-regulatory* tools and processes. The psychotherapist may also surrender to the wider mind, inviting the client into intersubjective spaces, where healing, growth, and regulation are done within the shared centre—at the *dyadic regulatory* fields.

Dyadic regulation is found at the heart of human relatedness. Shuy Grace, my youngest daughter, wakes up at night with a tummy-ache. She cries, tosses and turns in bed, unable to calm herself down. My partner, Tom, reaches out her hand and gently places it on Shuy's tummy. Tom's hand moves with Shuy's breathing cycles, and Shuy gradually relaxes. Another, slightly later example: Zohar is running outdoors, falls and hurts herself. She is bleeding, and starts crying. I run to Zohar, a little anxious and check that nothing is broken (well, I am Jewish after all), that the injury is superficial. She sobs loudly, and I turn my attention inwardly, calming myself down, it's OK. "It hurts and you are bleeding," I say and Zohar nods her head. "And it's frightening, but soon it will be less painful." I hold Zohar and she can sense that I calmed down, and at first it allows her to sob even louder (she need not care for me), and then she calms down too. Every parent who ever managed to calm a distressed child first attended to her or his own anxiety—we regulate the system by making inner adjustments.

At the heart of Allan Schore's groundbreaking research is the argument that infant–parent attachment is aimed at supporting both biological and behavioural regulatory systems (1994, 2003). Analysts Beatrice Beebe and Frank Lachmann (2002) similarly examined dyadic regulation (which they termed interactive regulation), proposing that it involved somatic attunement—bodily sensitivity to facial expressions, eye contact, head positioning, and more. This continuous bodily communication is not only found in mother–baby relationship but is also prevalent in other affective relationships, including therapeutic relationships. Such somatic attunement requires coordinated attentiveness to both self and other. Without such bodily listening, empathic failure is likely to occur. On the other hand, over-attunement could easily result in hyperarousal and anxiety in both parties.

Roz Carroll (2009) suggested looking at countertransference as a systemic regulation phenomenon—the therapist resonated with the client while regulating herself regarding both the wish for connection and the resistance against it. The more we were able to soften and melt our defence against dyadic regulation; the more we were able to surrender to the wider mind—the greater our capacity to create novel experiences and new types of relationships both within therapy and outside it.

I am proposing here that there are two distinctive types of dyadic regulation: *regressive dyadic regulation* and *generative dyadic regulation* (or *mutual regulation*). The regressive aspect of dyadic regulation correlates to what this section was dealing with: a process whereupon the therapist serves as selfobject, regulating the client "on his behalf" or together with the client, not unlike the regulatory examples I gave of my daughters. Body psychotherapists use skills for regressive dyadic regulation primarily when the client is flooded or retraumatised, or when working with regressive self-states. For example, in my work with highly dissociative clients, who are very disconnected from their bodies, a great deal of my therapeutic attention is directed at self-care, breathing, and supporting my embodied processes. I come back home to my body, and from there I am more able to help the client reclaim his body and feel it: I put on my own "oxygen mask" first before helping him put on his, as wisely recommended by emergency and security flight information.

Regressive dyadic regulation mainly includes inner work of the psychotherapist: strengthening her embodied presence, centring, and grounding. The body psychotherapist, who allows for or encourages regressive work, is required to cultivate somatic and emotional self-regulation as part of the dyadic regulation. As exemplified by Roz Carroll (2009): "The ability to regulate intense affect depends upon the therapist being anchored within their own body, able to bear and attend to sensation, and allow spontaneous autonomic shifts to occur. [...] Self-regulation does not mean being totally contained; however, it is a finely tuned flexibility in relation to oneself and another" (p. 102). When the therapist is able to attain such fine balance of self-regulation, she can afford to lose her balance occasionally, to be affected by the client or confused with her clients—she can survive herself and her client within the therapeutic relationship.

But not all dyadic regulation is regressive, and characterised by parental (or attachment) transference dynamics. Dyadic regulation could also be generative—one where wider mind powerfully (and mutually) operates on both parties as subjects—when I and thou becomes *us* alongside I and thou. Generative regulation in psychotherapy is an invaluable intersubjective space, whereupon *we* regulate us, only to discover that the *us*, which was created by us, is far more resourceful, flexible, and able to initiate novel dynamics, than the two subjectivities comprising it.

An example is one incident from my clinical work with Talya, following an unsuccessful intervention, when I offered her an exercise which I knew was inappropriate and would lead to a difficult knot between us. After our session I felt guilt-bound all week. I brought this to supervision, attempting to understand my motivation for this coarse and inappropriate intervention with Talya, yet we were unable to find any significant direction. I arrived for the next session embarrassed and confused. We sat next to each other and Talya shared the uneasy feeling, which had accompanied her all week, and her tendency to dissociate when it was too painful. We were both restless. We came closer to each other, our breathing slowed down a little bit. "You are tense too," said Talya. A new space opened up between us and from this place I could finally understand, with crystal clear confidence, how I tried to cause a friction between us for fear that Talya would dissociate and split, thus leaving me on my own. It was only from our togetherness that I could understand and give meaning to my clinical intervention, and my fear. I shared this insight with Talya. "I too can only understand my splits from within our relationship," she replied. Our wider mind was a platform supporting both of us and providing the two of us with opportunities to work together, and to process the therapeutic material together.

The therapeutic work with wider mind is in principle not a technical one, but it is nonetheless possible to navigate in it therapeutically and methodically. In fact, it is this very positioning, which could be cultivated, and which generates change and healing. Since body psychotherapy comfortably moves between verbal and affective, nonverbal and motoric platforms, it can offer a multitude of ways to open into the wider mind and work within it through *resonance*, sharing, and *embodiment*.

I see the regressive aspects of dyadic regulation as paralleling primary intersubjectivity, which includes symbiotic processes between mother and infant (Trevarthen & Aitken, 2001); transferential dynamics here are therefore primarily parental: between an infant and a parent. In contrast, generative dyadic regulation could be seen as parallel to the secondary intersubjectivity and the Buberian mutual relationship is far more important here. This notion will be expanded both in Chapter Nine (self and mutual regulation) and in Chapter Eleven (on resonance). Thus, while generative dyadic regulation is still done within an asymmetrical frame, it is characterised by mutuality, and could therefore be termed mutual regulation.

At the beginning of this discussion I used Gregory Bateson's poetic call to leave the forest alone so it may heal, letting the natural and organic forces of the forest do their work uninterruptedly. We may understand this as a call for self-regulation, following the belief that, as organisms, the resources for healing and growth exist within each and every one of us as individuals: that every bodymind is capable of self-healing and self-correction. However, if we look at Bateson's philosophy as a systemic and relational position, in fact—a seriously spiritual position—perhaps we can also understand his call somewhat differently.

When we are able to surrender to connection, to open to a wider mind—the resources that are available for us are richer and wider. Leaving the forest alone can thus be understood in almost the opposite way. Allowing the forest to become—by permitting the therapeutic dyad to become—is the most significant therapeutic act (perhaps the only one). According to this view, the major therapeutic task is not helping the other regulate his or her self, but instead encouraging them to become part of the system: an act of positioning and surrender and not one of skilful doing. Once we managed to surrender, we are then asked to let our shared space heal itself, including ourselves within it. The therapeutic relationship, inasmuch as it is an intersubjective phenomenon—a wider mind—carries regulatory capacities. Through these lenses, the self has lost its individual skin-bound definitions: it is no longer the client or the therapist, it is the dyadic dance, but this novel autonomous dance can self-regulate. This practice is not merely therapeutic; it is moreover a leap of faith.

To reiterate my position, therapeutic acts are intended to do little more than to support the creation of a wider mind, allowing it to become and pulsate. All we need to do is to surrender to become part of the forest, and hold our cultivated intent. More than that the forest does not need—we can leave us alone to heal.

Presence

> "Farewell," said the fox. "Here is my secret. It is very simple: It is with our heart alone that we see rightly. The essential is invisible to the eye."[3]
>
> —Antoine de Saint-Exupéry, *Le Petit Prince* (1943, p. 72)

Body psychotherapy is an affective psychotherapy which was incubated in humanistic nests—therapists are willing to work with highly affective emotional and somatic states with their clients, and might at times encourage affect or amplify affect. Thus, the emphasis on the here-and-now of the therapeutic experience is pronounced. Frequently, the body psychotherapist will invite the client to speak *from the experience* rather than to speak about it, since talking about something tends to dissociate the narrative from bodily sensations, from the emotions which emerge from it, and from allowing the experience to be present within the therapeutic relationship, here-and-now, and between us.

The concept of *presence* is deduced from the affective emphases on the here-and-now. The term is connected both with embodiment and flow, and it describes a therapeutic stance and positioning more than a therapeutic skill or act. There are, of course, techniques and practices to encourage somatic and affective presence—in Gestalt therapy, for instance, the therapist might ask clients to amplify and pronounce a movement they made during their speech; a focusing therapist might invite clients to bodily feel what they just said, here-and-now, in their own body. However, these important tools are derived from the therapeutic stance: it is the therapeutic position that defines these interventions and not vice versa.

We may wonder what are the conditions which enable us to be in relationships: particularly in therapeutic relationships. Or, as posed by psychologist Yorai Sella (Keet, Sella, & Ziv-Beiman, 2013): "How do we cross the divide between two people? Between the fact that I am present here, in my bodymind and somewhere over there—in space, on the futon, the chair, the couch, there is another person. [...] What is the right act for approaching the interface and crossing the divide?" Body psychotherapist Nick Totton (2003) suggested that in order for us to be open to connection and offer connection to another person we ought to be present to ourselves—to be able and willing to assume responsibility for our sensations, emotions, our capacities, and limitations—and accept these even when they are not pleasant. According to Totton, presence is therefore a precondition for offering a therapeutic relationship.

Psychologist Daniel Stern (2004) argued that affective psychotherapy—particularly modalities, which pay attention to bodily and nonverbal processes, are a more promising platform for presence and therapeutic transformation than merely cognitive processes (Ramberg, 2006). In fact, I believe that there is a gap between the depth of contemporary psychoanalytic and relational understanding regarding the importance of nonverbal and affective processes, and its clinical translation. Relational body psychotherapy may offer skills and practices that might be used to cross the divide between contemporary theoretical conceptualisation and the clinical practice.

To be fully present, we need to be available to our sensations and our sensations need to be accessible to us: to be present to another I need to be a body, and to manage to be in my body, I need another. Somatic presence is a position of grace and surrender: I submit myself to the onslaught of sensations, feelings, and thoughts of both my individual body and the dyadic body created between us. Philosopher, artist, and ecologist David Abrams (1996) phrased it elegantly: "The living body is the very possibility of contact, not just with others but with oneself—the very possibility of reflection, of thought, of knowledge" (pp. 45–46).

Embodied presence therefore requires surrender. Psychoanalyst Emmanuel Ghent (1990) eloquently expressed the quality of surrender to presence and flow. Surrender, for Ghent, was:

> An experience of being "in the moment," totally in the present, where past and future, the two tenses that require "mind" in the sense of secondary processes, have receded from consciousness. Its ultimate direction is the discovery of one's identity, one's sense of self, one's sense of wholeness, even one's sense of unity with other living beings. (p. 216)

Psychologist and aikido master Richard Heckler (1984) further elaborated on centre: "When we are connected with our body, the present moment comes more into focus and we can then begin to make decisions from there. [...] When we wonder about a direction to take, or an alternative to assess, we can consult the intelligence that resides in our body" (p. 12). Later, Heckler described the quality of such bodily presence within a relationship: "Contact can take almost any form as long as we bring an energetic presence to the form. Contact is how we are with somebody or something. Presence, which is our embodied awareness, is the mother of contact" (ibid., p. 119).

Somatic transference and countertransference

Anywhere we go, we take all our previous relationships with us; together with the knowledge we acquired through these connections. Within us we carry our mother and father, our siblings and our teachers, the heartbreaks we have known and the hopes for a better future, which we cultivated. Past experiences, particularly from our formative years, are the lenses through which we now view relationships. These lenses are not merely passive filters; instead these are active agents in contributing to the manner in which we create new relationships and position ourselves within them—both now and in the future. Psychoanalyst Harry Stack Sullivan (1954) illustrated it thus: "Even though only two people are actually in the room, the number of more or less imaginary people that get themselves involved in this two-group is sometimes really hair-raising" (pp. 8–9).

I believe that transference dynamics cannot but be part of relationships; that transferential dynamics are inevitable since we relate to the world through our previous experience of the selves we have partaken in—we were created in relationships and bring those remembered selves into any new connection. Psychoanalyst James McLaughlin (1991) presented a similar argument: "The transference ghosts of the past are never entirely laid to rest" (p. 613). As we are faced with new relational challenges, triggering affective and somatic activation, those "transferential ghosts", so argued McLaughlin, "return in fresh shape to revive shades of significance I had long forgotten I knew" (ibid.).

The transference of previous relationship patterns to new connections carries both pathological risks and curative potentials. The pathological aspect manifests in *repetition compulsion* (Freud, 1920g). At worst, transference prevents us from enjoying and benefitting from newly formed relationships since we only relate to our internalised models, creating these time and again in the present moment. For example, I may see my vicious maths teacher from primary school in every authority figure I meet, and hence fail to enjoy a good teacher or a good therapist. In discussing Jung's affair with Sabina Spielrein, Jungian analyst Gadi Maoz (2010) claimed that Jung confused the relationship with Spielrein, not understanding that even when they no longer defined their relationship as therapeutic it was always therapeutic de facto. "Psychotherapeutic relationships cannot completely terminate; therapy can naturally end but it continues in transferential terms in ways that are forever different from what we may call 'real relationships'." Jung, continued Maoz, like Breuer with his treatment of Anna O, did not know at the time how to deal with erotic transference without wounding his patients (and forced termination of therapy is wounding), engaging in repetition compulsion of the very injury the patient came to attend to and repair.

At best, transference dynamics provide us with therapeutic possibilities for psychic emancipation: a chance to work through and learn to relate differently to our past; to liberate the ghosts of our fragmented past from its repeated patterns: when even a momentary liberation potentiates genuine change. I believe that in every repetition compulsion there is a wish to tread new paths, and when we find supportive and facilitative relationships, which can concurrently contain transferential material and challenge it, we stand a real chance of changing some cyclical and wounding patterns and creating novel, new movements.

The paradox at the heart of the therapeutic relationship is a fertile ground for particular transference dynamics. On the one hand, therapeutic relationship offers deep and intimate relationship—we speak, in private, about our deepest wounds and injuries, our heart's yearning and fantasies. On the other hand, this is an essentially asymmetrical relationship, and only one side consistently shares its pains and needs. These aspects are anchored in an asymmetrical contract: within clear boundaries of time, space, and monetary reward (the Summary—The Relational Matrix, further expands on the intricacies of the therapeutic relationship). Indeed, every human relationship is subjected to transference dynamics, yet the therapeutic relationship is unique in its contracted commitment to place such influences at the heart of the work: to name them, work with them, and do so (hopefully) without shaming either party.

At the dawn of psychoanalysis, transference was seen as a unilateral event, whereupon the therapeutic dyad became a stage upon which the client acted her primary experiences and the reactions evoked her experiences. Thus, the therapist and client developed a relationship, which at some point repeated the same patterns yet was willing to learn, understand, and hopefully repair the distorted relationship (or, in Freud's (1914g) language—remembering, repeating, and working through). This complex phenomenon in which the client transferred past experiences (mainly with her attachment figures) to the therapeutic relationship became the basis of psychodynamic work.

However, it was already Jung who challenged the absence of the therapist from this transferential equation, when he portrayed the analyst as deeply involved in the therapeutic process (Field, 1996). Sándor Ferenczi (1930), too, argued that the transference phenomenon was bilateral: the therapist's biographical and historical transference dynamics inevitably influenced and shaped the therapeutic relationship as well as the client's. Today, different developments in psychoanalysis make extensive use in the way the therapist expresses her biography within therapy.

Relational psychoanalysis, and the modalities from which it emerged, related to transference dynamics very differently from Freud. In relational thinking, the therapist, the client, and the therapeutic dyad all became active players in a thrilling and unravelling drama, both genuinely attempting to come close to a subject-to-subject relationship in the here-and-now. I am not at all certain that attaining such a position is entirely possible, yet we can come close to it, and strive to work towards it. The relational premise is that emergent material in both client and therapist is relevant to both parties, as well as to the therapeutic relationship, or as relational body psychotherapist Michael Soth (Asheri, Carroll, Rolef Ben-Shahar, Soth, & Totton, 2012) argued: "Therapy begins with an enactment." Stephen Mitchell (2005), for instance, went even further to suggest that if the client could not "get under the therapist's skin", then the therapeutic horizon was inherently limited. In assuming such a position, relationalists follow psychoanalysts like Hans Loewald (1986) who boldly wrote:

> I believe it is ill-advised, indeed impossible, to treat transference and countertransference as separate issues. They are the two faces of the same dynamic, rooted in the inextricable intertwining with others in which individual life originates and remains throughout the life of the individual in numberless elaborations, derivatives, and transformations. (p. 276)

Transference dynamics are both limiting and enabling at the same time. Our previous relationships enable us to engage in our current relationships, yet at the same time they limit their scope and taint our current relationships with the shades of previous connections. How do we carry those previous relationships within us? How do these patterns of relating manifest inside us and in our contact with others? Are we only manifesting these as mental and emotional patterns? Could these relationships be internalised solely as cognitive or psychological structures? Body psychotherapy argues that transference is primarily a bodily phenomenon. Muscular armour in particular and bodily holding patterns in general *are* the way we embody the history of our lives and the history of our previous relationships. Nick Totton and Allison Priestman (2012) reiterated this position; they wrote: "Transference is thus, not only a psychological, but also a bodily process, a function of implicit procedural memories of childhood relationships, learnt complexes of physical response held outside consciousness and in part repressed from consciousness" (p. 39).

Surrender to relationship always takes place in a bodily context. Our bodily presence is at the heart of our positioning and relating to another human being. We give ourselves or withhold from giving ourselves first and foremost as embodied beings. Relational body psychotherapy claims that transference and countertransference, inasmuch as these are primarily unconscious phenomena, will express themselves also in body sensations, muscular tension, movement, temperature changes, proprioceptive experiences, and in other bodily dimensions (Appel-Opper, 2010; Asheri, Carroll, Rolef Ben-Shahar, Soth, & Totton, 2012; Rolef Ben-Shahar, 2008a, 2008b, 2009; Soth, 2005; Totton & Priestman, 2012).

Exploring the impact of trauma therapy on the therapist, relational body psychotherapist Elad Hadad (Hadad & Rolef Ben-Shahar, 2012) described the following incident:

> The uncomfortable bodily sensations began about two months after I started seeing Michele, an energetic woman who sought therapy following a chain of similar professional failures. A moment after saying goodbye to the previous client, my right shoulder blade started to hurt, limiting my mobility. The tension spread further and affected my breathing, which became agitated and flat, as well as my jaw muscles that tightened up; these patterns remained with me throughout the session and for a while after it too. I found myself feeling hypervigilant and very alert, confronting Michele too often, sometimes aggressively so. I felt that my responses were inappropriately proportioned and that I needed to better regulate myself before sessions, particularly as Michele claimed she felt neither anger nor resentment. It was only later that Michele disclosed that she was sexually harassed by her previous employer four years ago. Allowing ourselves to work more gently, Michele could feel her terror of potential violence, and later own her urges to hit her boss "till he bled" and "tear his flesh" with her teeth. My own tension soothed as she owned those bodily experiences. (p. 53)

Hadad and I related to this incident, writing:

> Understanding countertransference as a psychophysiological phenomenon might be both threatening and enriching. On the one hand, it gives an immediate and serious weight to the term "taking our clients home with us," thus demanding rigorous self-care and mindful self-regulation. On the other hand, it opens a window for the possibility of knowing our clients "from the inside." (ibid.)

Chapter Nine will provide clinical vignettes of working with somatic transference and countertransference.

Exercise: in the body I know—somatic organisations of emotions

This simple exercise is aimed at cultivating skills for increasing sensory awareness, and minding the way we organise ourselves somatically. It relates to the concepts of embodiment and somatic awareness which were discussed in this chapter. I recommend doing this exercise sitting or lying down. Additionally, I suggest you avoid choosing extreme emotional conditions, to prevent flooding and allow an appropriate learning environment. I have chosen here four basic emotions, and intentionally avoided working with fear, which requires different therapeutic skill. Naturally, you are invited to swap the emotions, add others, or alter the exercise to better fit the training or therapeutic encounter. I would also like to recommend that you complete the exercise with a pleasant feeling.

1. Close your eyes and allow yourself a moment or two of rest without doing. Direct your attention to breathing, and observe it sympathetically, without attempting to change it or influence it in any way.
2. Imagine a time in your life when you felt *angry*. Let yourself remember the context—what happened there? Who was involved? Etc.
3. Assume the posture and bodily gestures, which accompanied *anger*—not merely the visible movements, but also the inner, visceral ones. What happened to your breathing? To eye contact? Which areas of your body are you particularly mindful of now? Where can you sense tension? Where can you sense relaxation?
4. Let go of the *anger* bodily organisation by gently shaking the body, stretching your limbs, and taking a few deep breaths. Can you identify the cluster of bodily sensations comprising the emotional organisation of *anger*?
5. Repeat stages 1–4 with excitement, sadness, and joy.

Notes

1. Rumi's poem is reprinted here with kind permission of Coleman Banks, the translator.
2. Bateson's epigraph from *Milton H. Erickson—An American Healer*, is reprinted here with permission of co-editor and copyright holder Betty Alice Erickson.
3. Thank you to Miriam Nelken who helped with the translation.

PART III

CLINICAL

Teach me, god, to bless and pray
For the shine of ripened fruit, for a leaf in decay,
For this freedom: to see, to sense, to breathe,
to know, to yearn, to fail and stray.

Teach me tongues to sing your blessing and praise
For each cycle of moon, for renewal of days,
Lest my day today is as it was before.
Lest my life is spent in habitual haze.

—Poems at the End of the Road, *Lea Goldberg* (1973, p. 154).

Traditionally, bodywork and body psychotherapy were primarily recommended to clients for whom "talking" psychotherapy was inappropriate ("difficult" clients, or those who were uncomfortable with verbal therapy), or for clients with rigid defence mechanisms, for whom words easily lost their meaning. Contemporary body psychotherapy has become much more sophisticated, subtle, and updated with psychotherapeutic advances on the one hand, and somatic content on the other. New research, for example, suggests (Rothschild, 2000, 2004) that body psychotherapy is highly suitable for trauma work. Attention to body sensations, to breath, and even gentle touch might provide clients with a sense of safety, security, and grounding—all essential for recovery (Eiden, 2011). Body psychotherapy can also be the modality of choice for clients who could not speak or for those whose speech was not coherent (Zack, 2013). And it can even be a powerful modality for couple therapy (Keleman & Adler, 2000; Kessel, 2013).

The vertical (intrapsychic) entry point into body psychotherapy proved easier for many practitioners who were interested in somatic practices yet apprehensive about integrating these within their clinical work. However, relational interventions in body psychotherapy are more overreaching than procedural somatic exercises or effective trauma techniques. Body psychotherapy is an appropriate modality for a variety of clients who seek (want/need) to undergo a significant exploratory therapeutic process and wish to incorporate their bodily experiences within it; to engage in the language of the body alongside their cognitive and emotional engagement.

Part III (Clinical) opens a window into the body psychotherapist's clinic. Chapter Eight will allow us a rare glimpse into sessions of six experienced body psychotherapists, each bringing their unique voice and therapeutic style, demonstrating part of the theoretical and clinical richness offered in body psychotherapy. The other chapters in this Part will demonstrate some of the basic clinical skills of the body psychotherapist, through case vignettes accompanied by discussion. Part III (Clinical) exemplifies and brings life, body, and spirit into the theoretical discussions of Part II. You are cordially invited to engage with the material through thinking, moving, feeling, and sensing, and I hope you will enjoy getting to know my dear colleagues, and me.

CHAPTER EIGHT

Embodied therapeutic dialogues

Ich lebe mein Leben in wachsenden Ringen

I live my life in widening circles
that reach out across the world.
I may not complete this last one
but I give myself to it.

I circle around God, around the primordial tower.
I've been circling for thousands of years
and I still don't know: am I a falcon,
a storm, or a great song?

—*Rainer Maria Rilke*, (1996, p. 48)[1]

This chapter represents a unique attempt to engage in dialogue with other body psychotherapists, in light of their presented clinical vignettes and psychotherapeutic interventions. I have asked six experienced body psychotherapists to send me a short clinical vignette which described a single therapeutic session. Some of these encounters are from the beginning of the therapeutic process, others from the middle of a long-term psychotherapy process. I have chosen psychotherapists with different training backgrounds, different therapeutic emphases and styles, and different therapeutic skills. However, it was important for me to choose therapists who shared a psychodynamic understanding, even if their clinical orientation was not psychodynamic.

Each therapeutic encounter described in this chapter is divided into four sections: in the first part each therapist presents, in his or her own language, the therapeutic session. In the second part I shall offer a short analysis, explaining the therapeutic process through relational and embodied perspectives. The third part reviews the therapeutic skills unique to body psychotherapy as they manifested in the session. Last, the fourth part is a dialogue between the therapist and me concerning some key questions I had regarding the therapeutic interventions offered by him or her in the session. The names of all clients were changed, biographical details have been sufficiently changed and the therapists secured explicit permission to publish this material. Some of these case vignettes are amalgamations of a few clients. More than presenting the clients, the chapter wishes to allow you a genuine glimpse into six clinics of experienced body psychotherapists, so that you may appreciate the depth of the clinical work and the creative variety herein.

Body psychotherapeutic work within a therapeutic team: Guy Timor

Guy Timor is an EABP accredited body psychotherapist in private practice, as well as within the therapeutic centre, Kfar Izun (Balancing Village) in Israel.

The therapeutic encounter

Guy writes:
Tara is a twenty-two-year-old patient, who was admitted to Kfar Izun following a psychotic manic episode. Tara has been in psychodynamic psychotherapy for a few months. About eight weeks prior to termination of her treatment at the centre, her psychologist offered for me to accompany Tara's treatment with body psychotherapy in addition to her psychodynamic work. The main rationale for inviting me was Tara's boredom and apathy, which she was unable to shift. Her psychologist believed that body-oriented psychotherapy might mobilise Tara's apathy.

My clinical work at the centre tends to be different to my work in private practice, but the challenges of working with Tara began before even seeing her. I had to take into account many challenging factors: not only did I join the treatment team as a secondary psychotherapist and in parallel to her psychodynamic therapy, but it was also a short-term therapy towards its ending. Additionally, Tara's parents heavily pressured her to "improve and recover" while she was still in therapy.

These conditions, in addition to the manner Tara's complaint was presented to me by her psychologist, brought me to hold a therapeutic agenda before I even met Tara: an agenda, which is not representative of my current therapeutic style, but one which characterised my earlier training in body psychotherapy: I have made up my mind to work with Tara from a biodynamic body psychotherapy position, allowing bodywork to be the central therapeutic axis of our work. Excited, I planned on bringing into therapy mainly bodywork, movement, and breathwork techniques, encouraging Tara to experience herself and what emerged from the practices emotionally. I further planned that cognitive processing of our interventions will be done both with me, and with her primary psychodynamic psychotherapist. Therefore, before even meeting Tara for the first time, I already embarked upon therapy with a few inner splits: between opening to the encounter and having a set treatment plan; between different styles of therapeutic work; between psychodynamic therapy and technical work, and more.

Tara's body structure was muscular and hypertensive. She looked strong and present on the one hand, yet her chest and shoulders were inwardly pulled, contributing to a younger, almost teenage look. Tara complained of feeling bored and uninterested, and said that she needed stimulation to feel alive. She shared with me that during her mandatory military service she felt similarly, yet upon her release from service she was very dynamic and functional: she travelled abroad, came back to Israel and worked, travelled again for a few months and then came back due to her psychotic crisis.

When Tara spoke of the time she spent abroad and about her manic psychosis, she seemed filled with a sense of vitality: her tonality was amplified, her eyes widened, her chest opened and expanded, and her shoulders pulled back. Witnessing her power was exciting, and I felt jealous at this sense of liberation she experienced after her release and during her manic episode. However, when Tara spoke of her current feelings she felt and looked turned off, she lacked motivation or ambition to do anything at all. Tara wished to leave the therapy centre, just as she wanted to finish her military service, to liberate herself from a limiting structure and live in a world full of stimuli and possibilities. As I sat with her, I began to feel charged with ambition to act, wishing to help her retrieve something of the quality of presence and vitality, which I witnessed from her, and she claimed to have completely lost. "I only wish to be active again and do things so that my energy comes back," Tara said.

As Tara shared her wish to emancipate herself from the limiting structure of Kfar Izun, I noticed she was pulling in her shoulders. I made a link between the limiting and oppressing authority and the closed in and limiting chest, and asked Tara to close her eyes for a moment and direct her attention to her body following this statement. Tara reported sensations around her heart; she could sense her strong heartbeats and a feeling that something wanted to open up and express from the chest outwards, from the body upwards and outwards.

I was listening to Tara's description and wanted to offer movement practice, which would have allowed the front part of her body to expand and open. In my mind I planned quite a manipulative Reichian bodily intervention, where Tara would lie down on a chair supporting her back, in a way that arched her back, forcing the front part of her body—particularly her abdomen, diaphragm, and chest, to expand and open. While thinking about this intervention, I asked Tara to allow herself to feel the part of her that wished to open and notice what happened in her body. It was then that a shift in her inner experience occurred, and Tara reported that something in her told her to slow down and be more patient and less anxious; that the fire inside her burned at its own pace, and that this turned off feeling she felt would change too.

As I listen to the shift in Tara's experience, a powerful and quick shift happens in me too. First, I understand that the manipulative therapeutic intervention I thought of was inappropriate at the moment, and that Tara is in a sensitive and vulnerable place. My presence changes from a more masculine and dominant to a containing and feminine one. Her soft and gentle voice, which asks for time and calms down the speed, opens a deep understanding in me—I realise that I have identified with Tara's active voice, wishing to speed up and move forwards (a voice that could be seen as her superego, the internalised voice of her domineering parents). This voice was deposited with me as early as the preliminary conversation with her psychologist, and I came armed and prepared for active intervention that would help "wake Tara up" and push her forward to do and act.

Once Tara notices her softer voice, needing more patience and time, something in her body too softens and the tension in her shoulders eases. She opens her eyes and starts talking. Tara shares some of her current conflicts with me: should she hurry up and enrol for the next psychometric test (which is required by universities) despite the pressure and anxiety it creates in her life, or could she possibly consider enrolling for the following test, which will allow her to slow down her pace? Her parents expect her to enrol for the coming test.

Tara's short narrative and her body movements exemplified the psychopathic developmental stage she was at, reflecting an inflated character structure and its dilemma between being grown-up and big, and being small. Her parents pushed her to quickly grow up and become independent, and Tara could easily identify with their voice. As a part of the transferential enactment, I arrived in advance—full of goodwill to help her push forward and accelerate her pace. Luckily, a moment before we began our "catalytic therapeutic intervention", I invited her to close her eyes and tune-in. Tara discovered in herself a different voice, one which wanted her to grow in her own rhythm and pace without being prematurely speeded; a voice which could trust itself to be OK. This is the one-year-old toddler learning to walk, rejoicing in her discovery of her capacities and independence, yet still needing others to recognise her limitations, her pace, and the fact she was still young.

Later that day I met her primary psychotherapist who told me that, following our session Tara announced, both to the team and to her parents, that she had decided to postpone her psychometric test and to avoid stressing herself up unnecessarily.

The therapeutic process

Working as a part of therapeutic team in an inpatient institution poses many challenges to the psychotherapist, as well as allowing for collaboration and liberty of praxis, due to the strong holding potential in the teamwork, and the inpatient frame.

Guy described how his transferential positioning was created even before therapy began, as part of an organisational countertransference with Tara. He was invited in advance as the "Wizard of Oz" to enter an already established therapeutic relationship and intervene—with his body in "a place where words cannot reach". It was difficult not to be swept into the river of transference he was invited into, holding great risks for repetition compulsion and collusive enactment. Guy boldly and honestly shared with us the inner dialogue, which characterised the early days of body psychotherapy: an intense search for therapeutic interventions (what to do!). Guy's experience and skill manifested in his ability to recognise the enactment in time, severing the chain of collusive action and parental pushing.

Guy begins his description in a diagnostic position, including *body reading*: a somatic observation of Tara. He listens to the therapeutic narrative while also gathering diagnostic information—on the bodily-developmental level as well as on the muscular level. Guy illustrates how, alongside speaking he also looks for coherence or dissonance between the narrative and the resonant. This type of attention is a basic body psychotherapeutic positioning—of attending polarities—*between foreground and background*.

When Guy managed to establish a pattern of connection between the content of their dialogue and Tara's bodily expression (boredom, a sense of being turned-off, and needing stimulation to avoid collapse), he turned her attention to one of her sentences ("I only wish to be active again") and asked her to close her eyes and focus on the emerging body sensations when she spoke that sentence. Here, there are already a number of somatic interventions: *closing the eyes* was an invitation to tune-in and introspect, but it also involved letting go of control (seeing what's going on) and required trust in the therapist. Repeating the sentence inside and bodily focusing both helped Tara in establishing an affective experience, allowing for *focusing, embodiment,* and *affective amplification.* All these enabled Tara to focus on the relationship between the emotional patterns she spoke about and the bodily expression of tension *vs.* collapse. Closing her eyes also interrupted with the transferential bubble, which wrapped the therapeutic dyad, allowing Tara to establish connection with her true self.

Tara was able to report bodily sensations and identify her bodily impulse in them. She identified a wish to open up and expand, and in so doing was already able to bridge her somatic dialogue with her emotional narrative, even if this connection was only preliminary. Tara's eye closure and her sharing assisted Guy in recognising the paternal countertransference, with which he arrived—and this was where a novel and emergent dynamic began, different to the repetition that took place until that time. This impressive skill was a clearer example of contemporary (primarily relational) body psychotherapy, where bodily interventions derived from the therapeutic relationship and understanding of transference dynamics, and not as an independent agenda. Just as Tara "came home" to herself, so did Guy, in a parallel process, "come home" to his updates and attuned therapeutic identity.

The transition Guy exemplified between the primary wish to intervene and the inner process he shared with us, could be seen as parallel to the evolution of body psychotherapy: from a naïve discipline, primarily interventionist, where the body of the client was the centre of diagnosis and intervention, to a dynamic therapeutic approach where the three bodies (the body of the client, the body of the therapist, and the dyadic body) were present and analysed, as well as the somatic interventions and skill—but these stemmed from within the relational context, taking transferential complexities into account.

Guy considered offering a therapeutic *movement process with the thoracic segment.* Such intervention was another example of an *affective amplification.* It was also a classic Gestalt intervention: *externalising and amplifying* one aspect (or both) allowed for a dialogue to become more distinguished, as a means for *integration* (Houston, 1995). Such intervention was based on the assumption that an organised and educating dialogue could be conducted body-to-body without cognitive involvement.

As soon as one bodily aspect was properly expressed (the part which wanted a breakthrough and sought liberation)—the other aspect got a chance to be heard too and the dilemma arrived in therapy; for the first time, Tara was able to express another quality of feelings—she discovered a slower and less pressing pace. She was able to observe the pattern instead of merely participating in the movement between inflation (or mania) and collapsed deflation (or depression). Discovering her slower pace enabled Tara to establish a new transitional space, which she would indeed need to cultivate, but she not only understood it but also experienced it in her body.

It is important to note that Tara's new dynamic—slowing down instead of speeding up, being supported rather than doing it all on her own—appeared against all odds: the entire therapeutic system was deeply immersed in the countertransferential collusion of "advancing" Tara and accelerating her release and recovery. Eight weeks before termination of her hospitalisation, the psychologist felt that therapy had reached an impasse and invited Guy to join in and "shake Tara up" from her apathy and boredom. In my opinion, it was Guy's astute somatic attunement to Tara and to himself which made the transformative shift in therapy: for the first time Tara listened to herself and broke the spell of projective identification—allowing Guy to subsequently listen to himself and to her. This experiential integration received therapeutic processing and in the same week Tara managed to exercise her transitional space and changed her habitual position.

Guy identified the third developmental stage (between autonomy and support) and the inflated character structure (both presented in Chapter Six) as central to Tara's presentation, and appropriately directed his therapeutic interventions. He related to the information received from the body (a youthful inflated and collapsed body) as crucial to understanding the psychology and organisation of her psychotic crisis, and actively sought to encourage Tara's going into the world without giving up support.

Transferentially speaking, it is interesting to look at Guy as a "dad" who entered the system (while Tara was in therapy with a female psychologist, "mum")—at first colluding with wanting to push forward and accelerate therapy (by opening the chest through movement and touch). But he also allowed the other movement to take place (stopping, observing, waiting)—and mainly encouraged Tara to recognise how well internalised were her parents' expectations of her. Faced with kinder and more patient parents (the psychologist and Guy), Tara found her own voice.

Therapeutic skills

Body reading: The abilities to recognise bodily patterns, muscular armouring, and bodymind character structure are central to the work of the body psychotherapist. Body reading is a diagnostic skill, which accompanies the body psychotherapist throughout therapy. Attention is given both to large-scale body structures, such as character structure, body armour, and chronically held body segments, and to smaller-scale structures, such as minute shifts in breathing patterns, holding muscles and releasing them, and other somatic expressions. In fact, body reading is an important channel for receiving information throughout the therapeutic process. Chapter Nine exemplifies and expands on some clinical applications of body reading in psychotherapy.

Working with body segments—the thoracic segment: The therapeutic work with movement, which Guy considered offering, relates to energetic charge and discharge (see Chapter Seven). When a bodily pattern expresses itself, the associated feelings and thoughts often surface. Choosing to work with the thoracic segment was called for, since this was the somatic platform for externalising Tara's conflict—this is where she both inflated her chest and held it up, as well as the place she collapsed from. Additionally, through body reading, Guy identified an inflated character organisation, and one of the central corresponding places for holding chronic muscular tension with this character structure is the chest (and particularly the mobility of the sternum). We may compare Guy's considered bodily intervention to therapeutic enquiry regarding authority figures when the therapist notices power struggles in the transference dynamics. In both cases parallel processes will develop—the emotional and somatic power struggle in both cases would have invited the therapeutic dyad to attend to what was happening in the present moment, and to recognise that as familiar relating patterns of the past.

Working with somatic countertransference: Guy identified his preliminary wish for affective amplification. In accordance with the approaches presented in this book, body psychotherapy assumes that affective experiences allow for learning "through the muscle" (and through the flesh) and for cognitive-emotional internalisations and integrations which are qualitatively different to insights gained by processes, which dissociate from the experience and the body. We believe that learning through the body is a potent way of understanding and creating change. When sensations, feelings, or conflicts are insufficiently distinguished, the therapist might encourage amplifying them, to help and better understand the nonverbal undercurrent dynamics. In fact, *affective amplification* is meant to strengthen the dialogue between dissociated aspects of the self (or between different self-states)—between somatic, emotional, and cognitive processes. When Tara closed her eyes and reported strong heartbeats and wishing to leave, the parental countertransference was at its peak, manifesting in Guy's desire to be active and push Tara into action (and in his reported jealousy). Guy paused before intervening, and when Tara shared her wish for a slower pace, he was able to identify his somatic countertransference for what it was, and as a result abandoned the proactive physical intervention and prevented further enactment. In this case, processing transference material was primarily internal (inside the therapist). The sections with Ronen and Elad demonstrate different clinical use of somatic countertransference which is brought into the therapeutic dialogue. Further examples of working with somatic transference and countertransference are also given in Chapter Nine.

Foreground and background—in words and flesh: Confronted with a conflict, in which only one side of it is spoken or seen, the body psychotherapist might offer a Gestalt dialogue between the parts. A Gestalt dialogue is a dramatisation of internal dialogue—externalising and amplifying it for the purpose of cultivating intrapsychic relationships (between different parts of the person). The dialogue could sometimes be clearly stated and structured (for example, the empty chair technique), or more bodily—allowing one part to express itself, assuming that amplifying the conflict will create clarity for the entire pattern. While foreground and background are concepts from Gestalt therapy (Perls, 1969), working with polarities is common in many modalities of body psychotherapy. Many muscles in the body operate in pairs, holding polarities (for example the biceps and triceps muscles in the arm) and complementing each other's operation; some bodily rhythms also appear in polarised pairs (e.g., the autonomic nervous system, sweating and shivering, charge and discharge). There are varied tools in the somatic toolbox for working with polarities, including breathwork, movement, touch, somatic attention, and spatial organisation. Body polarity is a natural platform for working with foreground and background patterns of the Gestalt.

Externalisation and amplification: As I mentioned earlier, Guy's plan to work with Tara's background-foreground polarity was through behavioural and bodily amplification and externalisation. Externalisation and amplification are complex skills in practice, but are relatively simple to understand: they aim to amplify affect in order to clarify emotional contexts; a way of gaining insights through experience. Externalising as the means to internalise insights is an important movement in body psychotherapy, which places great emphasis on experiential bodily learning. Externalising an emotional tone until it becomes a conscious bodily behaviour, and inviting the client to "Show me" and not just "Tell me" is an important tool, which can increase body awareness and bring forth insights, which directly derive from the experience. Indeed, Guy did not exercise this intervention, but his mere planning of it, while working through the somatic countertransference, created—in my opinion—a similar process of externalisation and amplification in the therapeutic field, allowing Tara to find a new inner direction. Through externalising (of behaviour) the body psychotherapist endeavours to encourage internalising (of insights) and integration (between behaviour and understanding).

Shutting the eyes: Guy's invitation to Tara to close her eyes was seemingly a simple intervention; yet it was a powerful one. Closing the eyes asks of the client the confidence to let go and demonstrate her relaxation in her body—to show the therapist that she could, immediately and in her body, let go of control and trust the therapist and the therapeutic process. When the therapeutic relationship is stable enough, or when sufficient trust was established, closing the eyes may give the client opportunities to sense herself slightly independent of the other. Tara was so attuned to the environment's expectation of her, that closing her eyes provided her with a rare chance to feel her own body, her own rhythms, without attempting to read into Guy's facial expressions and posture, unconsciously extracting from these his wishes and acting accordingly. Shutting her eyes assisted Tara in decreasing what psychiatrists Lewis, Amini, and Lannon (2000) called "limbic resonance"—the deep, unconscious, and bodily attunement to the other.

Body focusing: Cultivating attention to the body and focusing on body sensations are skills common to most body psychotherapy modalities. When listening to body sensations and momentarily letting go of the attempts to understand complex feelings and thoughts, it is sometimes possible to liberate both client and therapist from defensive rationalisation, potentiating learning and change via experience. Developing a sense of our bodily self (or the felt sense (Gendlin, 1978)) is a valuable asset and resource for client and therapist alike.

Embodiment: From their very first encounter, Guy offered Tara bodily interventions which included attending to her body, noticing movement, exploring rhythms and movement, and shared processing of these. All these interventions included elements of familiarising with the somatic self, with embodiment—and indirectly—with getting to know the therapist. As we could see from the vignette with Tara, the somatic aspects of both her resources and her symptomatic behaviour were highly available to her, which made it possible to process emotionally, as well as advance cognitive change in a relatively short time. It is important to note that body psychotherapy is not necessarily quicker than other psychotherapeutic models, but sometimes somatic dialogues can offer direct and unmediated access to unconscious material, available to the therapeutic dyad which is willing to work with these.

Bodymind integration: The interventions Guy suggested to Tara were accompanied by psychotherapeutic conversation and processing—some during the session and some later (both with him and with her primary psychotherapist); the bodily experience went hand in hand with a therapeutic dialogue, promoting internalisation and integration. Thus, the client could attribute constructive and therapeutic meaning to the bodily interventions. Without such processing and dialogue, these experiences might have become interesting yet irrelevant experiential episodes, or unsafe and extreme experiences.

Embodied therapeutic dialogue

ASAF: Thank you for sharing this courageous session with us. Let us begin with your requesting Tara to close her eyes; can you explain the rationale behind this request?

GUY: This intervention rested on a basic sense of safety and security I felt with Tara from the first moment, as well as on the preliminary countertransference I arrived with, which directed me to treat Tara actively and in a matter-of-fact style, occupying a "doing" therapeutic stance.

However, generally speaking, closing the eyes allows the client to make a direct contact with his inner processes. He is less distracted by outside stimulation, or by eye contact with the therapist, and he can therefore turn his attention away from his thoughts to his sensations and feelings with greater ease. When Tara spoke of feeling boredom and apathy, we have naturally discussed it; but when she closed her eyes and examined what was happening in her body at the time, she noticed her heartbeat and desire to awaken her vitality and breakthrough. There was a movement from the belly upwards, which later changed—all these were easily identified by Tara and therefore available for therapy.

For most people, noticing this information is much harder with open eyes, particularly for a person like Tara whose centre of energy is outwardly attuned, and whose sensitivity is directed to the (perceived) expectations of the person she is with.

ASAF: I was very moved by the way you identified your countertransference and how you managed to avoid traumatic repetition. I wonder about working as a body psychotherapist next to psychodynamic therapists. Without sufficient understanding, it is easy to assume that body psychotherapy is necessarily more active (touch, movement, breath) than psychodynamic work. How do you manage to manoeuvre within this systemic transference and projective dynamics? Does inviting you to work alongside psychodynamic psychotherapy not always involve a fantasy (of the client, of the primary therapist, of the centre) of "the touching magician" who could move mountains?

GUY: Working in Kfar Izun is different from my work in private practice. The clinical work here is more focused, taking into account the point in time the patient comes into therapy. The initial stage of therapy is first aid: dealing with grounding, coming out of crisis, and beginning the recovery; the second stage is the heart of treatment, and here we deal with themes and content, which emerge from individual and group therapy; the third stage focuses on planning for life outside the institution and structuring a functional framework for the post-termination time.

As a body psychotherapist who often works alongside psychodynamic psychotherapists, I take into account the stage the client is at and the reason for choosing to incorporate body psychotherapy. Other alternatives exist here too, including art therapy, dance and movement therapy, or even therapeutic gardening.

Additionally, there are other factors influencing my work, like the interaction between the psychologist (or case manager) and the secondary therapists, and of course the information I receive and hear about the clients from therapists and guides in the village.

All these factors cannot but influence me as I commence therapy, and make a genuine attempt to meet the client from an authentic and personal place.

The body helps me meet the client in a manner that is more connected to what she feels at the time, rather than my preliminary agenda. When I direct her attention to her body, I also direct my attention to my own body. The sensations are never wrong (although their interpretations may be). They help us clarify the subject we speak about and arrive with at the meeting, and we can therefore discuss the emergent experience. My role as a therapist in Kfar Izun requires me to consider both information I acquired about the patient from other members of the treatment team, as well as the therapeutic stage she is at, and sometimes I try to connect the two.

Regarding the "magician" transference, working in Kfar Izun is a humbling experience. If magic does happen, it happens from a place of connection and a special relationship between the patient and the village (including the team, the patient, the patient's family, and the sea in the background). So today, even when this transference and projections are active, I am seldom activated by such countertransference, or I can identify it and change it quite quickly, as demonstrated in the work with Tara.

ASAF: You speak of your wish to offer a movement exercise very early on, and the processing you have internally done as a response to your transference. Can you elaborate?

GUY: My initial thought was to move from one end (inflated and collapsed chest) and provide Tara with the experience of where she wanted to get—and noticing what sensations and feelings would emerge in the interface between the two thoracic postures. But once I recognised that my wish was an expression of my parental countertransference, then my identification with the parental voice was broken. This parental voice was pushing, judging, and opposing Tara's real need at the time to slow down. My identification started as early as I was invited to join the team.

ASAF: Could you elaborate on your clinical considerations in balancing between talking and bodily interventions? For instance, how did you decide how much space to allow for conversation through words, and how much through body dialogue?

GUY: Tara came to see me for short-term and highly focused therapeutic work, and was already seeing a psychologist for biweekly psychodynamic psychotherapy. I entered the team as a secondary therapist, with an a priori bias towards experiential work, one which tended to have limited verbal exchange and cognitive processing. Tara was highly motivated to discover and work experientially, and dialoguing with somatic processes carried great potential for discovering the unknown. I was continuously attentive to Tara's words, as well as what I saw and received from the body, which helped me ensure we were working within her safety boundaries.

Bodywork did not come at the expense of conversation. We kept on talking and working verbally throughout the session. Verbal exchange accompanied the bodily experience giving words, images, and conceptualisations of feelings and memories which emerged for Tara throughout the process. But the verbal dialogue was not the leading agent of the process. As you have noted, Tara naturally and organically made connections between the bodywork and the relevant biographic material—the sense that she speeded up her growth (psychometric test) although she didn't really want that. The bodily experience provided her with an important insight, quickly, autonomously, and within her own processes.

ASAF: Could you tell us about the way you processed the bodywork with Tara? What kind of processing was done with the movement work? How was this processed with her primary psychotherapist?

GUY: The main processing resulted in Tara making connection to her psychometric test and deciding to postpone it. We checked if she was familiar with this pattern of behaviour, and I was curious to know how she felt about the voice inside asking to slow down. Some of the processing was done within the team and her primary therapist. When I shared my insights with her psychologist she could identify and connect with the themes we dealt with, and let me know it was one of the central aspects which emerged in the family therapy, where Tara's parents pressured her to terminate treatment quicker so she could commence her academic studies. As I stated, already that day Tara told her psychologist about her decision to postpone her enrolment in the psychometric test.

Holding the body in mind and embodiment: Ronen Levy

Ronen Levy is an EABP accredited body psychotherapist, working in private practice.

The therapeutic encounter

Ronen writes:
Craig, a thirty-five-year-old man, sought therapy to work with two prevailing difficulties in his life—emotional eating which manifested in overeating, and anxiety attacks. Craig's anxiety attacks increased in both frequency and severity whenever Craig was losing weight.

Craig is a tall and broad guy, his demeanour slow and gentle. He makes personal and warm eye contact, yet every so often his gaze seems suspicious and hesitant. His breathing is heavy and laboured, even when there is no seeming reason for distress or tension. His forehead is forever held in a frown, and it seems as if his lips move to narrate his thinking, as if Craig is rolling his thoughts in his mouth. Due to the distance and disgust he feels towards his body, attending the body and his concrete bodily experience are approached gently and cautiously. The following is an example of a characteristic session, from the second year of our therapy.

"I'm destroying my own body," was how Craig opened one of the sessions. "I've already managed to lose some weight, and here I topple into the same place … I fill it up with food, more and more, until I can no longer take it, and then I am left with a strong feeling of defeat—once more I've lost the battle to my body."

As I am listening to Craig, two questions pop into my mind: what made him lose his selfhood to such extent? What is he really telling me when he spoke of disappearing against this cruel desire which controlled his life? Also, how come I am sitting with this utterly pleasant man, who is able to establish such a comfortable and comforting relationship with me, who accepts my interpretations and therapeutic directions, yet I feel nothing at all? My affect is flat, and moreover, I am completely in my head—cannot feel any body sensations, except for some arbitrary associations about what I will have for lunch today: Craig's session takes place just before my lunch break.

Craig talks about a food-related experience, when he is faced with a table full of delicacies: "Everything looks so good; you can explode by merely tasting what's on it … and me? I cannot stop, it is as if in the moment there is food on the table I am trapped; I'm in trouble; there is no chance against this richness. I cannot say no, I cannot stop."

"Do you notice that when you talk about food, and generally about your body, you use a lot of military terminology—destruction, traps, defeat, explosion, trouble, battles?" I ask. "Yes, it is a real war," Craig responds. "Where else do you have such combative dialogue?" Craig speaks about his complex relationship with his wife, identifying the resemblance between his relationship and his mother's relationship with his father: "Dad was never at home or available for us. We always needed to walk on eggshells next to him, and my mother protected him fiercely. I had much more fun when dad was not around." Craig's father was critical and verbally violent towards his mother, and the mother was protective of the father even when he attacked her and Craig.

"You know, Craig, what you say is very interesting," I say. "It sounds like both your father and your wife are like this inner part inside of you, the one that dominates you, controls your life, and defeats you—not unlike the way dad defeated mum, disrespecting her or you, not allowing space for your feelings. Perhaps your father's controlling voice was internalised by you and is now controlling you, particularly around food," I suggest.

This demolishing paternal voice was joined by another cruel voice, which Craig internalised over the years; a voice which negated Craig's right to choose and weakened his sense of self. During his childhood, Craig underwent a brutal sexual assault of which he told nobody, since he was certain no one would believe him. Craig was not only left alone and isolated with this story, but the perpetrator was also a close neighbour and as Craig grew up the neighbour was a subject of Craig's admiration. How symbolic, I thought, excited by my insight; Craig is destroying his body just as it was destroyed before, and his own voice is unheard, evaporating and disappearing in thin air. Over the years, Craig sadly learned to identify with the aggressors in his life, enacting them in his relationship with himself, particularly in the way he nourished himself and ate.

Craig nodded and for a moment seemed far away. "Where are you?" I asked, and Craig replied, "Dunno, it's like I'm not really here today. I know that we are speaking about important subjects, but it goes by me, not touching me." I reflected what I heard to Craig: "So, we are touching on subjects which you can recognise as important to you, but you are not here, you cannot feel them." Inside me I thought for a moment that we were re-enacting Craig's relationship with his father—while I was excited by the insight of this unfolding drama of his relationship with dad (Craig and his dad were both alive in his body), Craig himself disappeared, defeated by my dominant presence. Instead of offering an interpretive response, it felt that Craig was really asking for me to see him, allowing him to take space. It seemed like an appropriate moment to attend to the body.

"And what's happening in your body, what can you feel in your body?" I asked. Craig's immediate response was confusion. "Body … I dunno … can't really feel it … you know I always struggle with these feelings about the body." "I know," I replied, "but nonetheless please try to return to the here-and-now. We speak and I feel that something inside really struggles to feel and experience what we're talking about." Craig agreed, and after a few moments of silence, where he looked concentrated and engaged said: "I feel heavy; I feel tightness and distress in my chest. It's sad, I was deprived of so many things." I suggested to Craig that we remained, together, with this sadness, but a few seconds later Craig continued: "And it makes me angry, how come they never saw me? Let alone dad, who was distant anyways, but mum, who I always thought of as considerate of me and close to me? Suddenly I understand that she too did not see me, I was so lost." "Let's stay there for a moment, Craig," I replied after a few more moments of silence, where Craig seemed to have regained his connection with himself. "It's true; it's very difficult to feel all this … but it's the way to reclaim yourself for yourself."

Like his body, Craig's feelings too were subjected to continuous onslaught. Providing space for his emotions was not a safe option for him. His greatest fear was of losing the control, which he had cultivated for years. Craig attempted to control his feelings too, and correspondingly attempted to control the spontaneous and involuntary muscular expressions. Craig's panic attacks represented it clearly, acting as an alarm, alerting him of forthcoming changes. It was here that Craig was unable to control. Whenever he felt emotional during therapy, his immediate response was withdrawal and dread. I, on the other hand, felt increasingly alive in my body. I understood that Craig's mind and body/feelings were polarised, and that his intellectual defences needed validation and respect; he bodily invited me to slow down, lest he had a panic attack.

Indeed, Craig is now feeling sad, and alongside the sadness he is angry too, and his body is uncomfortably moving as he expresses his emotions. I can identify the slippery slope of enactment, which may be embodied any minute: I invited Craig to feel, and he agreed and followed, despite the difficulty to come back to his body. And I was left wondering—was he placating now? Has Craig's domineering father, who is embodied in me, grabbed me again, from the very place where *I* felt safe, from my emotions? It seemed like an important place to check transferential dynamics with Craig.

"How slippery feelings are," I told Craig. "We feel for one moment, and then it slips way between the fingers." "Yes," Craig agreed, "I feel that too but I don't know why." I attempted to share: "You know, Craig, I thought that the moment where your feelings started to dissipate and you withdrew from your body and your emotions, was the moment I invited you to stay with the feelings and be with them."

"Maybe," Craig replied. He seemed interested, so I continued: "I thought that perhaps you experienced ambivalence towards my invitation—on the one hand it provided you with an opportunity to feel more, to be more present, and one part of you really wanted it; but perhaps it was also unpleasant that I told you what to do and how to be … I thought of your father for a moment … I felt his presence in the room, speaking from me." Craig responded: "I really didn't know why it was so difficult to listen to your request. Logically I knew you were OK, taking me to the right place, but inside me I resisted, something in me didn't want you to be right." "Can you feel this struggle in you now, in your body?" I enquired. "Of course," he answered, "it feels like the same struggle—with my body, with my father, with food, with my wife—a fight without winners—a lose-lose situation." This time, when it came from Craig, I believed him. I felt that the insight derived from the experience. Craig breathed deeply; "Wow," I said, "I can really feel you here now. There is something in this struggle, which protected you and helped you remain connected with yourself, even if it required you to remain stubborn and rebellious. I understand that you are telling me 'Ronen, a little slower if you please …'." Craig smiled, concluding with "Now I understand that you understand me … I feel relieved." I felt that we were, finally, together.

The therapeutic process

Psychologist and bodyworker Yorai Sella (2005a) listed five dimensions, in which the body psychotherapist's practice is focused. The first dimension was the possibility of mental representation of the body in the therapist's mind—*holding the body in mind*. Ronen's vignette clearly illustrated this dimension.

With painful honesty, Craig presented his violent relationship with his body—a battle of victories and losses, and mainly power struggles. Ronen allowed us a glimpse into his inner processing and mentalisation while listening to Craig: on the one hand Ronen was interested in Craig's violence and self-neglect and on the other he used his own sensations to better decipher the enacted dynamics. Ronen identified his flat affect—his lack of emotional responsiveness to Craig's story, and was curious about the gap between Craig's emotionally charged communication and the way it affected (or did not affect) him. Thinking psychodynamically, Ronen connected this gap to therapeutic dynamics, and appropriately considered it as worthy of shared exploration. In this initial internal dialogue we can already recognise skills of *embodiment, working with somatic countertransference, and mental representation of the client's (and therapist's) body in the therapist's mind*: Ronen was curious about the way his body and the client's body were alive and enacted in him and were expressed in his consciousness.

Ronen reflected to Craig the violent language he used to dissociate between himself and his body. This reflection presupposed the dialectic relation between bodymind and body–mind (see Chapter Five), that is: bodymind unity was where we started from and splits between body and mind deserve to be marked and enquired upon. When Craig was able to make connections between his relationship with his body (a body which defeated him) and the early patterns of relationships in his body, Ronen managed to bridge the interpersonal dynamics (Craig-his wife, mum-dad, dad-Craig, and later neighbour-Craig) with Craig's violent relationship between him and his body. Ronen understood this toxic nourishment (or internalisation of the bad breast, to use a Kleinian terminology) as organised communication: through the wounding nourishment, the body repeated the historical injury via embodied identification with the aggressor.

When Ronen offered this transferential interpretation to Craig, he mentioned that Craig seemed "far away". I consider Ronen's comment as an energetic and somatic evaluation, based on *body-reading, resonance,* and checking embodied presence. Ronen was interested in Craig's affective presence. Ronen demonstrated his psychodynamic skill by identifying the potential for repetition-compulsion of placating and disappearance in relation to an authority figure. In fact, by merely noticing this potential, a new movement was created in the field (in the intersubjective body), and Ronen offered a therapeutic intervention in directing Craig's attention back to his body: *somatic focusing* in the here-and-now as a way to attain bodily awareness and *affective amplification*. Craig struggled to feel his own body but Ronen encouraged him again and *shifting from thoughts into sensations* enabled Craig to gradually recognise his sensations. When Craig finally had some space to sense his somatic sense, new insights emerged regarding his internalisation of aggressive relationships. It seemed that the transference dynamic changed and Ronen too was more embodied as he empathically validated Craig's experiences.

Later on Ronen identified Craig's ambivalence in responding to Ronen's suggestions. Indeed, Craig accepted each of Ronen's suggestions and offers, but he did so hesitantly. When Ronen was passive, Craig was lost; yet when Ronen was active—Craig contracted and withdrew. Ronen and Craig together unravelled their transference dynamics (and homeostatic relationship); to make space for a new movement inside the enactment, Ronen allowed himself to "fail" and acknowledged his empathetic failure in being too quick for Craig. Assuming responsibility for "the failure" (inside the transference) and apologising was a significant relational intervention: following this intervention Craig was able to accept Ronen as a subject without placating him. We could feel how, if only for a moment, a novel and unfamiliar dynamic was taking place.

Therapeutic skills

In addition to Ronen's psychodynamic work, his empathy and interpretation, validation and reflection, we could identify in his presented work a number of body psychotherapeutic skills.

Embodiment: Ronen checks, time and again, his capacity to bodily experience his client's communication, as well as Craig's ability to do the same. Embodiment is used here both diagnostically and as in intervention. When Craig is emotionally flooded, directing his affect into the body allows for a more integrative and less overwhelming experience.

Working with somatic countertransference: This is arguably the central focus of the psychodynamic body psychotherapist. Ronen's work with transference dynamics begins with his identification of the flat affect. Through dynamic interpretations he suggests to Craig that his disconnection might be seen as an enactment. Ronen understands transference fields as somatically alive, and body attunement allows him to identify somatic countertransference and work with these with impressive speed and skill.

Holding the body in mind—mental representation of the body in the therapist's mind: Every session (and therapeutic process) requires us to make distinguishing and focusing choices: choosing where the therapist directs her curiosity, her attention, and her "therapeutic antennae". The body psychotherapist elects to pay attention also to the body, but this is not solely the concrete body she is faced with, but also the symbolic manner in which the body is held in the mind of the therapist—holding the body (client's and therapist's) in mind. Ronen holds Craig's body in mind as a significant aspect of Craig, not only his thoughts and feelings. Ronen accompanies Craig in discovering his sensations and reconnecting with his body; he identifies Craig's capacity to sense his own body (and to create an internal representation of his body) as central to the therapeutic process.

Body reading: The vignette allows us to see how the therapist uses bodily observation throughout the session, to check the client's presence, to monitor affective levels and the capacity to contain the session's material. Body reading provides the therapist with powerful monitoring and regulating tools.

Resonance: Resonance skills concern turning our body into an amplifier of the wider mind, the intersubjective body. When we resonate, we attribute each aspect of our experience, including sensations, as also relevant to the relationship and to the client. Ronen is highly attuned to his own bodily processes, and his interventions are guided by this listening to the body. For example, when Ronen fails to feel his own body, he utilises it as important therapeutic information. By self-regulating, the resonating therapist creates a change in the shared body (the therapeutic dyad) by offering dyadic regulation. Chapter Nine expands the discussion on dyadic regulation and Chapter Eleven discusses the therapeutic use of resonance.

Somatic focusing and shifting from thoughts and feelings into sensations: Throughout the vignette, we can see how Ronen refocuses on his own body and consults with the information retrieved from sensations; he also invites Craig to do the same. The invitation to shift from thoughts and emotions to sensations is not because the latter ones are hierarchically superior, holding "the truth", or because these are more accurate. Instead, sensations offer an alternative way in, through a less trodden path. Ronen aspires to establish a connected and integrated dialogue with Craig where thought, emotion, and sensation can all have their place. When Craig is able to turn his attention to his body and sensations (to tolerate the affect), his separated self becomes more distinct, and it is easier for him to identify his feelings and at the same time to surrender into connection.

Affective amplification: Amplifying a feeling or thought assists to create greater clarity, to foster insights, or to assist the client in acting differently in the world. Affective amplification is learning by experience, which characterises many therapeutic modalities and not just body psychotherapy. Affective amplification attempts to create integration and movement between witnessing an experience and associated and vital presence (being "in" it, and "outside" the experience). Ronen's initial reflection of the combative language created affective amplification, as well as his invitation to feel the body (and also, to stay with the "no body"). Affective amplification can be cathartic, but it is not necessarily so—it can also be expressed by merely agreeing to remain with whatever affective material is present, permitting its appropriate expression within the therapeutic relationship.

Embodied therapeutic dialogue

ASAF: Thank you Ronen for your open and vulnerable sharing. At the beginning, you describe feeling completely in your head. What does it mean and how exactly do you feel it?

RONEN: In a therapy session based on intimate connection, I strive to feel alive; emotionally, sensorily, and associatively present in my inner world. When a part of my inner world is suppressed or hard to sense I begin to question the quality of connection and its components.

When I sit with a client, I examine my style of listening and my presence in his company. To be in my head means to be intellectually present, as if I am in the middle of solving a complex crossword puzzle. Moments like these are characterised by tension in my forehead while my body from the neck down feels as if it was waiting; my vital levels and my capacity to sense myself are both low, and I am scarcely present in my body. In a situation like this, my motivation is much more understanding-oriented than affective; I am curious to know, but am less willing to experience.

Such dissociation calls for examining: is it a reaction to a client who somehow threatens me and therefore I emotionally withdraw (reactive countertransference, like Winnicott's (1971a) vindictive mother)? Sometimes, like in this case, the response is actually a part of the attachment style of the client, accurately corresponding to his intrapsychic and intersubjective experience in the world, and with me specifically.

ASAF: When Craig dissociated, you decided to invite him back into the body. Why did you choose to do this and not offer a transferential interpretation?

RONEN: My ability to foresee the value of transference interpretation rests on the client's affect in any given moment. If I notice a relatively flat affect, interpretation would not be my intervention of choice, as it is not supported by feeling and can therefore remain purely intellectual, thus perpetuating itself. In Craig's example: I would have remained the clever, knowing, and powerful authority figure and Craig the weak and defeated client/child. In a situation like that, interpretation can expropriate Craig's embodied feelings from the intellectual interpretation. Indeed, for some clients the mere interpretation can activate affect in ways which generate movement and change. However, from my experience with Craig, I have learned that he is able to generate greater value when a prior emotional infrastructure was established, into which we could later pour transference understanding. Additionally, it is highly probable that transference-related insights will spontaneously emerge from Craig during significant affective moments, with very little intervention on my behalf, as we noticed in the example above.

Furthermore, what I am most curious about as a psychotherapist is offering the client an opportunity to experience new interpersonal connection; transference interpretation is merely a means to that end, and is not a goal in itself for me. With Craig, it was sufficient to mark the undercurrent transference process. When this was done by owning up to my empathic failure, our relationship tightened.

ASAF: When Craig manages to sense his body, he reports distress and tension in his chest, and then speaks about his grief and anger with his mother. How do you connect these sensations with his insights?

RONEN: It seems only natural that when an emotion has more space, insight will follow. When we feel more alive, our inner world immediately reorganises, and the same happened with Craig. One of my premises as a body psychotherapist is that by giving more space in the therapeutic field to emotional content, we create a movement in the client's associative world and therefore increase the chances for emerging insights. As proposed by Daniel Stern (1985), when the sensations of the emergent self are validated in therapy, the entire experience of self is reorganised. The moment Craig felt sufficiently secure with me to let go of his isolated and intellectual defences, new and clear body sensations emerged. Following these body sensations, Craig could experience a clearer and fuller affect and meaningful insights proceeded shortly. Craig's emergent self was accepted and validated, and he was therefore able to renew maturation processes which were historically disturbed and arrested.

Additionally, Craig displayed a masochistic (or dense) character structure, and as a body psychotherapist I understand that recognition and validation of his emotional and bodily needs are of crucial importance. During moments of validating his emergent affect and sensations, he has a rare opportunity to adopt a more adaptive organisation, which challenges his previous form and fixated character structure. When the transition between one form and another is appropriately timed, as we can see with Craig, insight will spontaneously emerge.

ASAF: I was moved by the end of your dialogue, which was very complex. It seemed that you were locked in a catch 22: either you were a good initiative therapist (father) who therefore defeats Craig, or a hesitant and passive therapist (mother) who gave up on Craig. You managed to find a way out by allowing yourself to fail without being defeated, but paid a price of self-disclosure and deep sharing. How did it feel to expose yourself and your vulnerability with Craig?

RONEN: It felt like playing. It was not clear that I could play with a "heavy" client like Craig, but something in his pleasant presence helped me in entering a playful position. It was not always a fun and pleasant play, but a real play. I think of the session like building a sandcastle on the shore. Once the sandcastle is built, meticulously done and near perfect, a wave comes in and washes everything—and we need to start afresh. Playing with Craig challenged the predisposition of giving up and feeling that there was no hope in contrast to being full of dubious security and knowledge. I felt either helpless and hopeless or omnipotent and all knowing. Gladly, I was able to retain the insight, that my feelings and positions were mostly expressions of transference dynamics and projective identification, which I had to tolerate and survive.

In fact, I felt like the therapeutic holding process with Craig was a rite of passage of sorts, an affective test sent from Craig, which allowed me to feel aspects of his suffering. If only I could pass his test, I thought, we would be able to finally come closer. The last test of this rite of passage was, as you mentioned, self-disclosure—sharing myself, my vulnerability—my frustration, and my unwillingness to occupy the winning party of this game, and instead share my desire to play for play's sake; to play for connection. Sharing myself and my vulnerability with Craig, while maintaining my presence and therapeutic position was very moving for me, since I felt I have finally managed to provide him with a novel model of intersubjective connection, as well as with a different and healthier intrapsychic presence than the internalised attitudes of his previously relationships.

ASAF: Your work is very psychodynamic. What is your edge as a body psychotherapist?

RONEN: As a body psychotherapist, I enjoy a two-sided communication between my psychodynamic and my somatic understanding. On the one hand, I attempt to understand the dynamic processes taking place in the therapeutic space, and on the other hand make use of these understandings in the here-and-now and with the client also through bodily interventions, which validate these understandings and provide ample opportunities for emotional reorganisation in the body and vice versa.

I am influenced by dynamic thinking and theory as well as by bodily thinking. I search for bodymind patterns in my clients (in their behaviour, affective depth, thinking style, and bodily expressions) as well as for attachment patterns. Psychodynamic understanding assists me in gauging the parameters ahead and I initiate my therapeutic interventions accordingly. As a body psychotherapist I see the dynamics taking place in the present—and expressed not only in the narrative, but also in the body. For instance, I recognised Craig's body pressed into the armchair, his breathing held, and his difficulty to feel at ease in his body, which was particularly pronounced when his body responded spontaneously.

My therapeutic interventions can be psychodynamic or somatic. With Craig, for instance, I offered reflections and interpretations for his relational re-enactment; however, I also offered him a new arena to express his spontaneous urges: his affective, associative, sensory, and motor drives. When these drives become more conscious, the client will develop a stronger and more organised nuclear self, one which can experience oneself in the body in an established and secure manner.

During sessions, I feel as if I am invited to dip into the inner world of my clients. I take this dip with my body, mind, and soul. From this dipping, new therapeutic ideas and directions emerge, which are not limited to the verbal sphere but are instead enriched by other communication channels. Theoretical knowledge supports my diagnosis and my clinical decisions, as well as the interventions I offer to my clients—and by leaning against theoretical and clinical grounding I get to enjoy the two bodies of knowledge: the psychodynamic and the somatic ones.

Like a bridge over troubled water—building bridges: Ruth Ben-Asher

Ruth Ben-Asher is a senior clinical psychologist, offering supervision and individual, couple, and family psychotherapy, and specialising in trauma work with somatic experiencing.

The therapeutic encounter

Ruth writes:
Sylvia, seventeen years old, was a pretty and aesthetic young woman of average height and compact body structure. She came to therapy on her own initiative following her insight that she was running away from something, after she "ran away" from a relationship that lasted a few months, and from other opportunities.

At four and a half years, Sylvia accidentally swallowed a strong cleaning detergent, which burnt her oesophagus. She was immediately transported to the casualty department and from there to intensive care, where she was sedated and put on a respirator. A further attempt to save her oesophagus caused more damage in addition to an already spreading infection. Sylvia (together with her parents) had undergone a series of surgical operations in Israel and abroad, while throughout the years—until she started school (at six and a half), she expressed her clear opinion, made difficult decisions when her parents were hesitant (e.g., which kind of anaesthesia she would receive, intravenous or respiratory) and more. When I met her together with her parents it seemed that even though more than ten years had passed, her parents too were still post-traumatic and very worried for her.

To our first session Sylvia arrived in shorts, a pink vest, and slippers. She wore very gentle and natural make-up. I was impressed by a charming and delightful girl, highly motivated to do therapy. Sylvia asked for help in connecting her body with her mind and soul: she wanted to bridge the girl who underwent all these operations and the young woman she came to be, rather than looking at the world from the outside: "I always knew that I had plenty of surgeries, but it is like I have a cut in my life—there's Sylvia who had all these surgeries, and there's me. And there's a cut. When did I start? … I started in first grade …"

The following description is taken from our tenth session.

Sylvia tells me about Ted, a new boyfriend. He saw her scars and touched them. "He said that he wasn't bothered by them, but I don't believe him and I told him so," Sylvia continues. "It doesn't make sense that they don't disturb him." "And you?" I ask. "It happened to her, to this little girl. It didn't happen to me. There is a cut, a wall. When my parents told you what happened, you saw—I was all curled up, and when mum pointed at my tummy I couldn't listen anymore." "You really knew how to take care of yourself," I reflect to Sylvia. "Yes. Suddenly I realised it did not happen to some other girl. I realised that it happened to me!"

I choose to use Sylvia's image to see if we can gently approach the trauma: "It seems that there is a small hole in the wall, allowing for some information to come through and reach you." Sylvia nods. "And what does it look like, with that wall?" I carry on. Sylvia describes two rivers with a wall between them. Her parents, twelve years younger, are sat next to each other facing her as they tell her about the surgery. There is a hole in the wall. "Allow yourself to listen to their story," I suggest. Sylvia replies: "They're telling me but they speak far too quietly for me to hear. I get up and stand up, walking towards the hole in the wall and trying to listen. Mum still speaks ever so quietly, I cannot understand."

I try helping Sylvia: "Everything is possible in your imagination …" She describes how she stands high and attempts to shout to mum. Mum and dad cannot hear her. I gently encourage her, "If everything was possible … everything is possible in your imagination …" Sylvia is helped by Frances, a friend of her mother, who calls mum and lifts Sylvia so she could reach the hole. Time and again I remind Sylvia that everything is possible in her imagination, until, with the help of Frances, Sylvia manages to cross the wall. She reaches her parents, hugs her father and later her mother too.

"What's happening in your body?" I am curious. "My stomach begins to hurt," Sylvia replies. I invite her to check if she wants to return to stand behind the wall and Sylvia moves back. "What's happening in your stomach?" I ask. "There is a sensation there, but it's not activated, it's off. Turning itself off. My scar is painful, unpleasant."

I invite Sylvia to place her hand over the scar. "It's getting worse," she says, "my scar—an old grey lady wearing glasses—she talks to me—she preaches at me: 'I went through things in my life!' Like a really old person." Together we examine the inner relationship between the old lady and the girl. Finally, the old woman, ninety years old, agrees to tell her. "She tells me the story as if it was a war story." "And can you listen to that?" I enquire. "Yes," replies Sylvia. "The scar says: 'They came with their knives, like in a war, and they opened it up, and it was difficult and they took things out, and stretched it, and reconnected things', and then the scar has won the battle and they closed up the body and put everything back together."

"And what's happening to you right now?" I ask Sylvia, and she replies: "I feel in my body like a very strong medicine is poured into a test tube, filling up my scar just like you put something in a test tube, it's pretty and yellow, warm and pleasant, flowing downwards, like a magic wand it flows inside. My tummy is warm … it's nice."

I can sense my own stomach, and encourage Sylvia to stay with the pleasant sensation; she is calm and opens her eyes: "What I saw in my mind's eyes, like a computer game—I finished a level … I found … it was as if the scar was connected to my body … I can only see it. I cannot feel it in my body …" I am curious about the scar/old lady and Sylvia explains: "She was in a chapter that has just finished. She concluded her role in the book. At the beginning of the chapter I was a girl chasing her to tell me the story. In the end I saw a picture with me sitting on her lap. She was smiling and I could finally turn a page."

Sylvia says that she feels complete, "… as if all the pieces in my jigsaw puzzle are put together." There is a pleasant flow throughout the body, including the scar. As for me, I feel a lot of heat, I sweat and take off my sweater, inviting Sylvia: "Give yourself time to feel this flow … this is healing."

To check the efficacy of our work I ask Sylvia to go back to the river and the wall. Sylvia shares how she runs to hug her mother, and they bathe in the river: "The four of us are on the same side of the wall. Me, mum, and dad are in the water, and Frances watches from outside. She is part of the celebration even if she is not in the water." I check with her: "And when you see this image, what's happening in your body?" Sylvia shares an image of a pink cloud, which fills her body, breath which fills her lungs with positive air and she loudly exclaims: "Here I am! It's crazy! Fun!"

In the next session, Sylvia tells me about a new and unexpected connection with her body. "I used to never be able to look at myself in the mirror, or reflected in a shuttered window. It made me sick, or made me cry. I used to get angry with my image and now it's not the case, it just isn't! It's weird and it's really cool." I decide to check: "And what would happen if we spoke about the surgery?" "I really saw it last session," Sylvia replies, "how they reconstructed, what they did, how they stretched the stomach, how they stitched. I saw it all! And if the scar is a bit painful I just think of how they stitched me up and it calms. I can see it and it relaxes me. Now I am really curious to know if the organs inside are like I saw them."

When asked, and after slight hesitation, Sylvia says she has reached the goal for which she came to see me. I tell her: "I'm really impressed by you! It sounds too good to be true, hey?" Sylvia laughs, "Yes! That's why I was afraid to say it [having reached her therapeutic goal]."

The therapeutic process

As soon as Sylvia begins her therapy she clearly brings her history of traumatic dissociation. Ruth meets with her parents and indicates to the reader the gentle role reversal in the family system. Faced with parental distress, Sylvia took charge and made critical decisions. Among her many creative interventions, Ruth combines trauma work in somatic experiencing, with "internal family system", a therapeutic modality which allows differentiating between various self-states, working with their expression and assisting the client in internal organisation. The principle of *titration*, gently and gradually approaching the trauma, characterises all stages of therapy.

From the beginning, Ruth supports Sylvia in appreciating the advantages and resourcefulness of her defence system (e.g., "You really knew how to take care of yourself" when Sylvia described her inner split upon hearing about the surgery from mum). By so doing, Ruth is already *holding a bridge between dissociated parts* in Sylvia—she *establishes a kind relationship with the dissociated part*, which Sylvia labelled as pathological.

The *embodied guided imagery* work that Ruth did with Sylvia made extensive use of Sylvia's own images and language. The therapy mostly took place in a Winnicottian potential space (Winnicott, 1971a), where the bridges were lost, and Ruth supports Sylvia in re-erecting the bridges, connecting the two sides of the wall. The image is also a bridge between the world of thoughts (where Sylvia feels nothing) and the world of affect—body and emotion. Gently and carefully, Ruth helps Sylvia in *building bridges*, finding connecting paths between past and present, between Sylvia and her parents (and their inner representation), and between Sylvia and her body. The image of the wall is used to signify the dissociative defence and Ruth accepts the wall and its importance.

During the work, Ruth strengthened the transitional space where "everything was possible", thus allowing Sylvia to dare and seek external and internal resources for bridging the two sides of the wall. Sylvia's deep need for a responsible adult to hold her and her body in mind was clear, and although she wished it were her parents, she needed a third party. Ruth who was outside the wall (in the concrete world) took care of Sylvia as she entered an altered state of consciousness and Frances outside the wall (in Sylvia's inner world) also took care of Sylvia and assisted her in creating a bridge with her parents. This parallel process was a reparative process to other events of the altered state of consciousness—the traumatic surgeries where the entire family system was destabilised, and Sylvia had to act, to a certain extent, as the responsible adult.

Ruth was willing to *self-regulate and dyadically regulate Sylvia*, not allowing the girl to assume responsibility and do everything on her own, and therefore helped Sylvia to gradually reclaim connection with her body. Following this deep psychodynamic work, Ruth directed Sylvia's attention to the sensations of her body, which started to ache. Indeed, pain is one of the first sensations we encounter when coming out of surgery. Ruth invited Sylvia to *self-touch*, and an exciting *somatic dialogue* began with the scar (the old lady). The story was no longer disconnected and inner parts received their space without Sylvia's dissociation.

Ruth was attentive to her own *body resonance* as a source of information and compass for therapeutic intervention, and together they processed this deep experience. Sylvia experienced flow and Ruth checked the novel *bodymind reorganisation* by inviting Sylvia to speak about the surgery. Sylvia was bodily present and emotional, could tolerate the affect without dissociating, and was able to use the therapeutic work as a self-regulatory tool.

Therapeutic skills

Titration: Trauma work can easily flood the client, create helplessness, and loss of agency. As a chemist in a lab, diluting a highly concentrated solution, therapeutic titration is a slow, gradual, and gentle dance of coming close to the trauma and moving back, to the degree which allows the client to remain present and while considering defences, respecting them, and strengthening resources. Titration work with Sylvia allowed her, for the first time, to process her childhood trauma and the secondary traumas surrounding the surgeries.

Building bridges: The therapeutic work was skilfully dedicated to building bridges between split parts: within the family system, between body and mind, past and present. Each split and dissociation was reflected in the others, magnifying it like a prism. Similarly, each erected bridge strengthened the foundations for the following bridge.

Being a bridge: Ruth was not only helping Sylvia build bridges, she also held them inside herself. Unlike Sylvia's overwhelmed and traumatised parents, Ruth was able to hold Sylvia's body (and her own) in mind without dissociating; Ruth's physical presence provided Sylvia an anchor and a solid structure on which base the other bridges were held. Ruth's willingness to relate to Sylvia as a bodymind served Sylvia's early developmental holding needs and opened a possibility to remain in transitional spaces.

Liaising with the symptom/defence mechanism: When Sylvia spoke of her relationship with the scar/her body, the split between them was evident. She was judgmental of her dissociations, and Ruth on the other hand cultivated a kind relationship with the split. If there was a wall—there must have been a good reason for it, it did a good job—it protected Sylvia! Establishing a relationship with the symptom as an autonomous entity is characteristic of Gestalt therapy and is also found in other therapeutic modalities. The split, the scar, and the tummy all became important actors in therapy—and their respective voices were considered important. Ruth did not hurry to "break" defences. On the contrary, she respectfully positioned herself in a relationship with them and invited Sylvia to do the same. The therapeutic journey was therefore "around" the difficulty while respecting and considering its needs, rather than "into" the difficulty.

Embodied guided imagery: The imagery of the wall, the rivers, and the conversation from both sides of the wall told the tragic history of Sylvia, who on some level lost her childhood, and her relationships with her body, with her parents, and with her health all at the same time. This exploration was neither cognitive, nor was it concretely bodied—it was in the transitional space between the two. The guided imagery Ruth offered was completely reliant on Sylvia's inner world yet it invited, time and again, an expansion of both perception of agency and further possibilities. I relate to it as *embodied guided imagery* since Ruth was not merely aiming to enter Sylvia's intrapsychic world; instead, it took place intersubjectively, and Ruth kept emphasising its mutuality—the body was held in mind and the mind embodied in the body. Body movements, for instance, were translated into insights, interpretations, and emotions on the one hand. On the other hand, therapeutic processes were translated back into bodily experiences (e.g., a better feeling was tested by placing the hand over the scar and validating the different sensation).

Strengthening potential space: "Everything is possible in your imagination," Ruth kept reminding Sylvia, whose dissociation manifested in her difficulty to maintain a transitional space between inner and outer reality. A four-year-old child should not have to choose which anaesthesia would be best for her. Losing consciousness and being near death, anaesthetic sleep, the collapsing of her body and of her control, and lack of sufficient holding collapsed transitional spaces and made these frightening. Ruth held the space not only for Sylvia but also for her parents (both real and internalised), whom she kept in mind while working with

Sylvia. This aspect was particularly important, since probably the parents too had insufficient support during the frightening period of Sylvia's surgery, which might account for some of the dissociation. When the potential space was strengthened, Sylvia was able to feel her body again.

Self- and dyadic regulation: I am doubtful that any parent could tolerate such a shaking and destabilising drama of nearly losing a child and maintain appropriate regulatory functioning. The family system needed help, and Ruth—along with Frances (the internalised figure)—became the family therapist. When Ruth reported: "I feel a lot of heat, I sweat and take off my sweater," she demonstrated assuming responsibility for her self-regulation—which enabled Sylvia to use her. Ruth, just like Frances, was not as deeply involved as mum and dad were—both Frances and Ruth could tolerate her pain and survive it.

Self-touch: Ruth invited Sylvia to touch her scar, regaining connection between severed self-states. This invitation came only after the bridge between Sylvia and her parents, on the two sides of the wall, was established. With touch also came pain, but the possibility for a dialogue was activated. With much grace, Sylvia moved between narrative, imagery, and somatic dimensions. Ruth's love for Sylvia was almost palpable as Sylvia fought to reconnect the exiled aspects of herself through touch. Touching the scar helped Sylvia experience her body as self, and herself as a body.

Somatic dialogue: In traditional Indian films, it was forbidden to portray romantic touch between a man and a woman—not even a kiss. Instead, the woman would bite an apple, handing it over to the man who passionately consumed it. The apple was a buffer, which enabled a dialogue with the sensitive subject of sexuality. In therapy, too, particularly around trauma, there are areas where direct contact is too overwhelming and flooding. The guided imagery was one such buffer, moderating between painful materials and allowing a gentle movement between them. The somatic dialogue between the different parts of the system—between Sylvia and the old lady (the scar), was another mediatory process. The dialogue enabled Sylvia to internally validate her bodily reality and gradually reclaim her body. Sylvia engaged with the old lady, listened to her, and they formed a relationship. The dialogue was yet another bridge and when it was opened, a powerful somatic liberation of healing and flow followed—and vitality pulsated and moved through Sylvia uninterruptedly.

Resonance: Once in a while, Ruth shared her own body sensations, using resonance both for diagnosis and intervention. As an experienced body psychotherapist, Ruth was attentive to her body sensations, and could even deduce interventions and interpretations from these sensations. For example: "I can sense my own stomach, and encourage Sylvia to stay with the pleasant sensation."

Testing bodymind organisation: After it seemed that Sylvia was able to reconnect with her body and the past experience without dissociating, Ruth tested the stability of Sylvia's bodymind organisation towards the end of the session, and in the following one. She asked Sylvia to speak about the surgery and the scar. Together they monitored Sylvia's capacity to remain connected to her sensations, feelings, herself, and Ruth while communicating. This type of affective material was clearly dissociative in the past, but the bridges which the therapeutic dyad erected did not collapse and they stood firmly. Ruth fondly reflected to Sylvia her pride and joy, and they shared in celebrating her success.

Embodied therapeutic dialogue

ASAF: Thank you Ruth for this fascinating journey. You left me very curious. Did you continue to work together after that session?

RUTH: We met for a few more sessions. It was clear that there was still work to be done because Sylvia was apprehensive of hospitals. However, and particularly because of the stressful matriculation exams (A levels) we agreed to take a few months off and then continue. Despite this decision, and following a distressing event, Sylvia came back for a session shortly afterwards and one meeting was sufficient to strengthen her. We had some contact a few weeks later and she was completely fine. It is important for me to re-emphasise that Sylvia gave her permission for the publication of this vignette, with her details changed of course.

ASAF: What happened inside you (and in your body) in the dramatic session with her parents, when her mum talked about the surgery and Sylvia contracted and curled in?

RUTH: I found the story very painful to hear, and had many difficult sensations. I had to self-regulate throughout the session. I took care of Sylvia, but not only of her. Throughout the meeting I noted all the parties involved, checking who required my help—Sylvia, her mother, her father—and when we needed to slow down or stop. I felt empathetic to all of them and supported them. I reflected this distress to Sylvia's parents, but still asked them to notice and see—really see—Sylvia with her beauty, her capacities, her strength, and her aliveness. They were moved to tears.

This meeting might have provided the family, for the first time since the trauma (the event in itself and all the surgeries which followed it) with the support and holding the entire family needed. But moreover, perhaps the meeting planted seeds of hope and optimism, and recognising that the trauma was indeed over, and that Sylvia was now a teenage girl who behaved normally in an age-appropriate ways.

ASAF: You invited Sylvia to listen to the story from the hole in the wall. How did you know it was safe enough to do so?

RUTH: First, a moment earlier Sylvia shared her capacity to stare (to dissociate) if something was too much for her (she dissociated when the conversation with mum was too much). Second, the sentence "Suddenly I realised it did not happen to some other girl. I realised that it happened to me" hinted at her readiness. Third, I checked with her: "It seems that there is a small hole in the wall, allowing for some information to come through and reach you," and she simply responded affirmatively—all these were indicating readiness. If she was not ready she wouldn't have followed my request to elaborate on the imagery with the wall. The question "And what does it look like, with that wall?" was vague enough and very open. This is the beauty in working with gentle and slow work—there are ample possibilities to stop, breathe deeply, and move on or withdraw (which happened too when I asked Sylvia if she wanted to come back from the wall).

ASAF: I was very moved by your invitation for Sylvia to touch her scar. What made you offer it? Why did you offer it at that particular time?

RUTH: She said her scar felt unpleasant. When Sylvia came to therapy the scar was the most sensitive and disturbing part. My answer here is complicated: on one hand I didn't want the process to be too difficult for her. Perhaps I was worried. On the other hand, many times in therapy I offer to place a hand over a physically disturbing area to "converse" with it more directly, and then the sensations have space to "speak" their mind directly, or, as it happened with Sylvia, through an image or a figure—the old lady who spontaneously appeared and spoke.

ASAF: Towards the end, you described feeling heat throughout your body, which you interpreted as streaming and healing. How did you know it wasn't only "yours"? Why did you connect it with the therapeutic process?

RUTH: Let me remind you of the process: first Sylvia said that the jigsaw puzzle was completed, and then she described a pleasant flow throughout her body—including the scars. It was only then that I felt the heat inside of me. Where else could it come from if not from the healing process? Heat and streaming (alongside deep breath and other somatic signals) are clear markers of discharge taking place when trauma work is concluded. This is the energy which was held in the body (the trauma) and could now be released, allowing for the natural life flow of the client to resume. When such powerful work is done, as the piece described here, this energy does not only flow in the body, but is also released into the shared space.

Between self-regulation and dyadic regulation when working with anxiety and dissociation: Shai Epstein

Shai is an EABP accredited body psychotherapist, working in private practice.

The therapeutic encounter

Shai writes:
Maya, who is twenty-seven years old, sought therapy following a psychotic crisis six years ago and subsequent depressive episodes. After completing a few years of psychodynamic psychotherapy, she expressed a desire to continue her recovery process with therapeutic work which included her body.

Maya described her symptoms, which included floating feelings when she walked and a sense of no boundaries, as if the people around her could move through and into her. She developed social anxiety, had a few severe panic attacks, which caused vomiting and hospitalisation in the casualty department. Maya's sleep tended to be disturbed and fragmented, and she frequently awoke from nightmares with feelings of depersonalisation. Additionally, Maya reported long periods of dissociation, feeling generally flooded with intrusive obsessive thinking. Notwithstanding all these, Maya was intelligent and astute, arrived highly motivated, with impressive coping skills and highly functional, which also expressed in her postgraduate studies, working part-time, and her stable romantic relationship.

During the first months of therapy we mainly focused on grounding and centring: strengthening Maya's connection to earth and establishing boundaries. The following vignette was taken from one of our first sessions (therapy lasted about two years).

Maya entered the room with her head bowed low and her hair covering her face. Her movements were slow, conveying embarrassment and apprehension. She sat on the edge of the chair, looked at me and smiled. After a few moments of silence Maya started speaking. Her voice was faint, her breathing very shallow and concentrated in her chest, which seemed contracted and dense. Her diaphragm was held up, the stomach was full and with little breath. Her body seemed frozen, with little or no visible motion. Maya's shoulders were held in and up, and her lower body was fuller in comparison to her upper body.

Maya starts talking about an incident at work where she felt attacked. Her breathing pace is accelerated and in the resonant space between us I begin to feel tense, manifesting in my contracting chest, a slight sense of suffocation in my throat and a clearly identified anxiety. I ask Maya to stop her story for a moment and notice her body. At first, Maya is surprised by the unexpected disturbance to her flow of speech, and cannot understand why I stopped her. I briefly explain to her the concepts of regulation, slowing down pace, and working with body sensations as facilitative of self-regulation, slowing down, and connection.

Maya understands. For the first time she notices how she sits at the edge of the chair and, surprised, she shares it with me. I ask her to check if she can explore other ways, possibly more comfortable, of sitting on the chair; I offer her cushions and a blanket. Maya leans back, covering herself with a blanket. "What are you aware of?" I am checking with her. "How do you know that you are more comfortable?" Maya describes: "My back feels supported, and I feel warmer and protected by the weight of the blanket."

We establish connection with those pleasant sensations, and in parallel I feel that my own tension in the chest is decreased, alongside the anxiety I felt when Maya started talking. I invite Maya to carry on talking, and whenever I sense the beginning of hyperarousal, expressed through the resonant tension in my body, Maya's difficulty to maintain eye contact, accelerated breathing, or tears, I ask Maya to stop. With every break Maya notices her body sensations and searches for pleasant ones in her body: from the blanket, the comfortable sitting, and more. I encourage Maya to stay with these sensations for a while, before coming back to the constrictive sensations which appeared before the flooding.

Gradually, I notice that the amplitude of bodily symptoms of anxiety and tensions decreasing, both in me and in Maya. I take it as a sign that it has become safer now to explore the anxiety, and when Maya focuses on her contracted chest I ask her if she can demonstrate the tension with a movement. Maya chooses to make a fist, telling me that her contracted chest is like a tight fist, pressing from the inside and wanting to come out. I ask Maya to invest more energy in tightening her fist, and after a few moments ask her to gradually relax her fist. We repeat this process a number of times: amplifying the tension in the fist and relaxing it, all the while listening to her tense chest. Maya notices that this process has a calming effect on the pressure in her chest. "How do you sense this calming effect?" I ask, and Maya replies, "There's gentle warmth in my chest, and a kind of movement which wasn't there earlier." I ask Maya to go back to the work situation she started with.

After about thirty minutes, it seems that the process calms Maya down. Her body is more at ease, as if it finds the support offered by the chair more agreeable, and her breathing is easier and more expansive. Maya concludes her story without her familiar feelings of emotional overwhelming, panic, and helplessness. "How is it expressed in your body?" I ask, and Maya describes: "I am more relaxed than the beginning of our session, I feel the weight of my pelvis and legs, it's surprising—I am not used to feeling my legs."

At this stage I ask Maya to stand up on the floor. I, too, change my position, standing beside her and guiding her to notice how her body feels standing up. Her breathing is limited to the front of her body and is barely noticeable; it seems that her body weight is mainly focused in her heals and her toes are inwardly turned, as if trying desperately to hold on to the ground.

Maya shares with me her feelings of tension in her head, rigidity in the neck, and unpleasant fullness in her chest. She cannot feel her stomach, pelvis, and legs—her lower body seems to be split from her upper body. I gently guide Maya to pay attention to her feet, move them slightly, bend her knees, gently move her pelvic region—all directed at developing some sensitivity to her lower body through gentle movement. Maya is embarrassed to move these areas but I do not address her embarrassment directly, and instead guide Maya to follow a specific exercise: with every inhale, the toes are pulled upwards and with every exhale the toes come back to the ground and she relaxes. After a few cycles I change my instructions: with every inhale, her heels turn upwards and Maya stands on her toes, and with each exhale she brings her heels back to the ground. The exercise is synchronised with the rhythm of her breathing. The last stage of the exercise combines both movements in an alternating way: the toes come up with each inhale, and come down with each exhale; the heels come up with each inhale, and come down with each exhale. I ask Maya to pay particular attention to her experience in her feet and their connection with the ground.

When we finish, Maya speaks of feeling warmth and tension in her legs, and having a clearer sense of standing on the ground—she can sense the connection with ground more pronouncedly. I guide Maya to continue this exercise much slower for a few moments, and to my delight Maya feels connected with the movement work. She describes a pleasant feeling rising in her lower body: heat, strength, presence, and support. She is also more mindful of the weight of holding from the diaphragm upwards.

Coming back to our chairs, Maya says: "I feel more collected," and she further shares a novel sense of coherence with which she leaves our session. As a part of our therapeutic process, I suggest and Maya agrees to commit to practise this exercise twice a day and walk barefoot on earth or sand a few times a week while noticing the contact of her feet with the ground.

Over time, we developed this movement work until it became an elaborated sequence of daily practice, which accompanied the first months of therapy and helped Maya in establishing a more conscious connection with her body in general, and particularly with the lower part of her body. The exercise enabled Maya to feel the ground beneath her, strengthening her resolve to stand on her feet and feel her power and agency in coping with challenges: allowing the energy to once more flow in her lower body, which significantly contributed to Maya's sense of centre, stability, and capacity during the first months of our work together.

The therapeutic process

The last two decades saw increasing interest in the connection between dissociation and attachment style, with a commonly held presumption that extreme dissociative conditions correlate with disorganised attachment style (and appropriately, developmental trauma) (Jakoby, 2011).

Influential psychiatrist Giovanni Liotti (2004) dedicated a thorough research to the connection between dissociation and disorganised attachment, and demonstrated how disorganised attachment style (also resulting from unresolved parental issues) may result in dissociative coping mechanisms to trauma. Liotti wrote: "Whenever, from infancy to old age, human beings are called to cope with a traumatic stressor, their attachment system is activated" (p. 479). Liotti argued that psychotherapy with dissociative clients needed to emphasise security, slowness, collaboration and cooperation, and secure attachment. Stabilising the therapeutic relationship should precede any direct work with traumatic memories.

Shai's therapeutic work with Maya illustrates one of the basic ways of establishing security and grounding in body psychotherapy. The therapeutic relationship is established and deepens not only through conversation, but also with the shared experience of working below the threshold of flooding and retraumatisation. Shai's clinical decisions are guided by his evaluation of Maya's capacity for affective processing: he wants her to feel safe, present, and not overwhelmed.

Once Shai understands Maya's dissociative tendencies, he pays great attention to her bodily presentations and to the ongoing process of *body reading*. Maya begins to speak and Shai attends both to her narrative and to signs of neural arousal and activation—through observation and *resonance*—and stops her—*applying the brakes*—in order to direct her attention to her body. Maya's surprise exemplifies her default mechanism of charge-overwhelm-dissociation, which creates a familiar cycle of retraumatisation (but also serves as a powerful analgesic agent). Shai incorporates *psycho-educational explanation* about regulation, and then both move to *increase somatic awareness* to Maya's experiences. Her unexpected discovery about sitting on the edge of the chair leads to *attempts to find bodily comfort*, which is a central aspect of their work: turning the body into a potentially safe place. Shai uses resonance skills to test the possibility of continuing with the narrative and he regularly checks for early signs of flooding. *Working with flooding* involves learning to identify such signs, both by increasing Maya's self-awareness, and with the help of Shai who observes Maya and his own resonating body.

Maya takes concrete steps to feel safer: she makes changes in the room, covers herself with a blanket, and changes her posture. Together, Maya and Shai establish dyadic regulation through *embodiment*, attention to breath, and increased awareness of warning signs of hyperarousal. Working with the fist (open and closed) is a *somatic metaphor*. Tensing and relaxing forms an association between internal and involuntary (autonomic) sensations and the voluntary muscular system. This bodily association provides Maya with an immediate and available tool for regulating her anxiety and gaining more control over it. Maya is remarkably resourceful and committed, and making these resources accessible for her transforms her experience, allowing her a greater sense of freedom.

It is easy to see that Shai is fond of Maya and cares for her. Once they establish a warm "uterine" relationship (safe place, the clinical setting as womb, Shai as a mother), the transition into the archetypally paternal relationship (movement, coming out into the world, Shai as father) becomes possible, and later Shai guides Maya through a *movement exercise*, which is designed to provide Maya with a pragmatic and accessible tool for reducing terror and flooding. Maya's lack of connection with her lower body decreases her capacity to self-regulate, and the inwardly turned toes are a clear bodily sign for terror, which fits the first developmental angle (and the fragmented character structure). The movement exercise broadens the spectrum between bodily holding of fear and letting go, while increasing the awareness to bodily resources: *grounding* and *centring*. Additionally, the repetitive movement between nearly losing balance (standing on the tips of the toes or pulling the toes high up) and regaining balance (bringing heels down, bringing toes down) is a practice of *moving between challenge and support* without freezing in one state or another. Throughout the exercise, Shai stands by Maya's side thus *changing therapeutic positioning* (I am beside you, rather than in front of you)—a safer position for both, considering Maya's levels of dread and flooding.

Shai's relatively active therapeutic stance is indicative of early stages of working with dissociation (and trauma work in general)—Maya is invited to be an active participant in reclaiming and re-inhabiting her body: she can "take therapy home", and "do something". This vignette does not only illustrate Shai's impressive skills but also Maya's remarkable motivation, agency, and determination. Maya joins Shai as an involved and active agent to the therapeutic and recovery process and assumes responsibility, throughout therapy, for implementing the therapeutic process, which probably contributed a great deal to the therapeutic success.

Throughout the session, the therapeutic content and narrative was secondary to the capacity to tolerate affect. When Maya's bodily and emotional regulation became more stable and organised, the therapeutic work could become less tool-centred and more psychodynamic.

Therapeutic skills

Body reading: Throughout the session, Shai relates to bodily information he receives from Maya and adapts both his therapeutic interventions and his therapeutic positioning accordingly. Shai's body reading includes Maya's physical appearance, her bodily presentation, and the marked difference between her upper part and lower part of the body. All these assist him in recognising Maya's character structure, and furthermore in seeking potential resources and early signs of dissociation. Additionally, Shai checks for subtler movements and changes in Maya's somatic expressions, such as breathing, movement, her choice of physical positioning, and differences in bodily textures and temperatures. Shai is attuned to Maya's bodily information and relates to it with the same seriousness and curiosity as to her verbal expressions. His skilful somatic observation demonstrates the richness of therapeutic information which could be received through body reading, and I hope you are able to appreciate how useful body reading skills could be for psychotherapists working with trauma in general, and particularly with dissociation.

Resonance: Shai uses his own body (or, to be precise, his sensing of the intersubjective body) as an additional source of information concerning Maya's affective situation. Resonance, which is expressed here as somatic countertransference, is one of the main ways in which the therapeutic dyad Shai-Maya regulates itself.

Applying the brakes: Maya was surprised that Shai stopped her in mid-conversation. In working with traumatic flooding, and generally when working with overwhelmingness, the body psychotherapist endeavours to stop the client before entering a space where processing is not at all possible. This skill is common in most systems of trauma work, and is particularly identified with the work of Babette Rothschild (2004). Throughout therapy Maya experientially learns how these breaks (and her attention to precursors of flooding) could help her to process her experiences in a more organised and kinder manner, and without dissociating or overwhelming herself.

Psycho-education: This pedagogic positioning may look strange to the psychodynamically trained practitioner, but it is an important facet of working with trauma in particular, and also in body psychotherapy in general. Considering our culture, for many clients, especially those who are disconnected from their body, the directing of attention to their body could be experienced as weird and irrelevant to psychotherapy. Receiving explanations about trauma, regulation, and body can assist this initial connection between therapeutic conversation and the suggested bodily interventions. Thus, psycho-education is sometimes necessary as a contextual-cultural bridge between body and mind. Hopefully, when body psychotherapy becomes more integrated within the psychotherapeutic practice, such explanations will no longer be necessary.

Increasing body awareness: With attention and movement, invitation for body focusing and breathing, resonance and sensory curiosity, Shai encourages Maya to increase her body awareness and in so doing to assume more responsibility for her self-regulation. The therapeutic encounter portrays dyadic regulation (Shai's resonance, his extensive soft attention to Maya, seeking more comfort) from which self-regulation capacities are developed (for instance, Maya's adoption of the exercise and her disciplined practice).

Finding bodily comfort: Shai describes at length how Maya and he are looking for a way of her being comfortable in her chair. Staying with the sensory experience, expanding Maya's ability to check what feels good for her, establishing this, and taking an active stance in creating her comfort while the therapeutic safe space is created—all these are central to creating a sense of safety and security. Maya learns to feel bodily secure, to be in a safe space while she is embodied, and these are incredibly valuable resources for her capacity to deal with the world, with the other, and of course—with herself.

Working with flooding: The inside and outside movement, titration, recognising precursors, and applying the brakes, working with safe space and physical comfort, resonance and movement: all these comprise the therapeutic encounter with Maya, which focuses on working with flooding. Shai helps Maya to identify her involvement in her dissociative experience, which until then just "happened to her".

Body metaphor: Shai's request for Maya to demonstrate her chest contraction (of which she had no control) using a voluntary movement (Maya chooses to clench a fist) is a metaphoric demonstration. Working with metaphors is valuable in changing limiting patterns, and this body metaphor provides a powerful experience of control which helps Maya to regulate her flooding. Once sufficiently practised, the association between the autonomic experience and the voluntary chosen movement is established, and then Shai makes use of this established association (I rather look at it as a metaphoric association than as conditioning) to relax the fist, which helps relax the contracted chest.

Movement exercise: grounding and centring, between foreground and background, and between challenge and support: The movement exercise Shai offers to Maya is an elaborate intervention. Maya describes (in words and without words) her bodily splits, which parallel other splits in her life. The exercise strengthens her centring skills—establishing her somatic self and finding a relaxed and present centre inside her. The movement, synchronised with her breathing, enables experiential learning of the way to establish habitual patterns and to change these, and Maya learns to reorganise herself in connection with ground and gravity. This is a very grounding exercise. Shai invites Maya to tell him about splitting (unbalancing, abandoning her body, depersonalisation) and the connection and depression (regaining balance, coming back to the body), and all this through the body and without reaching the extreme conditions: between the two extremes of dissociation and depressive collapse they discover a spectrum, and this movement exercise demonstrates this range. This exercise is an un-conceptualised application of the Gestalt therapy movement between foreground and background, working with polarities. Maya learns how to receive support (from the ground, through her legs and earth, and alongside Shai) and allows space for challenge (destabilising connection to ground and earth), both in a regulated and soft way. The exercise she takes home loosens a firm bodymind organisation around these two choices (depression or disconnection) and introduces mobility, flexibility, and non-binary choice.

Changing therapeutic position: During the exercise Shai stands alongside Maya. This intervention, mentioned in passing, is of great therapeutic significance. The body psychotherapist is extensively sensitive to his bodily position in relation to the client, and may offer shared bodily exploration of this (changing) positioning—both to examine its impact on the transferential relationship, and to monitor its impact on the here-and-now connection. Being positioned in front of the client may be perceived as confrontational or threatening (against), while being alongside the client—as it was in this case—eases the exploration. The body psychotherapist may move away from the client or come closer (or offer the client to be more active and explore the appropriate distance and positioning in space), change sitting angles, postures (standing, sitting, or lying down), as well as the quality of presence in choosing touch, eye-contact, or buffers (such as the blankets). This dialogue enriches the therapeutic dialogue, diagnosis, and intervention and moreover allows both parties to discover and cultivate the appropriate conditions for kind, deep, safe, and mutually enriching therapeutic relationship.

Embodied therapeutic dialogue

ASAF: Thank you Shai for your rich embodied vignette. You begin your vignette with an elaborate body description. What did you deduce from it?

SHAI: Maya's body taught me about her systemic and energetic organisation: where blood, emotions, and movement can easily and freely flow and where such flow is limited. With Maya, without even going to character structure, I could see high energetic charge in her upper body, an attempt to create stability in the world by tensing muscles in her upper body, while the lower part of her body was present but meaningless, distant. Maya could not establish connection with her lower body, which expressed in its relative fullness a heaviness of movement, a sense of stagnation, or energetic impasse. In short, Maya's dissociative tendency was clearly visible in her body.

The diaphragm represents our capacity to move between our lower and our upper parts—between the earth and the sky, the child and the adult. In its movement, the diaphragm connects the worlds and allows a flexibility and movement of emotions, while establishing a consistent connection with the earth. When the diaphragm is held high up it may be indicative of a high level of anxiety, great fear of losing control, and disconnection from the lower centres of the body, avoiding a conscious connection with these which was also expressed in difficulty to breathe into them. Diaphragmatic contraction creates a pseudo-balance, an illusion of stability and in Maya's case—her tensing of her upper body, when in fact our organic and natural experience of stability should be felt through establishing connection with earth by relaxing into ground, allowing the pelvis and legs to establish our stability in the world through contact with the earth beneath our legs. Initially, Maya's body expressed her disconnection from the ground—from a sense of stability in her very existence. All these manifested well in the symptoms she described, as well as her psychotic crisis and the acute panic attacks in her past.

ASAF: When Maya told you about her incident at work you reported feeling tension "in the resonant space" between you. How could you tell if the physical tension you experienced did not belong to your own biography and was your material? What helped you in making this diagnostic differentiation?

SHAI: Working with the wide variety of body sensations which I can feel during a session is one of my central therapeutic skills. Many times I am uncertain whose sensation it is, and whether it is "mine" or being somatically picked up from the client, but I endeavour to be mindful enough to identify that this sensation was not here earlier on; or perhaps it may become clear that a particular body sensation (usually accompanied by a feeling, a repeating image, or a movement that my body wants to do) recurs every time I meet this particular client. I am attentive to how this sensation makes me feel or what it moves me to do, as well as mindful of the way it affects my relationship with the clients. There are certain therapeutic situations where I would choose to share with the client what happens in my body, and check if it corresponds with the client's feeling. In this particular case with Maya, I chose not to share and check what was evoked in me, and instead I used my sensations as internal barometers for our dyadic state.

To some degree, the question of "whose sensation is this?" is less relevant: resonance appears during the meeting with the client and is therefore connected with this meeting. Body resonance parallels here somatic countertransference and I relate to it in the same way I relate to countertransference—I endeavour to identify it, to be mindful of it, and to use it in order to deepen my understanding of the client-therapist dynamics. Additionally, over the years of practice I learned to recognise body sensations which emerge during a session, distinguish them (and between them) and process these "live". What is taking place in my body before, during, and after a meeting with a client is an integral part of our relationship. As a body psychotherapist, part of my training concerned cultivation of skills for identifying body sensations and processing these, reclaiming a conscious relationship with my body in general, and within the therapeutic encounter in particular.

ASAF: Once Maya manages to find a comfortable position on her chair, and covers herself in a blanket, you speak about establishing "connection with those pleasant sensations". How do you establish connection with sensations and why?

SHAI: Establishing connection with pleasant sensations means directing our attention to these and staying with them mindfully. I have invited Maya to notice one of the sensations she mentioned: back support, the warmth of the blanket, the sense of security which came from the weight of the blanket (which strengthened her sense of boundaries). I asked Maya to describe the sensation and allow it to expand, spread, and receive conscious presence in her bodily experience. When that happened, I invited Maya to attend to the different and varied occurrences taking place while she stayed with the pleasant sensation, such as involuntary diaphragmatic breathing which appeared, slight tremor in her hands, leaning deeper into the chair. When Maya managed to direct her consciousness to these events, she noticed the regulatory process taking place: a discharge of the autonomic nervous system and pent-up energy which got freed up.

Attending to pleasant sensations is a resource, which I am aiming to cultivate in therapy in general, and particularly when working with trauma or dissociative processes. When a person is conscious of these pleasant sensations, such as warmth, streaming, expansions, pleasant shaking, etc., he or she in fact activates the parasympathetic branch of the autonomic nervous system, encouraging calming down and down-regulating. The client can experientially and bodily learn that there is no immediate threat at that moment, no need to be activated, and it is possible to let go and relax, allowing different systems to enter a state of relaxation.

When working with trauma or flooding, I place great emphasis on connecting to benevolent sensations, which allow the bodymind systems to retain its self-regulation—moving from survival mode to relaxation, from (mostly unconsciously) interpreting the world as dangerous and threatening, to gaining other possibilities of encountering reality. As clients experience these transitions and the accompanied changes in feelings during therapy, they understand that the process takes place through them, and that they can control it to an extent. This is a highly important experience considering the sense of helplessness and loss of control which usually accompanies flooding and trauma. In so doing, clients remind themselves—their bodies and minds—what they might have forgotten but have never lost—the capacity for functional self-regulation.

ASAF: At the beginning of the movement exercise Maya felt embarrassed. There was a precious possibility for working with the therapeutic relationship and her embarrassment, yet you chose to avoid directly relating to the embarrassment and lead the exercise. Could you share your clinical judgment in making this choice?

SHAI: Relating to Maya's embarrassment—to what was taking place in the therapeutic space between us at that stage—was premature at the time. During this stage therapy was not yet focused on examining our relationship consciously. Later, a few months into therapy, I began to incorporate psychodynamic and relational interventions. During these initial stages of therapy I was a benevolent figure, caring and protective, constant—and I did not wish to undermine my role for her before Maya felt secure and safe between us and within the therapeutic relationship. I consciously avoided entering this transferential affect which could have activated further flooding or destabilising, even if it seemed minor. There are some clients for whom moving their body in general and in therapy in particular is a new and unfamiliar experience, which easily brings up embarrassment, and I do not always dwell on such feelings immediately, through directly relating to these. Embarrassment in itself could be a marker, a place to come back to and check what it holds.

In Maya's case, her embarrassment did not stop her from connecting to the exercise (which, for me, was an indication that the exercise was appropriate and accurate for her). Had her embarrassment been paralysing, we would have touched and attended to it then. Later on in therapy, her embarrassment returned in a variety of forms when we addressed Maya's body and our relationship during sessions, and it became an entrance gate into our relational dynamics.

ASAF: Towards the end, Maya accepts your invitation to continue with this exercise slowly and to your delight she connected to the movement work. I was surprised to find the phrase "to my delight" in the description. Could you explain?

SHAI: I am personally very connected to therapeutic work in movement, but there are but a few clients who surrender to regularly exercising movement at home. Naturally, this depends on the client's personality but also on me—and my ability to suggest the right exercise at the right time. When Maya began the exercise, it fitted her perfectly, and it was a special feeling which appears when I witness a client exercising a precisely tailored movement sequence. Appropriate movement exercise can serve the therapeutic process and meet a deep bodily need; in Maya's case—loosening the upper body, connecting with the pelvis, the ground, and strengthening her capacity to move up and down safely. I felt excitement mixed with satisfaction. Therefore, I was delighted when Maya seemed to have connected with the movement work and was able to surrender to it, to explore it and to sense the qualities it could help her develop. Additionally, Maya's willingness to practise at home was a significant step in her active partnership in the process. Strengthening her sense of power and agency in facing life on her own, without constant support from her surroundings, was a central theme in our work. By taking upon herself to practise at home and exercising disciplined practice for a long period, Maya managed to leave behind a passive victim position and cultivate an inner position of capability and agency which was independent of outside forces. Maya has taken notable responsibility for her process from its very beginning. This was an expression of her seriousness and commitment, her power, and her willingness to fully use what body psychotherapy could offer her.

Focusing with a post-traumatic client: Liora Bar-Natan

Liora Bar-Natan is a body psychotherapist, working with individuals and couples. She is the founder of the Institute for Focusing Oriented Therapy in Israel. Liora trains and certifies therapists in focusing oriented therapy. Her training is recognised by the international Focusing Institute.

The therapeutic encounter

Liora writes:

Jonathan, a thirty-three-year-old man, married and father of three, came to therapy following a serious car accident he was involved in two years previously. Since the accident he suffered from severe and debilitating pain. After the accident Jonathan stopped working and his family moved in with his in-laws since they were unable to support themselves financially. All major attempts—both medical and psychiatric—to diagnose his medical complaint failed. Jonathan arrived in therapy in a difficult state, which was threatening his already shaken marital life. Any hope for change for the better and recovery was faded, and instead Jonathan was sad, helpless, despairing, and depressed.

Physically speaking, Jonathan looked like a boy, short and small-bodied. As a result of his accident, his pelvis seemed as if it was paralysed, his right leg kept shaking vigorously even when in rest; the upper part of his spine seemed frozen and rigid as well. Occasionally, in unexpected and unforeseen frequency, Jonathan experienced debilitating headaches which left him paralysed and immobile for a few dreadful and intolerable minutes at a time.

The session below took place about seven months into therapy, and was a climax of a slow and prolonged process.

We came back to the day of the accident. Jonathan recalled the sequence of events that morning. This time, when he reached the crossroads where the accident took place, he felt a stabbing pain in his back and sharp pain in his stomach. Inside the stomach, he said, was fear. Fear of the unknown, of something unclear. The feeling was vague. It rose towards the chest, where the fear was clearer. It was like a black mass. Jonathan was frightened that something bad was going to happen. Once more, he felt this sharp pain in the stomach. Jonathan literally curled up with pain in his chair. I directed his attention to his stomach:

JONATHAN: "I can see a vortex."
LIORA: "Can you describe this vortex?"
JONATHAN: "It is a very powerful vortex, it pulls in everything."
LIORA: "Is there any sensation coming from that vortex?"
JONATHAN: "Fear. Fear that I'd be pulled into the vortex. I must get out of the vortex, but I feel that I can't."

I could sense Jonathan's distress in his tone of voice. I felt the trauma-vortex strengthening. In myself, I tuned in to Jonathan's resources, his strengths and determination. During these moments I felt that, as his therapist, I was holding both recovery and hope on his behalf.

LIORA: "You say you must get out of the vortex, but you feel that you can't. Can you move away from the vortex to a safe distance or move the vortex away from you?"
JONATHAN: (after a few moments of silence) "I can move away from the vortex and look at it from a distance; from a safe distance."
LIORA: "You are now in safe distance from the vortex. Can you look at it now from a distance?"
JONATHAN: "Yes." And after a few moments, "I feel I am pulled in again, I won't be carried in again. I have to get out."
LIORA: "Just notice if there's anything there that could help you or anything external? Try looking at yourself from the outside for a moment, and see what could help?"
JONATHAN: "I don't want to use any external help. I can do it by myself, I can let go of the vortex's pull on me."

LIORA: "What's helping you?"

JONATHAN: "I am pulling myself upwards."

LIORA: "How are you pulling yourself? What with? Can you look at your hand; what is it holding?"

JONATHAN: "It's like a rope."

LIORA: "And what is it like in your body now?"

JONATHAN: "I feel that I can pull myself out of the vortex and that it slows down. It's not as powerful. Gradually it becomes less powerful."

LIORA: "You feel that as you pull yourself out of the vortex it slows down; less powerful. And what's happening in your body? What are you sensing?"

JONATHAN: "There is less fear; much less fear."

LIORA: "There is less fear, much less fear. Can I invite you to breathe into this sensation?"

JONATHAN: "Yes," (a few moments of silence). "I see myself sitting in my car, feeling the back pain and the feeling of uncertainty, but the fear is not as strong. I see the blue car approaching very fast. I see it about to bump into a pole and then the car is changing its angle and is moving towards me. There is a gap ahead of me, the car which was there moved and I wonder whether I should move too. If I will, the blue car will bump into my door. I stay put. I feel a horrid pain in my back. The blue car crashes into the side of my car and I can feel another car crashing me from the back."

Tears, Jonathan is crying. After a few moments of silence, Jonathan continues: "I feel a terrible backache. I think I might be dead, and I am moving my fingers to check that I am not dead. The backache is horrible. I remember that the first thing I've done was to call Dana. I told her that somebody crashed into me and asked her to come quickly."

The therapeutic process

The following therapeutic encounter is an excellent account of gentle body psychotherapeutic work with trauma. Liora invites her client to go back to the day of the accident, to allow for a non-dissociative processing which is still within the bounds of his capacity to tolerate it without emotional flooding. Liora invites Jonathan to focus on his sensations when he arrives, in his mind's eyes, to the place of the accident. This invitation incorporates *bodily focusing and transition from thoughts and feelings to sensations*. Jonathan uses the image of a vortex, and Liora joins in to work with and around his image. Therapeutic work with the visual image is less emotionally overwhelming for Jonathan than looking at emotions. It is interesting to note that the vortex image is a basic metaphor in somatic experiencing (Ross, 2003), which describes the healing and recovery process as moving from the trauma vortex to the healing vortex.

Liora *stays with the client's spontaneous body movements* (e.g., wriggling in the chair) without judgment, and *relates to movements and sensations as communication* in a direct fashion—she invites Jonathan into his stomach. When Jonathan reports a potentially flooding affect within the vortex, Liora suggests he either moves away from the vortex or moves the vortex away from him. This offer makes use of a few skills: *focusing on resources, applying the brakes*, and emphasising agency. Apart from this, as Liora indicates, she holds the healing vortex for Jonathan—there is a degree of *somatic dyadic regulation* as well as *holding the client's body in mind*.

Time and again, Liora both reflects and validates Jonathan's experience, using his own language and re-inviting him to search for internal and external resources, while holding the belief and faith in their existence, to create a movement within his learned helplessness. She assists Jonathan in *creating inner representation of the healing movement*, and in *anchoring these representations in the body* (the hand holding the rope, breathing into the sensation).

When Jonathan manages to be less activated, he is spontaneously able to process the moment of impact—and despite the pain, he remains present and not overwhelmed. Jonathan manages to maintain a coherent and consistent narrative while remaining connected to himself and to Liora, to his feelings as well as to his body.

Therapeutic skills

Holding the body in mind—mental representation of the body in the therapist's mind: Throughout the session, Liora holds the client's body in mind as a reliable source of information, a diagnostic tool, an intervention, and a compass for gauging the volume of affective activation. Not only does Liora keep a mental representation of Jonathan's body in her mind, but she also holds the "healthy body" in her mind, presuming its organic agency and capacity. I believe that Liora's holding capacity assisted Jonathan in entering those terrifying spaces and finding there some relief for his pain. Liora relates both to Jonathan's narrative as well as to every bodily communication he offers her.

Bodily focusing and transition from thoughts and feelings to sensations: Liora is a highly experienced practitioner of focusing oriented psychotherapy (Gendlin, 1998), and it is easy to see that her recurring invitation is to focus inwardly. This emerging space, which is unfamiliar and scary, also holds the potential for healing and recovery. What Liora offers to Jonathan is to simplify the information processing schema: from thoughts, images, and feelings, she encourages him to notice his sensations, which are less loaded and overwhelming. At the same time, once Jonathan is able to process his sensations without dissociating, Liora offers an opposite movement: embodying those thoughts and images (from sensations—to images, feelings, and thoughts). When sensations are used to guide the pace of imagery, the image becomes embodied and enables a monitored and safe self-regulation.

Staying with the client's spontaneous body movements and relating to movements and sensations as communication: Psychologist Yorai Sella (2005a) describes the two skills above as important dimensions within the body psychotherapeutic practice. Liora is willing to be with Jonathan's spontaneous body movements while maintaining safe boundaries—she does not ignore Jonathan's body wriggling movements, for example, but she is not threatened by these either; instead, Liora views these as an integral part of the therapeutic work and directly addresses the contracting stomach; she naturally and organically engages with those sensations and movements. Liora's suggested communication is gentle and cautious throughout, to avoid flooding and retraumatisation.

Focusing on resources: Similarly to other trauma work methods, focusing oriented therapy emphasises the importance of focusing on resources when doing therapy with a post-trauma client. Jonathan arrives for therapy prone to despair, helplessness, and ready to give up. These have already led to functional and interpersonal deterioration and depression (Seligman, 1975). In order to recover he needs to reprocess his experiences and attribute different meaning to them from the one he had given these, time and again, during the last two years. Liora's frequent invitations to Jonathan to look for resources assists him in changing the focus of his observation, but moreover challenges him and encourages him to become an active agent in his recovery, after he has been a passive medical patient for months on end, thus changing his dissociative and helpless position.

Applying the brakes: Body psychotherapist Babette Rothschild (2004) emphasises safety as the most crucial element in trauma work, and has coined the term *applying the brakes*. When doing trauma work, when there is a danger of emotional flooding, the therapist becomes much more proactive: she may stop the client and prevent him from being sucked into retraumatising vortexes. Twice during the session above, when Jonathan describes the seduction of being pulled into flooding spaces, Liora stops him, inviting him to look for resources. The titration movement of going in and out, focusing inside and outside, creates a movement which defrosts the traumatic freezing and allows for narrative processing.

Somatic dyadic regulation: Liora reports how amid Jonathan's vortex she senses his distress and holds the recovery and healing vortex for him. In this affect-laden encounter between Liora and Jonathan, her inner work (self-regulating her autonomic nervous system arousal) affects the intersubjective body. Chapter Eleven, dedicated to resonance, expands and exemplifies ways of working therapeutically with the intersubjective body.

Creating inner representation of the healing movement, and anchoring it in the body: Liora seamlessly and skilfully moves between symbolic (spoken) dimensions and subsymbolic (bodily and metaphoric) ones. When Jonathan begins to narrate his emergence out of his trauma vortex, Liora is not satisfied with solely emotional descriptions, but instead asks Jonathan to anchor this transition with imagery and sensations. The hand holding a rope becomes an anchoring station to which Jonathan would be able to return both within therapy and outside therapy as a symbol for resources, and as inner representation of healing and resourcefulness. Just as Liora uses body processes and images to extract mental and emotional processes, she now brings emotional processes back into the body—into body images and body sensations (breathing into the safe sensation, for example), thus assisting in bodymind integration.

Embodied therapeutic dialogue

ASAF: Thank you Liora for a vignette full of hope in our human potential. I wish to begin by asking what did you feel when Jonathan started contracting with pain in his chair?

LIORA: When I looked at Jonathan wriggling and contracting in his chair I could sense his distress, which manifested in his bodily motion and contracting. I sensed his emotional activation—the fear in his stomach giving rise to bodily impulse and movement in the legs. The movement stopped in his pelvis amid the contraction. These survival impulses—fight, flight, and freezing, which are centred in the brain stem, are primarily expressed in the limbs. Jonathan's survival instinct (as we noticed in previous sessions) was to run and escape from the place of the accident, getting away from the threat.

This impulse was arrested in his pelvis. The reasons for that could have been either physical or emotional. Throughout the process I noticed Jonathan moving his body, thus expressing those previously unexpressed survival impulses and sensations by moving; at the same time in my countertransference, I noticed these sensations in my own body.

ASAF: You described how you tuned into Jonathan's strengths and determination; how you held the healing vortex—can you explain how exactly you have done that?

LIORA: As Jonathan was pulled into the trauma vortex, I could have found myself drifting with him into this vortex. Since the accident, Jonathan lost his self-esteem and confidence, his sense of worth, agency, power, and determination which he used to feel before the accident. The lack of these feelings was stronger in the presence of fear, helplessness, and distress, which he experienced during the process. It felt like trauma was controlling his life and managing it. That the difficulties "were winning".

As a therapist, I was holding for Jonathan what he could not access during these moments—his strengths, his resources. In a very real way, I felt his capabilities while he could only sense his helplessness. I called forth the way he managed his life prior to the accident, personally, socially, and professionally. I remembered his warm feelings towards his wife and children. I could sense my own body relaxing; I could sense my centre.

In such moments I bring my attention back towards myself. I check my body and sensations, making sure that I breathe, calm, and relax myself. I sense my faith in our relationship and in the therapeutic process. My tone of voice is calm and low, I look straight at Jonathan, and my heart is very open towards him. Jonathan could sense that.

ASAF: Thank you. I am very curious about your offer to Jonathan to move away from the vortex or to move the vortex away from him. Can you share what brought you to offer these two possibilities?

LIORA: Jonathan reported being swept into the vortex and was unable to exit it. The offer to move away from the vortex or move the vortex away from him facilitated the creation of distance between him and the traumatic experience. The position of observing something, in contrast to "being in it" allowed him less identification with and greater distance from the force of the traumatic experience, and enabled him to exercise more control and choice of response and action.

ASAF: When Jonathan told you he was pulling himself up, you invited him to check what he was pulling himself with and look at his hand. What prompted you to make such a specific suggestion, why the hand?

LIORA: As Jonathan was talking about pulling himself up, I noticed a very gentle move in his right hand. The move prompted me to ask about the hand's bodily impulse. The entire body was an active participating agent in the process, and was responsive to the images and visualisations from Jonathan's imagination.

ASAF: While the therapeutic relationship could be sensed during the vignette, it was not spoken of. Could you share your stance regarding the therapeutic relationship in general, and specifically in your work with Jonathan?

LIORA: The therapeutic relationship is the basis for the whole process. In his childhood, Jonathan grew up in an environment where he experienced lack of trust and insecurity in his relationship with his significant attachment figures. He never felt that anyone took account of his needs, saw these, or was willing to meet his needs. The most important aspect of our work together was building trust in our relationship. Jonathan could sense securely that I was with him, seeing his needs, giving space to the difficult feelings he never had legitimacy for, being unthreatened by his feelings, and allowing their expression. Jonathan needed to feel that I was with him; that he was not alone.

Therapeutically working with the intersubjective body: Elad Hadad

Elad Hadad is an EABP accredited body psychotherapist, working in private practice.

The therapeutic encounter

Dinah, a thirty-nine-year-old divorced woman without children, has been in therapy with me for about a year. She sought therapy wanting to find a good relationship and have a child, after she experienced a few abusive relationships. Dinah has a characteristically dense structure, with accompanied physical symptoms of breathing difficulties and constipation. In her relationships, Dinah tended to be placating. She needed relationships, yet she tended to be passive and reactive in her relationships. She was very loyal, yet seldom showed her vulnerability or explicitly expressed her wants or needs.

About two months prior to the session below, a new and sweeping romantic relationship began. In the sessions, Dinah expressed great joy and satisfaction with how "different" this relationship was and how "different" her own behaviour had been, as well as the fact that he was "different". Dinah felt the fruits of her therapeutic labour and ours—finally as the relationship which she had waited for. She thanked me frequently, and wondered what we shall do in our sessions, now that her goal was achieved. At first, I was happy for her, but very quickly I recognised that the joy I expressed felt fake; that my body was heavy, my breathing was short, and my back was aching.

My attempts to clarify with Dinah her body sensations and her feelings regarding the pace of this forming relationship were bluntly rejected, spiced with further gratitude, which already felt like "bribery" meant to get me to turn a blind eye. I was ashamed to offer her this interpretation, I felt traitorous, puny, pathetic, and needy in comparison to Dinah's liberation and openness. I thought I was experiencing paternal countertransference, re-enacting her controlling father, who resisted letting Dinah grow up. I felt that we were drifting apart, and kept smiling (with pain).

During one of the sessions I was sitting with Dinah, and a presently common theme with her recurred: tiredness and sleepiness took their comfortable place in my body. Dinah's face, in contrast, was beaming as she told me enthusiastically and with a broad smile that something amazing happened: her partner offered her to join him for two years relocation in the US. "It's a dream come true and a genuine validation of his love. It's also good for me, an opportunity to get to know a new place, to learn, and to develop," Dinah continued. "I am so thrilled and I've so waited to share this news with you." She looked at me with yearning eyes, desperately seeking my recognition and approval.

I am sitting with her, listening to her words, and so dearly wish I could join in her happiness, so much so that I find myself imitating her sitting position and facial expression, yet my main experience is a growing contraction in my chest and shoulders, throbbing pain in my throat and dried lips, all accompanied by a sense of losing balance. Faced with Dinah's eager look and scrutinising expectation I cannot smile; on the contrary, I can feel my face frozen and pale … I've been caught. At loss for an escape exit, I choose to share with Dinah the incongruity I feel between my genuine desire to share in her happiness, and my body's sensations, my body which refuses to participate and is shutting down.

Dinah waits, suspended for a few moments, then her eyes gently close and her mouth is starting to quiver. A soft wail of crying comes out and tears flow down her cheek. Dinah's eyes open and are focused on me, with worry and dread. I can breathe deeper, and for the first time in two months, I sense my body expanding and the wall between us slightly removed. "Yes … it's all happening far too quickly, ahh …," Dinah mumbles. Suddenly her eyes look stern again, the tears and shaking stop; my own breath too is yet again heavy, pulling me down. "What has just happened, Dinah?" I ask. Dinah places her hand over her mouth, as if preventing it from speaking and she looks away. "I thought, here I am ruining the only chance I have for love with these resistances of mine." "How exactly are you doing this?" I wonder. "It's this traumatic body of mine," she answers, with unfamiliar insult and wrath, "it doesn't allow me to go with this flow and adventure. I am really trying hard to do this—telling everybody, happy and enthusiastic, but it wouldn't come with me. I've been constipated for a week, and every night I need an inhaler to fall asleep," Dinah says, defeated. "Perhaps it's worried about you, the body," I suggest, "after all, you do have a full and rich life here, which you are willing to throw away in an instant, and it is all so fast …" "Yes," replies Dinah, "the problem is there's no communication. We are like two strangers, me and my body, a power struggle, each pulling in her own direction."

I notice a repeating terminology, me and my body. It is clear that Dinah does not identify with her body, and I suggest an experiment: "Could you test an alternative declaration to 'my body holds me'? Something like 'I am holding myself from the stomach and chest'?" Dinah tries out this sentence, first in her mind and then aloud. "Sounds weird but true," she says, and for a moment seems slightly more grounded and less struggling. "It's not easy, holding me … I am stubborn," Dinah says smilingly. "I think I need some help with that."

"If everything was possible, who or what could have helped you?" I ask. After a short silence, Dinah's gaze wanders downwards, and then she takes a breath and looks at me: "If you could have helped me hold me, perhaps that would have helped," she says rather embarrassingly. "Perhaps I can," I answer. I ask Dinah to show me how. Dinah moves with her hand; attempting to demonstrate the inner holding, she places one hand over her lower stomach and another on her back, "Something like this." I ask for her permission to replace her hands with mine, and ask her to correct my holding so it matches her needs as closely as possible, and she does it for about a minute, whereupon both of us laugh out loud and there is a strong sense of intimacy. "Check if you'd like to keep your own hand there so that you could continue to regulate this holding according to your changing needs," I suggest, and Dinah remains.

"Wow," says Dinah. "What a relief. Finally I can breathe. I feel like I haven't breathed in a month, everything happened so quickly … too quickly … it's not my pace at all. Shit, I've lost myself yet again." Dinah finds it difficult to remain in this expansive body and "comes up" to her familiar critical thinking. [In the Reichian levels of awareness, as described in Chapter Seven, sensations are "lower" and thoughts are "higher". This is not hierarchically so, but a spatial metaphor, which is also in accord with the philosophy of yoga—the chakra centres. Sensory centres are lower in the body, while cognitive centres are higher—ARBS.] "Yes," I respond. "But this time your body insisted on you staying … or perhaps it would be more accurate to say that you have insisted on yourself through your body, and this time you might have slowed down in time because of it." Dinah is drawing another deep breath, her chest softens as well, and her face too. Tears are streaming now. "I am not sad, I actually feel happy now; I feel complete right now. It is such a new feeling. I think I can hold myself on my own now … you know what, I'll hold the front and you'll help me with the back, if that's OK." "It's perfectly OK," I smile at her. "This way I can feel that I don't need to make a rush decision, that I can take the time that I need. I feel like I am on my side despite his pressure."

Towards the end of the session, I ask Dinah to find a way of marking and anchoring her sensations. "It's as if I am not alone inside of me," she says. "My back is stronger, more stable, and I can breathe." "You know, Dinah, I can breathe now as well. I found it difficult to breathe lately during our sessions. I felt unable to be with you, as if I was holding you back and not supporting you. I felt we weren't together. I can now breathe again. Perhaps I felt like your body, as if what I had to say was not interesting, I felt rejected. Not anymore, though. I feel that I have space, and I feel close to you and together again …" "Me too," says Dinah. "I feel that I am back in myself, in my body, and in our relationship. I feel that I want to apologise and say thank you to me in the body and to myself in you, thank you for waiting for me."

The therapeutic process

In his excellent book about Jung and Reich, psychoanalyst and psychotherapist John Conger (1988) argued that Western culture tended to turn the body into the shadow—the aspect of us onto which we projected all our characterological rejected aspects, those we did not wish to acknowledge or identify, as *I*. Elad's session with Dinah was such a journey for retrieving the body from the land of shadow, the wasteland, and an example of relational body psychotherapy in practice.

Elad portrayed a therapeutic process in which he served as Dinah's selfobject. Elad's false-self (Winnicott, 1960a) was far less functioning than Dinah's, and it was this very deficiency which became his major therapeutic advantage. Confronted with Dina's dense character structure, placating and self-defeating, Elad was fighting for himself and for Dinah, and the intersubjective body came to life. Where Dinah found herself sleeping and swallowing, Elad was contracting with pain, becoming vulnerable; where Dinah was quietly faking, Elad was unable to fake, choosing to share. Gradually, Dinah joined Elad in fighting for herself—by repossessing and owning her body, freeing Elad from the role of body-shadow he adopted. Relational psychoanalyst Lewis Aron (2013) argued that much of the analytic endeavour concerned the constructing and deconstructing of binaries (dichotomies), which the therapeutic dyad inevitably entered and got itself entangled with, and opting for undecidables—aspects of thirdness which helped, if only for a moment, exit the binary see-saw dance. The therapist's vulnerability, his willingness to asymmetrically yet mutually surrender to his raw and pounding vulnerability, inviting the client to join, was one important way of achieving this awesome task, for Aron; and Elad was demonstrating this motion of leading through and with his vulnerable and fragile authenticity.

The session began with *identifying the therapist's empathic failure* in relation to the client's happiness through bodily attention. Elad shared his painful and difficult countertransference material. In retrospect, we can see how the therapist *embodied*, with resonance, his client's neglected body. When his somatic countertransference was amplified, Elad chose to share with Dinah his sense of incongruity. This *self-disclosure* created a stormy therapeutic drama. The resonance seemed to be accurate, since Dinah succeeded in assuming responsibility over her effortful and rebellious self-state, which was represented by (and held by) her body.

Shortly afterwards Elad identified a bodily-energetic change in himself and he checked with Dinah, and then the split was more fully exposed. Dinah presented the split between foreground (herself, her cognitive self) and background (the "underdog", the bodily self, the shadow). Dinah's "traumatic body" surfaced and arrived in therapy, and Elad welcomed it—*holding the healthy body in mind, and speaking for the body and on the body's behalf*. Whereas Dinah was used to a violent relationship with her body, Elad demonstrated a *kind relationship with the three bodies in the room*—his own body (who chose not to tolerate unnecessary suffering), Dinah's body (which took care of her), and the intersubjective body (whose information was invaluable for Elad).

Following the split, Elad offered *a reorganisation in the relationship with the body*. At first with words—an organisation which *repossessed the bodily self* (moving from "I have a body" to "I am a body"). Dinah identified her need in help and expressed it, despite her difficulty to do so. Elad assisted Dinah in expanding possibilities by *inviting her to transitional space* ("a world where everything was possible") and Dinah asked for physical holding. The dense character finds asking for help a real challenge, and Dinah's request must have been a moving step. Elad asked Dinah to *demonstrate and calibrate physical contact* before joining in to provide her with *physical holding*. The intimacy reported by Elad was, for me, a testimony of the strengthening of the intersubjective body and the occurrence of both *self and mutual regulation*, and Dinah began to assume responsibility for aspects which were, until that time, represented mainly by Elad.

Touch helped Dinah in marking her boundaries and feeling herself, for the first time in many weeks. But this relief quickly shifted back to her familiar intellectual defences of self-criticism. Here Elad insisted on *connecting to resources* (your body insisted on you)—and presented the body as an active agent, a part of her which supported her, thus inviting Dinah to a kinder and less violent relationship with herself. Connecting to her body was followed by tears, and insights concerning centring, which Dinah described and felt.

Elad asked Dinah to *anchor her feelings*, making these more accessible for her. Dinah observed her body and was able to connect the feeling of centring, grounding, and breathing with her emotional experience. Elad shared his sense of identification with her body and Dinah was able to recognise the wider mind which opened between them and to appreciate its significance.

Therapeutic skills

Identifying the empathic failure: active work with negative countertransference: The case vignette begins with a description of unpleasant sensations and feelings, and generally moves along the edge of discomfort. Elad's willingness to reflect and introspect on his bodily experiences as belonging to a shared field allows for creative and deeply therapeutic work with Dinah. These body sensations are the markers which allow Elad to identify the empathic failure and incongruity within him, setting the substrata for his later sharing of his countertransference material.

Embodiment: Elad comes back to his bodily presence like an anchor in the stormy seas of transference dynamics, and uses his embodiment as a compass in those waters. The sentence "At loss of an escape exit, I choose to share with Dinah the incongruity" tells us of the suffering which accompanies the bridge between sensations and thoughts. Without consistent embodiment, this latent "sleepy" self-state could have lasted for far longer.

Transferential sharing: Choosing to share such a complex set of countertransference material requires clinical judgment, and further—a relational position. Elad shares his vulnerable dissociative states, which reflect within Dinah and in their relationship. Such disclosures expose him as a subject and allow Dinah, gradually, to relate to him—as well as to herself—as subjectivities and not merely as objects or part-objects (from "my traumatic body" to "thank you to me in the body and to myself in you").

Speaking for the body and on the body's behalf: Elad speaks for Dinah's body, defending its intention and presence. He establishes a kind relationship with the neglected self-state, appreciates this part's contribution (inside him as well as in Dinah) thus allowing the therapeutic dyad to take this screaming body-communication more seriously. This kind relationship echoes in the room and is later adopted by Dinah.

Establishing kind and benevolent relationships with the three bodies in the room: The attempts to ignore the body resulted in many splits: between Dinah and her body, between Elad and his body, and between Dinah and Elad (and also between fantasy and reality). Elad was "the weakest link", the less masochistic party (less able and willing to suffer unnecessarily), who challenged this denial and made benevolent connections with the three bodies in the room. At the heart of contact which Elad offered rested an opposite understanding of the Freudian impulsive id: the body was good, and connecting to it served us well. When Dinah adopted this benevolent approach, connections between those aspects were made and the system relaxed (in Aron's (2013) language, they found a third).

Reorganising in the body: How could such gaps be bridged? Through three levels of interventions—linguistic (affective, cognitive), somatic, and relational—Elad encourages Dinah to consider a different bodymind organisation. First, they practise *embodied language*, in which Dinah is called to identify with her body (repossessing her body) through words; second, *contact intervention—self-touch*, demonstrates to Dinah a different possibility of being with her body sensations; last, *the physical holding* offered by Elad (alongside Dinah) reorganises them differently in the relationship. It is no longer necessary to do everything on her own. Chapter Ten expands the discussion on touch in body psychotherapy. Elad offers two types of touch—one which supported Dinah (touch as comfort) and another which strengthened their relationship (touch as relational affirmation).

Inviting and cultivating transitional spaces: In a world where everything was possible there was no need to severe emotion and thought from the body, dissociate myself from the other, split fantasy from reality. When the client's sense of agency (or possibility) was limited and limiting to start with, it meant that transitional spaces were narrow, and the invitation to open fantasy space deepened the connection to transitional spaces and the intersubjective body, allowing Dinah to get in touch with her wish for support and express it, helping Dinah in slowing down and in connecting with her authentic needs.

Self- and mutual (dyadic) regulation: The physical contact portrayed by Elad exemplifies touch which is not done *to* the client or *on* the client, but rather continues the therapeutic dialogue and enquiry. The image of Dinah supporting herself and alongside her Elad who supports her physically is a climax of mutual and self-regulation. We can witness the mutuality of the intersubjective body (Elad is supported by this intimate connection as well) and its asymmetrical nature (Dinah is not called to support Elad, and he holds the responsibility for the boundaries of mutuality).

Connecting to resources: The last two interventions were meant to strengthen integration between cognitive, emotional, and somatic processes. The possibility of viewing these uncomfortable body sensations as resources was a result of a long therapeutic process, and Elad offered a way of exploration which might allow Dinah, over time, to cultivate a more benevolent dialogue with the narratives of her body.

Anchoring the work in sensations: Elad asks Dinah to mark the therapeutic process and anchor it in her body. The bi-directionality of bodywork is expressed here well. Body sensations facilitate the maturation of insights, and those are now returned back into the body, making these more accessible to the client. This anchoring invites Dinah to assume an active position within the therapeutic process.

Embodied therapeutic dialogue

ASAF: Thank you Elad for sharing such an honest relational engagement. You begin by describing very painful countertransference responses, shame, and bodily discomfort. I am curious about the point of no return where you stated: "I've been caught. At loss of an escape exit, I choose to share." What happened there which was too much? And why did you have to get to this "too much" before you could share your incongruity with Dinah?

ELAD: Christopher Bollas (1987) recommended that the therapist should get lost within his countertransference for prolonged periods of time before the processes of identification, sharing, and disentangling could take place. My relationship with Dinah challenged the significance of my own somatic narratives and the place I usually allowed them. Projective identification of loneliness, shame, rejection, and desire to leave the body, in conjunction with Dinah's continuous rejection of my offers throughout our work together to explore the relevance of somatic narratives in the room, all these led me to experience *an empathic failure* with my own body, in which I was lost for a while. It is important to note that in my own biography, I treated my body with mistrust for many years and learning to trust in my body was acquired as a foreign language over the years, so the sense of dissociation found a resonant familiarity in my history.

You may say that for a while, during the sessions with Dinah I had "forgotten" this re-established trust in the body; a forgetfulness which later allowed me to authentically remember it—I believe that this remembrance assisted Dinah too in her authentic remembrance. But this forgetting was not as complete as it was in the past—both with

Dinah and myself (in retrospect, I was happy to discover that I was no longer capable of such an extent of disconnection), and in that moment there was a climactic peak of a struggle, activation of the conflict between the true self (which was in the body at that time) and the false self, motivated by shame and sense of failure. At the peak of the conflict my shame dissipated and I was clear about the dissociation, and with it inner support (in my back) helped me. I no longer needed Dinah's approval that "what I had to say was important enough". This organic processing, which was allowed in my opinion because the conflict was held long enough without splitting it or resolving it, enabled a relatively simple possibility for sharing which was not there earlier. Reflecting on timing, I believe that sharing this earlier would have forced me to be a therapist who "does what needs doing", overcoming the feelings of shame and self-doubt by dissociating from these. Thus, it was actually the capacity to tolerate these feelings over time which brought the organic maturation, a non-violent containment of the conflict, and subsequently a possibility for Dinah to do so herself.

ASAF: After Dinah places her hand over her mouth and rages against her body, you speak for it: "After all, you do have a full and rich life here, which you are willing to throw away in an instant"—and I was thinking of her willingness to throw away you in an instant. Where were *you* there?

ELAD: Following the sharing of my body sensations (which was initially autonomous, without conscious awareness of the conflict), a rupture and repair took place in me, and then Dinah's holding mechanism re-establishes itself—in both of us, really. Only this time, the holding is less "tight", hence she can be mindful of the conflict. Dinah, experiencing her body as almost demonic, once again threatens to abandon herself and therefore the intersubjective body, too, and therefore me as well. There is a threat here, but it is not as violent as it was, and less muted too. I do react with holding against the threat of abandonment, but it is less grasping: I am not overwhelmed by it; my heart and mind stay clear. I am quieter and therefore not identified with the abandonment. For a moment, I feel lonely again, but I do not leave myself behind; the selfhood in my body which is reacting to this abandonment in the shared field remains intact. Therefore this time shame, guilt, and doubt are no longer clouding my experience. I can choose to remain present and once again feel the body (bodies) as benevolent.

ASAF: So, you say that even if Dinah "threatened" to leave you, you did not abandon yourself so it was more tolerable. It connects me to another question. When and how did you realise that you have become identified with Dinah's body?

ELAD: After sharing my feelings with Dinah, and her body responded with shaking and tears, I felt a huge release and was increasingly curious about this mutual influence. I understood that I was her body when my body, yet again, responded with similar sensations to her more explicit reservation (hand on mouth) a few moments later.

ASAF: The description of touch felt highly intimate. What did you experience there? Was there an erotic charge? How did you know it was appropriate, particularly in light of the therapeutic goal?

ELAD: The physical contact was indeed very intimate, but it wasn't sexual. Sharing in the holding felt more like partnership and strengthening of Dinah's parental selfobject. I felt within an interesting transference dynamics, as a "half parent" alongside Dinah.

However, since I am also a man representing for Dinah the world of men in relation to which Dinah attempts to establish herself, I held in mind the importance of withdrawing from the physical holding when Dinah managed to sufficiently strengthen the inner symbolisation and the resource of holding in her body. Indeed, later in therapy this positioning allowed her to position herself differently against me as a man and we were able to work with issues of eroticism and sexuality between us.

ASAF: Your countertransference disclosures, throughout the session but particularly in the end, felt exposing and made you very vulnerable with Dinah. Could you share some of your motivation for such sharing? Wasn't it frightening?

ELAD: Yes. It was frightening. Frightening and enlivening. In working with most clients who come to me a theme is becoming clearer over time, and I am mindful of how significant my capacity to tolerate my vulnerability in my encounter with the world is for me and my clients. I truly believe that my monitored disclosure and vulnerability is the most powerful and softest therapeutic tool I possess. I invite myself, time and again, in accordance with my resources and the resources available to the shared field, to bring myself into the therapeutic relationship with my raw openness, my vulnerability, and my apprehension. I do so in a regulated, gradual, and examining manner, without abandoning myself or burdening the client with my material. I have chosen to demonstrate good enough attachment, and encourage the client to perceive herself or himself as well as me as subjects. The extent to which I can offer myself like this, if at all, and the fullness of this feeling (its somatic quality) is also an important diagnostic tool for me, indicating the aspects of character structure and current positions in the client's life and in our relationship.

Note

1. Rilke's poem is reprinted here with kind permission of translators Anita Barrows and Joanna Macy.

CHAPTER NINE

Body psychotherapeutic skills

> "I can't believe that!" said Alice.
> "Can't you?" the Queen said in a pitying tone. "Try again: draw a long breath, and shut your eyes."
> Alice laughed. "There's not use trying," she said. "One can't believe impossible things."
> "I daresay you haven't had much practice," said the Queen. "When I was your age, I always did it for half an hour a day. Why, sometimes I've believed as many as six impossible things before breakfast."
>
> —*Lewis Carroll,* Through the Looking Glass: And what Alice Found there (1871, pp. 83–84).

In the last chapter we looked at six body psychotherapeutic approaches, and were able to appreciate their different theoretical and clinical richness. This chapter focuses on eight body psychotherapeutic skills, which are presented here through clinical vignettes (except one) and a short discussion. Two other skills, touch and resonance, are expanded upon in separate chapters. Client names and identifying details have been changed, and permission to use these vignettes was given. Some of these descriptions consist of an amalgamation of clients.

Embodiment

Throughout the book, and particularly in Chapters Five and Seven, I wrote about the centrality of embodiment in body psychotherapy. We could also see in Chapter Eight how different therapists used this skill as a part of the therapeutic process. The following vignette demonstrates how embodiment could be used to support recovery processes from addiction.

Nigel came to therapy after his recovery from heroin addiction (smoking, not injecting) and following a suggestion from his Narcotics Anonymous (NA) sponsor that he sought psychotherapy which included his body too. Nigel was a bachelor, a handsome and impressive man in his early thirties; his upper body was broad and well-developed, his shoulders strong and well-shaped. Contrasting with these was his lower body which nearly did not exist; thin and unsubstantial legs continued the back with no buttocks.

Nigel "came from money", an upper middle class background, the eldest son of wealthy parents, a very influential English family, and was the future heir to an important family and political business. Hard work and high achievements were important values for both parents, who sent Nigel to a prestigious boarding school when he was seven. Nigel described the sorrow he felt when he left home: "I wasn't really sad to leave my dad, 'cause I never really saw him anyways, but I missed my mum and my au pair who was made redundant the day I left for boarding school." His busy parents never gave Nigel any boundaries, and he started smoking at nine, and drinking alcohol and smoking marijuana at eleven: "… in the boarding school too but mainly at home. Friends would come to our house during the weekend, and we would party." The motif of rebellion and "partying" was central in Nigel's life.

Nigel's drug habit expanded as part of his lifestyle, and when Nigel graduated from one of the most esteemed independent schools in England he was sent to study political sciences at Oxford University, where he met his first true love, heroin. From that moment onwards, Nigel's degradation was a common path of hard drugs addiction, moving through theft and begging, through being expelled from his parents' home, uncontrolled and unprotected sex with men and women for a hit or for money, and interweaved in all these—ample doses of self-abandonment. Nigel said that "One day I woke up in the morning and I saw myself from the outside, having reached rock bottom, begging for money, stinking and filthy, wondering who I could offer a blow job to for a hit, [and then] I managed to persuade my parents to help me and send me to rehab." Nigel came to see me after a year of being "clean". "I still want to smoke all the time," he said, "and I know that I will never stop missing heroin, but I have a hole in my stomach, and I always had a hole in my stomach, and I want to understand it."

Nigel worked part time, was financially and emotionally supported by his parents (for the first time in his life, really) and lived next to them. Although he despises his dependence, he knew (and I concurred) that he still needed close support and gradual, lengthy, and gentle recovery and rehabilitation.

The twice weekly therapy with Nigel was exciting and frustrating at the same time, oscillating between slow and authentic tiny changes and "revolutionary insights and grandiose climaxes" which expectedly turned out to be short term and temporary. In my countertransference, I sometimes felt like an outside observer, looking at an exciting yet dangerous adventure, sometimes full of envy, and at others grateful for my "boring" life. We had sufficient shared spaces to allow for our connection to deepen, and we were sufficiently different to not be swept too deeply into his dangerously addictive places. Therapy with Nigel felt like fighting for his life, a fight which was not merely symbolic.

After two months of establishing the therapeutic frame and getting to know one another, I invited Nigel to look at "the hole in his stomach". He looked at me with dread: "Are you sure it's a smart move?" he asked. Immediately, I was filled with fear and doubt. What if we open a can of worms? What if this bodily enquiry into the void will send him into the streets again? "I am not at all sure, Nigel," I replied. "At the moment, I am not sure about anything here—it's frightening to touch and frightening not to touch. But perhaps you are right, perhaps getting into this hole is too early. How about looking around it?" Nigel stretched his arms behind his head: "The no-man's-land around my belly button," he laughed bitterly, "where I keep all the junk," he said and patted his stomach.

"So, allow yourself to be this no-man's-land for a moment, inside your body, feeling yourself from the inside. What's happening there?" Nigel looked at me as if I had just come from a different planet: "It sounds interesting, but I have no idea how to do that." I proposed he place a hand on the area of his body surrounding the hole in the stomach. Nigel placed his hand there, and breathed. I felt restless. "I fancy a fag," he said. "Can I smoke in here?" "No, you cannot," I replied.

Together we sit for many long hours, session after session. The body awakens and shouts. Nigel is processing his grief and is mourning, and the body tells us about his losses. Cigarettes soothe the pain only a little, alcohol a tiny bit more, but the real craving is for ultimate silence. "It pains me to be in my body," he tells me after a month. "It always did hurt. When I was a really young boy at school I'd go out into the cold with as little clothes as possible until my feet no longer felt anything, and then I'd scratch myself with sticks and stones and take delight in not feeling any pain."

A week later I put my own hand on Nigel's lower back. "Can you breathe into this place?" I ask. Nigel breathes; I feel an unpleasant contraction in my diaphragm. He speaks of the blows he regularly got from his classmates "every morning in the let's hit Nigel ceremony". "In the first months I really did hurt, then I started laughing—nothing touched me." I contract with pain, and so does Nigel: "Suddenly the back of the boy that I was really hurts; there is so much pain in me."

Nigel religiously arrives for his sessions, is never late. Week after week he discovers his body and I am filled with doubt. What is so precious about having a body when it harbours so much pain? Why not help Nigel dissociate less dangerously? Who am I to decide that "being inside the body is good, being dissociated from the body is bad"? To supervision I bring concrete debates, technical questions. I keep my true inner heresy to myself, swallowing the pain, just like Nigel.

One day Nigel arrives for therapy in a storm. He knocks on the door before the session while I am with another client. In the last moments of that session my mind is busy with Nigel; my client is insulted by my lack of attention: she is right, of course. "I had sex yesterday, for the first time in my life," Nigel storms in excitedly when we begin. I look at him with confused eyes. "What?" Nigel reiterates: "Yesterday, for the first time in my life I had real sex. I was in it. I didn't smoke before, I didn't drink alcohol. We were simply together." He looks so moved, and I begin to get excited with him and for him. "Well, what was it like then?" I ask. "Truthfully?" he answers. "Pretty shit. I was nervous, I couldn't really get it on, and when I did I came within a minute or so. But we were together, and we talked, and I could feel myself and her—and we have a way to go, we can grow together."

I share my heretic thoughts with Nigel and he laughs at me: "This valve is not selective, Asaf. When I turn off the pain—joy, pleasure, and connection to God—these too are blocked away, do you get it?" I nod. For a moment we seem to have swapped roles, and Nigel carries on: "I feel that for the first time since I was five or six I am inside my life, not seeking to live alongside my life but really am inside it. And my life is not always fun, but it is mine, and I can do things in my life, I have me."

During the next years of therapy Nigel approaches, in narrowing circles, the void in his stomach. At every step of the way we discover pain and courage, and he reclaims another dimension of his being; his presence and existence strengthen together with our relationship. And the homeostatic dynamic between faith and heresy continues to accompany us: we swap roles—at times it is my role to hold faith and trust in the process, and at others it is his; sometimes I question and doubt the need for mourning, and at other times it is Nigel who doubts. And as we play together, Nigel finds a partner and leaves his parental home, and goes on to study gardening, where he is contented.

Sensory attunement

> Nonverbal attunement creates the original space of thirdness in which the free flowing back-and-forth does not appear as a reaction to the other's demand but as the partners' mutual creation of a dance—the first form of mutual recognition. This space later becomes that of dialogue, in which it becomes possible to create meanings that transcend those of the singular person …
>
> —Jessica Benjamin (2000, p. 49)

I loved Phil from the beginning, but felt slightly apprehensive towards him. We met in a workshop I gave, and Phil was an active and dominant figure there: asking questions, participating, and generously sharing of himself. Two years later he came to therapy. Phil, forty years old, was a talented psychotherapist, divorced and a father to two sons, handsome and tall, and a self-made man. He was born in Glasgow to working class parents, full of inferiority complexes. His father was a bitter taxi driver and his mother, who was half Indian, was temping all her life. Phil, forever alien, graduated from high school and moved to London, where he studied psychotherapy in college and worked to support himself. He sought therapy because of violence—both internal and external. "I seem to attract violence to me," he reported sadly. "I get stressed by that and then disconnect from my feelings and experiences."

The first months of therapy were stormy for us both. On the one hand, we shared a deep sense of coming home—we both felt somewhat comforted in the mere knowing that the other existed in the world. We had an immediate connection. The fact that I was Israeli was central for Phil—being foreign in England dictated my class—I was, to a certain extent, outside the British class system: I was not "born into a class without ever being able to get out of it" as Phil was. My Israeli nationality was, for Phil, a declaration of being unclassified, and allowed him to explore his relationship with me and with himself in a purified way. However, alongside the ease of connection it was also difficult for me. Sometimes—and inconsistently so—Phil would attack me: raising his voice, using harsh words or hand gestures, which I experienced as violent. I usually reacted to this violence in one of two ways: I either found myself inwardly withdrawing (and feeling like a victim), or analytically withdrawing, which concealed a sadistic wish to hurt Phil, particularly with knife-sharp words and uncompassionate interpretations (where I would abandon him, "victimising" him, sacrificing Phil to the shrine of understanding the process).

The experience of attack was mainly sensory, including irregular breathing and discomforted stomach.

These fluctuations exhausted me, and alongside looking forward to seeing Phil and genuinely enjoying our meeting, I found myself anxious and apprehensive towards them. Our dynamic was tense: moving, but tense. Slowly, I learned about Phil's mother, who had clear borderline and exploitative tendencies, and about his physically violent father. Mum "sacrificed me to dad in order to save herself". One day Phil spoke of an experience, which "demonstrates how people in authority positions respond to me". Phil arrived for his group supervision, and after he presented his client, the supervisor invited the group to "kick Phil's arse" with criticism. I felt nauseated and contracted when I heard this description, and was filled with anger, guilt, and fear. When Phil asked his supervisor why she was cruel to him, she responded: "Because you can take it, you're strong." "They don't get it," he protested, "that I am weak too, that I too need softness. Somehow I only show one side of myself."

After some deliberation, I shared with Phil that I, too, knew this movement, of wanting to "kick his arse" because he could take it. We also talked about my fear of him. "It saddens me," he replied, "but it's nothing new—it always happens to me." We were both disappointed with our enactment, inevitable as it might have been.

This session changes something in me, in my readiness to examine my reactions and Phil's. I prepared for the next session by centring and grounding myself, and made a vow to use my violence and fear as a source of information and a compass, and to make an effort not to shame myself for feeling these feelings. We started talking and Phil told me that he experienced splits throughout the week and had a real urge to call me and speak with me during the week. I started moving uncomfortably; feeling a claustrophobic suffocation, as if I was expected to give more than I was ready to give—as if by meeting Phil's needs, he will only want more and more. When I found myself feeling aggression towards Phil I stopped him. I could feel my hands wanting to clench into fists; my eyes following Phil's movements, even the tiniest motion; my jaws locking. "I feel a lot of aggression inside of me," I told Phil. He was angry with me: "It's because I'm opening up to you. I allow you to come closer and share my vulnerability and need, and you want to hit me."

Was he right? Was it projective identification, and was I activated by Phil's neediness, moved to attempt to destroy him (the weak) like his father? While this felt like a possibility, something in it felt inaccurate for me. The next time I felt this aggressive urge I asked us both to slow down. I wanted us to examine the roadmap paved by our bodily sensations to better understand our emotional processes. We "rewound" the film and in "slow motion" explored our body-to-body communication: Phil talked about wanting to send me a text message, and a moment later my fists began to clench. Perhaps he was right after all! We were trapped in a loop of violence. But then Phil interfered, saying: "I'm telling you about the text message, and noticing that my jaw is locking." A memory surfaced, and Phil's eyes moistened: "Dad couldn't bear my softness. Every time he felt I was too weak he would smack me like a carpet beater, perhaps hoping to rid me of the dust of neediness with enough smacking." As Phil spoke, I noticed slight movements in his hands, chest, and shoulders. He shared an experience of hurt and immediately inflamed his body and his hands clenched into fists: "I'm awaiting the blow," he responded when I asked him about those fists. "I won't hit you, Phil. I will not kick your arse or destroy you."

Thanks to our bodily tracking of the process of projective identification, we were able to exit (for a while, at least) this unconscious transferential lattice and engage with it more consciously. Sensitivity to sensory information and using it as a compass to our work supported the therapeutic progress and the more Phil and I were able to notice our bodily defensive mechanisms, the better able we were to relate to one another—our relationship changed, gradually yet consistently. The ambivalence in our connection faded away within a few months, and from the cycle of violence we were hooked in came a great neediness, which Phil expressed for the first time clearly and without restrictions. Our love intensified too, and alongside the erotic challenges it brought with it, it also created a safe space which enabled both of us to change.

I was no longer fearful of Phil or his angry outbursts. I could mostly foresee them, and not feel personally attacked. The sensory attunement completely transformed our aggressive transference dynamics, and Phil shared a novel feeling: "I no longer repeat previous relationships here with you," he said. "We are building something new. It frustrates me to realise that these enactment loops exist in nearly every relationship of mine, but at least there is one place where they are stopped in the act—and then you can see me, and I can see myself." From the violence emerged deep mourning, which Phil managed to feel for the first time—grieving over the neglected child that he was, the violence which surrounded him, the inevitable repetition compulsion in his relationships with others.

Phil's stormy relationship patterns began changing as well. From short-lived and dramatic sadistic-masochistic relationships, with women who fell madly in love with him only to later behave violently towards him, and Phil himself being violent and aggressive, he found a stormy woman in her own right who consented to stay. Annabel still struggled to see Phil's aggression as neediness, but unlike past relations, Phil insisted on showing her—bringing his softness and neediness into the relationship. And she opened towards him, accepted him, and chose him.

It seemed that the energetic and emotional reaction to the violent father and borderline mother, which activated Phil and subsequently his environment, softened a little. The sadness which replaced the dissociation can sometimes give way to joy, connection, and true mutual witnessing and validation. Phil married Annabel and they had a girl. The sensory attunement skills which we have developed and cultivated in our work together still help Phil in living more consciously and acting more mindfully in his life, creating, from the old bodymind patterns of the past, a novel movement of connection, faith, and love.

Body reading

In Reichian body psychotherapy modalities, body reading could be a formal skill: the client stands naked or minimally dressed while the therapist examines him, gathering anatomic information and analysing the somatic and emotional contexts. Character structure analysis through body reading may provide accurate and important information about the client, his beliefs and fears, pains, and defence mechanisms.

Needless to say such type of observation, beyond the dread it may evoke in many clients, could also perpetuate rigid transferential patterns, which would later be difficult to transcend—primarily authoritative doctor-patient ones. This type of body reading could at the same time cultivate saving fantasies with the client who surrenders to the omnipotent and expert therapist. The painting presented in Chapter One, *A Clinical Lesson with Doctor Charcot at the Salpêtrière*, portrays such a pathos laden-context, which may create a myriad of transferential distortions, which unless tended to, would complicate a collaborative and shared-agency process of psychotherapy.

However, body reading can provide the therapist and client with invaluable information about the client, the foreseen difficulties, and the prospect of therapeutic work—sometimes much more than words (Rosen & Brenner, 2003). Additionally, many psychological diagnostic tests face the same problem, and still these are occasionally administered. There are some forms of body psychotherapy where formal body reading is still practised, but this is done collaboratively and in a more humanistic fashion. In postural integration, for example (a method established by Jack Painter and presented in Chapter Three), the therapist stands alongside the client adopting her posture; together they look at bodily patterns and muscular holding which they notice. The body reading process becomes a position from which client and therapist deduce (together) therapeutic interventions (Painter, 1984).

For example, Brandon is standing up and I stand beside him. "Let yourself stand in the most natural and comfortable way," I ask, "and scan your body with your attention. Notice where you are attracted to, where you feel yourself present." Perhaps there are areas which are more relaxed, or contracted; there could be differences of temperature or texture; heavier sensations in some areas; left and right differences, up or down. While Brandon is scanning, I adopt his body posture and observe my own. My left foot turns outwardly (the toes are looking to the left) and I feel that, in order to maintain this position, I need to tightly tense my buttock muscles. "What are you aware of?" I ask Brandon. "A dull and uncomfortable pain in my lower back, on the left side." I draw his attention to his feet: "Could you amplify this outward position of the foot, a little bit like Charlie Chaplin?" Brandon tries and loses his balance. "And what would happen if you exaggerated the opposite movement, if you turned your feet inwardly?" Brandon tries. "My backache completely disappears," he smiles, but a moment later continues, "But I feel very exposed." This body reading becomes the basis of psychotherapeutic work with these two movements which we bodily explored: Brandon felt either tense and safe, or relaxed and exposed.

Regardless of whether formal body reading is practised or not, the body psychotherapist continuously observes the body of her client and the somatic expression which reaches her clinic (as well as those which are left outside). She may, for example, be curious about body segments which may indicate bodily holding, or attempt to define character structures; but moreover she relates to her client's bodily organisation in her presence (and her own organisation in the client's presence) as a central source for information, diagnoses, and therapeutic intervention. The following vignette will demonstrate using body reading both as a diagnostic tool at the beginning of a session (assessing the foreseen therapeutic work) and as a supportive agent for reaching clinical decisions:

Diana was depressed and lacked any motivation for change. She came to therapy because "There's no choice, it must be dealt with"—but she did not really believe in her capacity to change, or in her language, "to improve". Her body structure was dense, with distinct muscular holding in her buttocks, jaws, diaphragm, shoulder girdle, and back. She was firm and strong, and felt like a rock: unmoveable.

Because of her dense body structure, and especially due to her frequent, if indirect, expressions of anger, I expected anger to become a major therapeutic issue, but only in later stages of therapy. As for Diana, she denied the existence of anger in her life. "Can't you see I'm depressed? I am not angry, just very sad," she insisted.

One day Diana sat in a characteristic position: she took a big cushion and put it on her knees, thus creating a big buffer between us, and started to laboriously portray a story about her work partner and lunch sandwiches. For years Diana brought sandwiches to work and Geoff had never brought any. Every day Geoff "… was ordering himself a sandwich, and I soon realised this was the case so I made him food too. Last week," Diana continued, "Geoff arrived to work. for the first time in years—with food! He received a big box of pastries from a happy customer and he brought this box to work. I sat next to him as he took out the cardboard box and reached for a pastry, without even thinking of offering me one. I was so insulted." Naturally, Diana said nothing, not even when Geoff took his daily sandwich, without flinching.

Hearing the end of the story I found myself feeling infuriated with Geoff and angry with Diana's placating passivity; nevertheless, I was no longer bored. Looking at Diana, I noticed that her entire body changed: her face was crimson red, her shoulders were pulled to the back, and her legs were swinging restlessly. But my attention was actually drawn to her hands. I was looking at her hands as Diana spoke—she pinched the cushion, slapped it, and scratched it. "As I'm hearing you speak of Geoff, Diana, I get angry and irritated, it is infuriating." Diana looks at me bewildered: "It's not infuriating, Asaf, it's insulting and saddening." I attempted to draw her attention to her hands—"Your hands don't seem to be insulted, actually." Diana threw the cushion on the floor, "You and your silly things, analysing everything. I was just playing with the cushion."

I asked Diana to stand up and she complied (as always). The cushion was there, just in front of her. "Here's Geoff," I said. "Just notice your bodily impulses." Diana was shaking, trying to retrieve her balance with a breathing exercise. "Stop your meditation, Diana, please. Stay with me."

Diana is looking at me, and I at her—a volcano. "Don't let anything out," I ask, "keep it all inside." She asks if she can sit now, it's tiring for her to stand up. I ask her to stay standing just for a little longer. Her legs begin to kick the cushion. Small kicks, so that neither of us will notice. We continue to talk and her kicks grow stronger and more forceful. Only when she kicks so hard for the cushion to fly to the other side of the room does she notice her power. Spontaneously, we give some space for cathartic work with anger: Diana kicks the cushion time and again. In my mind, the sandwiches are now spread all over the room. "I am not angry, I am just doing what you've asked me to," Diana is shouting while kicking. Only after long minutes, when she sits down breathing heavily, she smiles: "I hate him, and why could I not ask for a bloody pastry?"

In the following week Diana does not bring Geoff sandwiches, and she delights in her expression of anger and in Geoff's placating flattery during the week. We spend a few sessions working in front of a mirror, and Diana is astounded to discover her bodily expressions of anger. Gradually, she learns to express her anger directly and her bodily tensions ease. Together with these, her victim position softens as well and the depression, which accompanied the pain and tension, is also relieved.

Breathwork

Reich's biographer, Myron Sharaf, drew similar parallels between the psychoanalytic free association technique and Reichian observation of breathing patterns. In psychoanalysis, the patient was asked to say whatever is on her mind, while the analyst pointed to resistances in the free flowing nature of association. "Correspondingly," wrote Sharaf (1984), "in Reich's therapy, the patient is asked to lie down and to breathe. Then attention is called to a variety of ways in which he or she 'resists' natural inspiration and expiration" (p. 236). The following vignette will demonstrate breathwork as part of a psychodynamic therapeutic work. While the presented skill is not Reichian breathwork, it nonetheless rests on the assumption that breathing and breathwork serve as a useful "door in" to affective and dyadic spaces.

Marian, an interior designer, was thirty years old when she started psychotherapy. She was a petite woman, with bright hair and eyes on fire; searching for herself, wishing to explore. During the initial phone conversation she was upfront and open: "I'm fed up with my life. I get into depressive periods which last a year or two at a time and then come out of them. I begin new initiatives and new life, then get depressed again and leave everything behind." Marian is married to Garth, a businessman who "doesn't like talking, doesn't like sex, and doesn't like being with me". Garth's parents are good friends with Marian's parents who introduced them to each other about ten years ago. During the initial phone call Marian warned me that "I am a difficult case." She described herself as lacking the capacity to love or express feelings in a relationship, "... which is why I make do with such a pathetic relationship." She told me that she was in many psychotherapeutic relationships and had exhausted all her therapists, just like she exhausted Garth in their marriage, and her parents since she was a young girl. Marian came to see me through Joyce, a massage teacher who I knew. Marian studied massage; for her, "Touch always helps me connect me to myself, even if it never lasts." Her train journey to my clinic was about three hours long.

At that time, about three years after we moved to England, I had difficulties breathing. It was hard for me to breathe in, and I experienced bodily anxieties and fear, although I could not recognise any significant emotional difficulties at the time.

We met for an initial session about a month after our conversation. In this first session, Marian went into the room, sat in front of me and told me that her sleeping was very fragmented last week, and that she had many distressing and invasive memories. For about twenty minutes Marian told me about her dreams, highly exposing and sexual, painful, and full of graphic details. Marian spoke without a break, and with great speed. She seamlessly moved from speaking about her dreams to describing her marital life, which was boring and unsatisfying, came back to some dream imagery, then once more followed an association to speak of how her life was void of meaning, lacking any focus or real passion, and her terror of change. I felt split and confused. On the one hand, Marian described a near-dead world, turned off and pale, yet she was vital as she spoke, her language rich and colourful, and Marian beamed with beauty, which was childish but still moved me.

It took me over fifteen minutes to notice my discomfort. My heart was pounding and I barely breathed; I was leaning forward with interest and my neck was hurting. When did I manage to compromise my posture like that? How come I did not notice? I sat cross-legged, frowning and not breathing—yet I felt vital and excited. It was a very strange experience for me. I decided not to change my posture. On the contrary—I exaggerated it a little, contracting my body even more, and looked at Marian. She talked and talked, her eyes gleaming and her pace was quick and stormy. My mind wandered to Joyce, the teacher who referred Marian to me. Joyce would move as she spoke, as if she was massaging the ears of her listeners. Once more, I was with Marian, feeling slightly guilty for my reverie. If you were looking from outside at her monologue and my response, you could have thought that two people were intimately and affectively speaking with each other, while being attuned to one another. But from the inside it felt very different. I did not know her at all, it was our first session. I felt tempted to just let things be, to allow her to go on and on talking. I thought to myself: "We're nearly halfway through our session; soon she'll finish and I'll get my money and could then rest a little …" I did not want to make any more effort, just to let go and rest. And I wanted my reward.

Yet another part of me began to rebel against the contraction and incoherence I sensed. I sat up straight. Marian, who seemed oblivious to my inner turbulence, carried on talking. I asked her to stop for a moment. "Marian, we don't know each other yet—it is our first session, and you share yourself with so much honesty and openness, talking about important and deep material," Marian nodded. "It must be at least a little bit scary or embarrassing to share so much of yourself to somebody you don't even know, isn't it?" I asked. Marian's chest moved subtly; she took very little air (I imagined her trying not to breathe too much) and said: "Not at all, why would it be? I'm used to it, as I told you—I've seen many psychotherapists, and it feels the easiest place in the world, and I feel that you are really listening to me and present with me and it makes it easier still."

I felt guilty, as if I was deluding her. And I started to resent Marian for the dissociations I felt, and the efforts I have made, for my sense of misery. Notwithstanding this storm, a part of me managed to witness these storms and smiled, compassionately, at both of us. I placed my feet on the ground and sat down again, inviting Marian to stop and breathe. I attempted to reflect to her what she said: "You have seen many experienced therapists, and you're used to talking about your feelings, your past, and your discontentedness, your hopes and your difficulties; you know this position well. And you've been referred to see me by Joyce your massage teacher, and on the phone you told me that your body helps you reconnect with yourself," I spoke slowly, and with the measured words felt that my body was returning to me. Marian nodded. I offered her an experiment: "Let's see what will happen if we found a pleasant breathing rhythm, one that allows you to be present to yourself, your sensations, and your feelings, but does not overwhelm you." For twenty minutes Marian breathed. At first, her breathing was small, chesty, and quick. Gradually it slowed down. "I'm really surprised to see how my natural rhythm is much slower than I thought," she said. The session was about to end, and I sent Marian home with a task of practising her breathing in the mornings—reconnecting with the rhythms of her breath. I suggested that our next sessions should be ninety minutes long, to enable us to slow down her pace as well as because of her long ride (three hours in each direction).

As a body psychotherapist, I look at breathing patterns as expressing particular (if idiosyncratic) emotional positions. Change of breathing patterns fosters affective change, and breathwork becomes a highly valuable tool for regulation and calming down, amplification, and connection, embodiment, and attunement (Heller, 2006). Knowing all this, I felt smug with the breathing interventions I offered. But when Marian left the clinic I had a minor panic attack. I firmly held on to the chair, breathing slowly, trying to calm my fear. At first I connected my anxiety to Marian and her emotional flooding, when I suddenly realised that my own breathing difficulties during the past few months finally received their due place, when I slowed down to demonstrate the work to Marian. Slowing down enabled me to feel the depth of our conflict about being in England—missing Israel on the one hand, and wishing to remain and live in England on the other—a debate which I was not allowing myself to fully feel for several long months. My panic attack slowed down, my breathing softened, and I smiled when I thought of my patronising intervention—of "the expert" and of the lesson I was given by Marian.

Marian arrived for the next session excited and wanting to share with me how significant she found her homework. Within moments she was carried away with her free association at a rapid pace, which formed into a narrative that reminded me of our first session. I found myself leaning towards her, tensing my eyes, brows, and forehead, while my breathing was gradually but surely disappearing. This time I stopped her after merely a few moments. I briefly shared my sense of anxiety and breathing difficulties—and how the attention to breathing was important for me too. With my bodily subjectivity reclaimed, Marian was excited to hear this, and had to quickly check that I was not leaving for Israel any time soon; then she calmed down and we resumed talking while noticing our breathing.

The following intervention accompanied us for eight or nine sessions and, for me, marked the transition from enactment to forming novel movement. I limited Marian's stormy pace, to the extent that allowed me to remain present. We repeated the breathwork exercise time and again, and Marian slowed down. As her rhythm changed, my dissociative and resentful countertransference softened as well and I was better able to be present—to feel my body and take an interest in Marian. "I want to offer something a bit unusual, Marian. I'll mark the rhythm of your breathing by gently tapping on my knees, like a metronome. And I want to suggest that whatever you wish to say today—you say in the pace of the marked rhythm of your breathing—and only when exhaling." I thereafter used my body as a metronome, which was in accord with Marian's slow and connected breath, as well as dictating the rhythm of our conversation, which made it hypnotic for both of us. Marian was enthused by the idea, and told me about a dream while we both kept this slightly artificial pace of her breathing, speaking, and tapping. Within two minutes her eyes were filled with tears and she stopped: "It feels too intimate," she said. "I nearly don't know you at all and I'm sharing my erotic dreams with you." I sighed with relief. "It is truly too much for today, Marian. How about telling me something simpler? Can you match what you are talking about with your capacity to maintain this breathing?" The session continued bathed in this trance quality, characterised by slower rhythm than our regular ones, extraordinary muscular relaxation, and openness to ideas and possibilities which Marian did not consider before. Every so often she stopped and moved to a less charged topic. Despite the fact that the content of her sharing was less interesting, I felt more present and kinder to myself and to her.

Breathing exercises are among the most ancient ways of changing states of consciousness. In many cultures, breathing is identified with spirit (and soul), and breathwork is seen as a way of inviting the spirit to dwell in the body—feeling god within our body (Hendricks, 1995). Breathing is forever with us, one of the most constant forms in our life, yet at the same time, breathing is always dynamic and changing. Breathing is one of the most efficient ways to regulate emotions, and many powerful and simple meditations use breathwork—focusing on our sensory experience serves as a bridge to the vitality principle and the pulsating nature of the universe. Often it is sufficient to return our attention to our breathing in order to open a fertile affective field, ripe for inner work or therapeutic work. When we breathe together, as I breathed with Marian, we share in the breath, and so partaking in the intersubjective body receives yet another dimension and depth.

To my surprise, Marian brought a metronome to our next session. Having established her breathing rhythms, she used a metronome to be reminded of it. This time her sharing was a tad more intimate, but still miles away from the unregulated sharing of our first session, and it was accompanied by stopping and checking with me—that I understood, that I was there. The slow rhythms allowed Marian to stay attuned to herself and also to notice me. However, she was frustrated with her slow pace: "When I breathe slowly I don't really trust you enough, and I feel that I need to test you all the time. At this pace therapy will never ever end …"

I shared with Marian my excitement about the tests she put me through. These tests actually relaxed me much more than the implicit uncensored trust of the first session. I could increasingly trust myself in her presence, and therefore I was more able to trust her. Marian learned to tolerate emotional charge without always splitting, and in so doing enriched her bodily presence with substantial emotional presence. She no longer exhausted me and reported an awakening and enlivening of her friendships. "It still annoys me that as soon as I slow down I feel so many feelings, but I guess that most times it's better than not feeling at all," she said during our eighth metronome session. "Perhaps", I suggested, "there's a place for both of them—for feeling deeply and for dissociating from the feeling and easing the pain, only your capacity to choose adds a little more freedom …"

Over our three years of psychotherapy, breathing was an important guide to our capacity to regulate affect, not just for Marian but also between us and between Marian and the world. Intense listening to her natural breathing rhythms (which changed over time and according to circumstances) enabled Marian, after a while, to identify early markers for depression, which were always present but she was previously unable to recognize, and to cultivate an appropriate support network around these depressive ways. Thanks to identifying those markers, and her capacity to answer her needs during these early stages, Marian managed to sometimes avoid turning her lower moods into full blown paralysing depressive episodes.

Working with somatic transference and countertransference[1]

I met Jennifer when she was thirty-six, working as house doctor in an NHS hospital. A year into therapy I still felt that I nearly did not know her at all. In her presence, I was surrounded by a sense of great emotional complexity which I could not disentangle, a kind of fog. I made tremendous efforts to remain centred without being pulled into self-criticism or dissociation; I lost my sharp thinking. Over time, I found ways of overcoming this lack of concentration and it seemed that the fog dispersed a little. During this year Jennifer underwent real changes in her life—she was more assertive in her workplace, her relationships with her parents and sister improved, and she managed to slightly liberate herself from recurring obsessive thinking patterns. Only sexually nothing moved and Jennifer felt frozen and completely disinterested. She found her almost daily intercourse with her partner Michael a real wonder. "He seems to truly enjoy himself while I try to think about food or work so I won't get too bored." Our attempts to trace the sources of her dissociation, or alternatively establish reconnection with her eroticism and passion were futile. Jennifer learned to feel her body and listen to it, but ultimately remained asexual. To survive the fog, we "did" things; it was as if much of my psychodynamic thinking and practice were left outside the room. Additionally, my countertransference surprised me: although Jennifer was a pretty and attractive woman and I "should have" been attracted to her, she evoked in me only anatomic, mechanical curiosity.

After two years of psychotherapy with Jennifer, where working with touch was a central connecting agent, a curtain of heaviness and sadness enveloped our process, yet it lacked any narrative content. For a good few weeks, and during every session with her, I suffered from stomach cramps, and if I were not so uncomfortable showing it, I would have contorted in pain. Jennifer would speak, and I was cramped with pain and gas, trying with much effort to conceal my suffering; I felt ashamed of my pain and terrified by the prospect of her noticing it. I found myself in a familiar position; a shy teenage boy, trying to conceal his fear and loneliness in the hope that nobody would notice him and reveal him.

Interestingly, my contorted pain corresponded to Jennifer talking about her father, or thinking about him. Regardless of the content, whenever her father came up in our conversation, my stomach tensed with pain. At the time, I was able to recognise the context and connection, still, the thought of farting was so shaming for me that I was unable to look at these connections therapeutically. We both colluded with the pretence that nothing happened—inside her, inside me, or between us. Then one day, Jennifer asked me to touch her back and, as I crouched down on the mattress, I farted; a loud and very smelly fart. We both froze.

At the time, I could not see anything funny in the situation, let alone harness it therapeutically; I just felt ashamed, deeply ashamed. Trying to regulate my breathing I looked at Jennifer, neither of us could deny the reality of the stench in the room. "It stinks in here," I finally said. "Let me open a window." I felt like someone had just died, like I broke every written rule in the holy book of psychotherapy laws and that our fate was doomed. I heavily sat next to Jennifer.

After a short silence, and while we were sat on the floor, Jennifer started speaking about her father and her apprehension of him. "I've always felt sexually threatened by him," she said, as if following an interrupted strand of conversation, "and I wanted to bring it up for a while but felt ashamed, because I didn't know whether he actually did anything to me." Jennifer felt guilty by merely thinking, let alone disclosing, her subjective sexual experience as a teenager, since she had no clear-cut evidence or concrete memories of abuse or sexual contact with her father: "I know that he never touched me inappropriately or raped me, but I never felt safe to be a girl or a woman next to him; I used to feel that he stripped me with his eyes, that he looked at me more like a man would look at a woman than a father looked at his daughter." Jennifer started crying, and something in me calmed. I was able to restore myself. "Neither of us could hold this stench in any longer," I said, and Jennifer nodded, and we smiled.

I no longer suffered from stomach cramps with Jennifer and the paralysing body shame dissipated as well. "The stinking session" became a landmark for both of us, marking a more authentic commitment on both our parts to bring ourselves into the sessions. The fog between us disappeared as well, and I could clearly think again. We spent many sessions validating Jennifer's subjective experiences without having to produce objective behavioural proofs for her feelings. I too had to honour my own subjective experiences and my vulnerabilities and give these aspects of me space. At the same time, Jennifer brought up her sexual fears with her husband: "Every time Michael touches me, I need to remind myself that these are not daddy's hands, but my first response is always pushing him away."

The type of countertransference, which I have experienced with Jennifer, was described by body psychotherapist Michael Soth (2005) as a parallel process, where the client's conflict became the therapist's conflict: "Not only the client's awareness is fragmented: as the client's conflict has become the therapist's conflict, there is a tendency for the therapist to be drawn into similar denials and avoidances" (p. 51). Soth argued that in order to disentangle those transferential patterns which limited the client, the therapist should allow herself to partake in the therapeutic dyad, which might include embodying the conflicts and enactments. Soth acknowledged the risk in enactment and repetition, but argued these were inevitable; hence the therapist should foresee enactment and be mindful of early signs of it in the transference dynamics. Bodily attunement was an excellent way for bringing awareness to these enactments.

After our "stinking session", therapy with Jennifer became intense and sometimes more difficult, but the unspoken undercurrents were now part of our dialogue, both between us and in her real life. The fear that she had finally allowed herself to feel took over for a while yet she did not abandon herself this time. Jennifer stopped, for example, her placating and dissociated sex with her husband and resumed sexual relations after almost a year—but was then more connected and present (and sometimes was able to enjoy sex). In our relationship, I too started seeing her as a sexual woman and our erotic tension was a blessed surprise for us both—we validated it and were able to gently work with it. If our first therapeutic years were characterised by many sessions of bodywork, the arrival of Jennifer's father into the clinic brought with it caution and bodily tentativeness. We felt that touch held a dangerous edge, and we needed to discover one another afresh, much slower this time. This edge, despite the discomfort it brought into therapy, was a tolerable price for the emotional wealth which opened in Jennifer, in our relationship, and—gradually—between Jennifer and her partner Michael too.

Chapter Eleven will expand, present, and exemplify the clinical use of somatic countertransference through looking at resonance.

Therapeutic regression

> Therapeutic regression offers a powerfully transformative analytic experience, a new way of re-experiencing, reliving, and restoring longed-for, long-lacking, traumatic, and inadequate primal bonding because of an early environmental-maternal failure. Therapeutic regression postulates a return to the point where psychological growth was halted and enables a living breakthrough.
>
> —Ofra Eshel (2005, pp. 719–720)[2]

Eileen came to see me for focused bodywork and stayed for three and a half years of moving psychodynamic work. Fifty-eight-year-old Eileen was a surgical nurse, divorced and mother of three mature boys. She was seemingly functional and connected, organised and happy. She had been through many psychotherapeutic processes, was an experienced client and well versed in psychotherapeutic language. Eileen's GP recommended her to explore the emotional and biographical sources of her lower back pain, and she came to see me to attain some therapeutic insights into her pain. "I don't think I want another therapeutic process, just some tools for bodywork and meditation." Eileen suffered from debilitating backache which limited her physical mobility, her choices in life, and her capacity to properly function.

During one of these initial sessions Eileen lay on the therapy table and I asked permission to touch her diaphragm, to encourage abdominal breathing. As soon as her breathing deepened, Eileen started to sob—a heart-wrenching cry which lasted almost the entire session, leaving us very little time to reorient and process. In the week between sessions I thought of Eileen a lot, and felt detached, confused, and fearful. My body ached when I thought of Eileen, and I waited for our meeting to find out in her presence (either with myself or with her) the meaning of these sensations. Eileen came in and surprisingly sat under the writing desk in my clinic room, covering her entire body (including her head) with a blanket. I sat next to her, checking if she needed any contact. A hand, which looked very little, came out of the blanket, holding my hand firmly. She spoke very quietly, with a voice of a young girl, and told me her story.

Eileen's mother died from complications while giving birth to Eileen and dad was overwhelmed with shock and grief, blaming Eileen for the death of his beloved wife: "Within six months he remarried my stepmom, the only mother I knew. He was always helpless with me as a father, never knowing what to do with me; and the more I grew up, the more he hated me. I became the familial dustbin, the source of pain and suffering. My stepmother joined in with daddy's violence. I never felt safe." Eileen was sobbing, completely soaking the blanket with her tears. "Daddy's right," she whispered, "mum is dead because of me." The detachment, confusion, and fear which I experienced were validated and made sense to me now. "Can I stay here?" Eileen asked. "Under the table?" I checked. "No, here in therapy with you," she replied. "Of course," I answered. "How old are you now?" Eileen sniffed hard and responded without hesitation, "I'm three."

Touch, which functioned as the first language we learned, may encourage regressive states of consciousness. Attention to the body in general, and particularly working with touch may indeed potentiate regressive therapeutic states (Rolef Ben-Shahar, 2002a, 2002b). The connection between touch and trance (or altered states of consciousness) was known for ages, and was used and developed into both traditional and contemporary therapeutic techniques (Rolef Ben-Shahar, 2008a, 2008c).

Regression holds a risky potential for repetition compulsion and perpetuating infantile states, and at the same time it holds the possibility for reparative work. In his seminal work, psychoanalyst Michael Balint (1968), who was influenced both by Winnicott and by Ferenczi, differentiated between benign and malignant regression. Benign regression allowed for reprocessing of frozen developmental processes, or deconstructing pathological bodymind organisation and re-forming: going backwards to allow for moving forwards, if you will. In contrast, malignant regression perpetuates maladaptive patterns and it may poison the therapeutic relationship rather than support it (for example, when satisfying expressed regressive needs of a client simply awakens exponentially greater needs which threaten the therapeutic boundaries and become increasingly uncontainable). While benign regression could help easing symptoms, malignant regression tends to create further symptoms, out of the wish to have further needs met, needs which seem to stack up and which are frequently accompanied by hysterical signs.

Winnicott (1954) spoke favourably about the healing potential of regression: "The organisation that makes regression useful has this quality distinct from the other defence organisations in that it carries with it the hope of a new opportunity for an unfreezing of the frozen situation and a chance for the environment, that is to say, the present-day environment, to make adequate though belated adaptation" (p. 283).

Body psychotherapist Rachel Shalit (2011) explored the efficiency of therapeutic practices which incorporated altered states of consciousness. She wrote: "When regression is needed, on any level—be it psychological or spiritual—we should allow it to happen. [...] I suggest to allow regression when it's required and to encourage growth and development when there is sufficient ego strength to allow for it" (p. 97).

As we saw in Chapter Six, which dealt with bodymind character structure, lying down horizontally may encourage an infantile bodymind organisation, particularly in relation to gravity, and Eileen spontaneously regressed as soon as she was positioned this way and noticed her breathing. I was neither encouraging regression nor inviting it, but I certainly allowed it to happen—and felt it was a constructive and useful regression, not physically contracting or dangerously perpetuating dysfunction. For long weeks, Eileen would come to therapy and sit under the table to cry. Surprisingly, I felt very calm. The relationship between this young girl and me felt more real and consistent with my experience of Eileen, while communication with the woman often felt confusing. Week after week, the blankets got soaked wet and changed, the room was darkened. We sat together under the table, Eileen covered with a blanket with me next to her. With time, her breathing eased without any further intervention. Eileen's pain eased too, and she was more physically active; she could walk—she explored—and her pain attacks were less frequent and their intensity lessened as well.

And then, about two months after our sessions went under the table, Eileen asked to lean against me. I rested against a wall, inviting Eileen with a gesture to lean against me, and to my surprise she rested her head on my chest. I recall feeling like a newly born baby was handed over to me. She breathed ever so gently and I had a big impulse (which I did not follow through with) to take off my shirt and let us have skin-to-skin contact. In retrospect, these sensations were very similar experiences to those I had had with my two daughters shortly after their respective births, but the experience with Eileen happened a few years before my first daughter was born. Yet the pleasant trance-like feeling with Eileen had also shades of heaviness and sadness. I felt old and solemn while I stroked Eileen's head, and she—who for the first time in months stopped crying, looked at me with huge eyes. I wanted to say to her "I'm here Eileen," but instead found myself saying "Daddy's here."

After some time, Eileen's look changed. Suddenly, our close physical cradling which was anything but natural until that moment became a little awkward. We both responded by changing our posture, sitting up. "You've grown a little," I remarked. "Yes. I have," Eileen responded. "I can't believe that I heard your heartbeat. It was the most amazing thing I ever felt in my life. Suddenly everything felt in its place. I exaggerate, not everything—but I felt my right to exist. I felt that I have a place in the world." Once we left our place from under the table she added: "And here I am and the bodywork techniques I came to learn," and we both laughed.

During the following months we carried on talking. Crying under the table stopped, but our conversations continued with me cradling Eileen in my arms with her ears against my heart. When these father–daughter moments were therapeutically activated, touch felt important and natural, and when we felt awkward or dissonant, we learned to identify those moments as changing of self-states: an older part showed up. For two years of therapy Eileen "was growing in my hands" and together we experienced a different developmental process to the one she had. In the opening quote for this section on regression, psychoanalyst Ofra Eshel described a benevolent return to the place of deprivation, where reparative "living" breakthrough is enabled thanks to the re-enacted transference dynamics in psychotherapy. Despite the fact that there were other transferences in our work together, including homicidal, violent, terrified, and erotic, these mostly resided alongside our physical contact which was, by and large, comforting touch, and a stronger and deeper base of benevolent parental transference. I loved her very much. At the end of these two years, Eileen smiled when she described "my second childhood". Her back pain significantly eased, as well as some of the fear and anxieties she had suffered from for years. We carried on in non-regressive psychotherapy for eighteen more months before concluding and terminating psychotherapy.

Joseph Breuer (Freud & Breuer, 1895), who collaborated with Freud in *Studies on Hysteria*, believed that trance was a regressive state of consciousness holding a great curative potential. Freud (1900a) himself later distinguished two types of regression: topographic regression (in space) and temporal regression (in time). Topographic regression represented for Freud a reversal of the desired information processing and responses to stimulation: instead of the transition from primary to secondary processes, the movement went backwards from secondary processes to primary ones. He understood this regression to be grounded in the neurology of the reflex arc, reversing psychic movement "from the region of thought-structures to that of sensory perceptions" (Freud, 1905d, p. 162).

In contrast to Freud's conceptualisation of primary processes as counterproductive for the therapeutic process, psychoanalyst Hans Loewald (1977) identified mental processes as incorporating and requiring both primary and secondary processes. In fact, he saw psychoanalysis as attempting to bring patients closer to primary processes by encouraging them to free associate. He wrote: "The process is primary in a deeper sense insofar as it is unitary, non-differentiating, non-discriminating between various elements or components of a global event or experience" (p. 196).

Nick Totton (2003) concurs with Balint's warning against adopting an omnipotent therapeutic position, which could sweep the therapeutic dyad into malignant regression. Even if the therapeutic situation might foster a facilitative environment for reparative regression, a therapeutic promise (be it explicit or implicit) for saving the client from her regressive spaces would burden the client and the therapeutic process with unnecessary difficulties. Perhaps this is the place to reiterate, that choosing to work with affective psychotherapeutic tools invites states of high emotional charge anyway, thus alongside the potential there is always a risk. The more the psychotherapist is mindful of psychodynamic and clinical complexities, of her capacities and limitations, the risk could be more calculated and the potential for healing and growth higher. Nevertheless, is anything worth exploring not also risky?

As a child, I remember my dad telling me that "A clever person knows how to get out of situations that a wise person doesn't go into in the first place." I have to admit that I was always drawn to this saying, yet I tend to be clever rather than wise—I can get out of complex situations more than avoiding them in the first place. Perhaps this is why I found attachment theory (and the relational approach which was influenced by it) so befitting, as it describes the ongoing movement between ruptures and repairs at the heart of relationships (including therapeutic ones) (for example, see D. N. Stern, 1985). However, there is a spectrum between cleverness and wisdom, not a dichotomy. There is a degree of wisdom (foreseeing risk) without which the psychotherapist would be irresponsible. At the same time, to paraphrase Winnicott's views of mothering, "too much" wisdom (avoiding therapeutic risks at all costs) could also harm the therapeutic process in general, and therapeutic attachment and progress in particular (Rolef Ben-Shahar, 2013e). Examining regression under the cleverness-wisdom scale, we may suggest that working with regressive states is predisposed to entering situations from which the therapeutic dyad would have to get out (enactments)—but that these very states (and the process of getting out of them) may prove an invaluable source for healing and change.

As I mentioned before: "In its whole strategy of turning the client's attention to their body—it seems reasonable to say that body psychotherapy has an inherent tendency to be regressive" (Totton, 2003, p. 124; also see Rolef Ben-Shahar, 2002a, 2002b). As for Eileen—although she has spoken of these experiences in her previous psychotherapeutic work, the sensory immediacy of her experience and the physical holding provided Eileen with a very different kind of processing to her previous therapeutic experiences.

This enhanced risk for regressive states (at least at the beginning of therapy) requires the therapist to understand the price of working regressively (primarily transferential prices) as well as being sufficiently trained and proficient in working regressively. However, this statement seems to be true for every therapy which allows for and works with affective states. The choice of clinically working with affect-laden material bears with it risks, thus requiring precautions to enable taking calculated risks: appropriate command of theory, clear boundaries, sufficient supervision, capacity for introspection, and personal therapy.

The psychotherapeutic work with Eileen liberated blocked and life-threatening bodymind patterns and allowed for bodily, emotionally, and relational reorganisation. The regressive transitional space in our work soothed my own fears about the possibility of becoming a father. Working with regressive clients (and regressive processes) was a true and deep preparation for my parenting, and had contributed to my ripening and readiness for the process more than any other therapeutic work. I am indebted to Eileen and other clients who allowed me, among other roles, to be their father and mother. It seems that alongside the risks of working regressively, affective psychotherapy in general, and within it body psychotherapy, also holds great potential which justifies, in my opinion, taking those calculated risks.

Deconstructing rigid forms and encouraging flow[3]

> Life makes shapes. These shapes are part of an organizing process that embodies emotions, thoughts, and experiences into a structure.
>
> —Stanley Keleman (1985, p. xi)

Melissa: body psychotherapy with boundaries

Melissa and I had been working together for eighteen months when she arrived one day in a particularly fragile state, both physically and emotionally, telling me she had scarcely left her home that week. At thirty years old, married without children, Melissa was a highly talented classical pianist. Mel sought therapy following a complicated history of familial incest and blurred familial boundaries, which manifested in her life in addictions (mainly to physical activity), depressive episodes, limited sense of agency, and splits. Our transference dynamic was similarly complex, with recurrent shifts between paternal, sibling, and authoritarian relationships, all the while dancing to and fro with erotic charge and the dread of her childhood history. We learned, slowly and by stumbling, to create safety in the non-sterile environment of our therapeutic relationship.

In my countertransference, I was often washed into my own history of body shame, dissociation, and terror, and it was difficult at times to distinguish the two enmeshed stories. Expectedly, my personal psychotherapy and supervision were a significant and central part of my work with Melissa.

During one session, Mel complained about her inability to form stable boundaries, primarily at work and with her partner. She tended, so she claimed, to give up too quickly, to let go and accept other people's boundaries. Mel connected her fragile state with the unregulated impact her surroundings had on her. I felt that alongside our psychodynamic work around boundaries we could use a concrete experience to facilitate change in these patterns, and offered Mel to do some boundary work with strings. We each chose a string, marking our respective boundaries on the floor. Boundary work with strings is a common and very useful technique in body psychotherapy.

The boundaries each of us created fairly represented our bodily, cognitive, and relational organisation of that moment. Melissa's string was spread all over the floor—exposed and chaotic, and while it made an aesthetic picture it left her exposed and unprotected. In contrast, my brown string was tightly fitted and completely solid: an impeccable closed circle. I felt at home in my boundaries, and Melissa expressed her envy when she saw my perfect and distinct boundary: "I wonder what it would be like to live in your world," she commented.

Following her comment, I suggested that we swapped places to experience the other person's boundary and learn about our own boundary in the process—and about the other. Melissa sat in my boundary and immediately could breathe better and make eye contact. I, on the other hand, felt insecure and confused in her boundary/non-boundary. Inside, I felt a patronising self-righteousness, and was happy with the pedagogic opportunity to *teach Melissa a thing or two about healthy boundaries*.

Let it come

What happens to us when a client experiences a deconstruction of rigid organisation? What happens when we experience such deconstruction? Can we stay there, with the unclear and uncomfortable stream of ourselves and the other? The body psychotherapist, who chooses to open herself to sensations and resonance, is often flooded with body sensations which are at times meaningless to her, and she might feel defenceless against them. Having no choice, we become aware of our primordial anger, passion, shame, and dread through body sensations. The foaming stream of resonance is not only unavoidable, it is moreover a first-rate therapeutic tool: we may use our bodies to open to a universe which manifests before us as a stormy river of raw energy, and we might surrender to it, or try, in vain, to swim against it. Somehow, I always attempt to swim against the current before I am able to surrender. Gertrud Stein (in D. B. Stern, 1983) said: "It will come if it is there and you let it come" (p. 96), but how do we let it come?

We then returned, each to our own string. I breathed with relief, and offered Melissa that we each made a small change to our own boundary, to reflect our learning from the experience of the swapping boundaries. I offered this mutual formula, not because I believed, at that moment, that I could learn anything from Mel's boundaries, but to avoid shaming her.

Mel tightened her boundary and made it slightly more ordered. The main change was that her boundary was no longer open, it felt less exposed and not as vulnerable. Her breathing slowed down, her face became less flushed, and her entire posture seemed calmer. As a perfunctory courtesy I decided to loosen my rigid boundaries a little, and gently untied the end of my string, thus leaving a tiny opening in my string. Almost immediately, I froze, as if all my blood washed away from my body. I could not look at Mel at all, and an early memory surfaced. I was five, reluctantly being placed naked in a paddling pool with two girls, I was angry, felt exposed, shamed, and screaming "Take me out" (inside my head ...). Mel took my hand and held it firmly; my breathing relaxed, and I no longer felt activated and flooded, but I felt very guilty for this momentary role reversal. However, and despite the fact that our two life stories surfaced in the room and got entangled, we both experienced a sense of hope—and of newness.

Stanley Keleman and Sylvia Adler (2000) described the stages of forming, the creation of new organisations:

> The first stage is an ending, the disassembling of an established form. This ending is actually a conceiving stage. Disorganization is accompanied by intense somatic emotional excitement. This excitement catalyzes the possibility of new behavior. This intense period is followed by a second stage, a middle ground between what was and what is not yet. Middle ground is an unformed or porous state, a womb for new form. The last stage is one of stabilization, a form which emerges with a feeling of competence to perform and to contain new behavior. (p. 51)

For me, a significant aspect of the psychotherapeutic challenges in deconstructing rigid organisation and encouraging flow concerns a long stay a long stay in the transitional space, in the formless land, in the unformulated biblical *tohu bohu*—this is where new bodymind organisations brew. According to a famous pronoun: "Enlightenment is an accident; practice makes us accident prone." Indeed, cultivating our capacity to remain in this potential space fosters a more accurate capacity to move between organisations, not merely choose more adaptive forms.

Our string incident was similar to Melissa's repetitive narrative, but it was not the same. Incidentally, the shaking of my boundaries (and the subsequent loss of therapeutic positioning) intensified our transferential tensions and brought our enmeshment to the fore, yet it also allowed space for a new scenario. The unsettling of our boundaries which I experienced and both of us had to survive as a therapeutic dyad, encouraged change. For a moment, it was Melissa who regulated us. She experienced how my own bodymind organisation (and ours) changed and how, instead of getting lost in this transferential vortex we managed, together, to survive our formlessness.

This joint survival was a cornerstone in our therapeutic work and it can account, in my opinion, for many of the changes in Mel's life, including a tightening of her boundaries, both at work and in her relationship. As for me, my own dialogue with boundaries changed following our work—my therapeutic organisation became more flexible and less defensive. This therapeutic encounter provided me with important material for my personal therapeutic work.

The "us" created between us needed to be formed outside our therapeutic position, which was saturated with rigid organisations as part of our transference dynamics. This intersubjective connection enabled us later to deepen therapeutic work and assisted Melissa in strengthening boundaries in her life, and moreover to position herself less as a victim against the repeated transferential enactments she experienced in her life. This intersubjective connection took place in a space which seemed outside the therapeutic frame, or—to be more exact—outside our habitual therapeutic frame.

Jungian analyst Ernest Rossi (1973) portrayed the process of organisation of liminal experiences, which we could say are the inhabitants of potential space:

> A creative moment occurs when a habitual pattern of association is interrupted; [...] there may be a psychic shock, an overwhelming sensory or emotional experience; a psychedelic drug, a toxic condition or sensory deprivation; yoga, Zen, spiritual and meditative exercises may likewise interrupt our habitual associations and introduce a momentary void in awareness. In that fraction of a second when the habitual contents of awareness are knocked out there is a chance for pure awareness, "the pure light of the void" to shine through. This fraction of a second may be experienced as a "mystic state," satori, a peak experience or an altered state of consciousness. (p. 461)

My unexpected distress following the flexing of boundaries, and the manner in which we retrieved our balanced and constructive therapeutic work was such a moment for the two of us. As soon as our bodies were differently organised, we could speak another tongue. Our string work, my freezing, and Melissa's ability and willingness to support me there (be my selfobject), together with the fact we survived it as a therapeutic dyad, all these created an anchor, a fulcrum we frequently revisited in our mutual endeavour to soften rigid muscular holding positions, dogmatic thinking patterns, or relational organisations which were no longer appropriate for Melissa's life (or mine).

This session symbolised a significant shift in organising the three levels of self explored in Chapter Four: somatic, linguistic-cognitive, and transferential (the field of relationship). Although our therapeutic relationship held a potential for growth and change, the culture of relationship between Melissa and me turned into a shaming impasse in our work. To avoid paralysis by the spaces of shame and "stuck-ness" we simply avoided going into these. Melissa came to therapy as a practised victim, and I locked myself in the patronising and self-righteous fortress of the kind and loving therapist. Inside this therapeutic position, very little movement was possible.

Until that meeting, our therapeutic work with boundaries was mostly psychodynamic. We painfully tried to save ourselves from the quicksand in which Melissa trod all her life, with very little success. Even when we did incorporate body interventions, they involved rigid relational organisation (I was "doing something to Melissa" or "was showing her the way"), and their therapeutic horizons were consequently limited and limiting. But the help Melissa offered me, even if it was very painful for me at that time, positioned us differently. Melissa took responsibility for a different organisation against me, I submitted and let go of my convenient position, and change occurred on all levels. We both changed. This change and novelty characterised our later work where we could more easily get lost, let go of dogmas and beliefs, and open to a creative and generative relationship.

Therapeutic deconstruction of organisation is not merely technical. It represents an understanding that bodily, cognitive, and relationship organisations are intertwined, and the therapeutic relationship is richer when there is more than a single door in. Body psychotherapy presents the therapeutic dyad with a door into experiences which are inaccessible to other modalities. Changing somatic organisation is neither the only door in (not even in body psychotherapy) nor the best, but it opens possibilities which enrich the therapeutic relationship. I believe that other modalities of psychotherapy may learn a lot from the knowledge gained in body psychotherapy regarding somatic organisations and ways of flexing these.

Fairy wings and the psychotherapeutic act: self- and dyadic regulation[4]

In a nature reserve we saw a Lanius perching on a branch.
My daughter remembered the dog that my sister used to have, who died
"She is with god now, isn't she?" "You also had a baby who went to god, didn't you mum?"
When my daughter will ask me where god is
I shall take her to the mirror,
I shall ask her to stare deeply into her own eyes
"Here is god" I would tell her "right inside your eyes"

—Asaf Rolef Ben-Shahar

Finding an "OK" foot: selfobject and resonance

Biosynthesis body psychotherapist Gil Arad (Arad, Askarov, Gihon, Lieblich, & Medina, 2013) presented a client who, despite his wish to engage in a meaningful relationship with his girlfriend, could only feel terror and dread whenever their relationship deepened. Even though the client acquired some intellectual understanding of the origin of his anxiety, his bodily and emotional responses were nonetheless paralysing. Arad described his resonant experience of paralysis and tension, yet he insisted on searching for sensations and feelings other than the terror and paralysis. The client was unable to relate to his therapist's request—nowhere in his body could he sense anything other than pain, tension, and sheer panic. But Arad insisted and looked for other aspects by observing his own resonating body. "After a while, and much weaker than the tension I could sense that my feet were OK," said Arad. Feeding this information back, the client too could acknowledge that his feet felt OK. Slowly and gradually, with the use of somatic resonance and feeding it back to the client, the therapeutic dyad was able to regulate the dread and limit the extent of the panic. The client reclaimed his body with the help of Arad who sensed the generative aspects of the client's body before the client could do so himself.

The concept of selfobject was coined by psychoanalyst Heinz Kohut (Bacal, 1995; Kohut, 1959) to describe relational regulation. When the child was young, he or she were yet unable to contain certain feelings or affect; the mother or father "held it on the child's behalf", feeling what the child could not feel, experiencing unformulated and flooding experiences until the child was able to reclaim these as her or his own.

The therapeutic act frequently involves similar processes: we feel for our clients aspects of themselves that they are unable to yet feel, either because these are too much (like fear, anger, sexual arousal, or neediness), or because these clash with their belief and value system and are in conflict with their defence system, like the example above. Arad's client was unable at first to notice or tolerate the OK sensations—it would have confronted him directly with his avoidance behaviour. One of the most common and important roles of the psychotherapist is to serve as selfobject for the client (Lichtenberg, 1991), and the example given by Arad is an excellent one, demonstrating that serving as a selfobject may involve holding generative and resourceful aspects as well as painful ones. This task is often somatic and energetic in its nature and is not symbolised in therapy until the client can respond to and work with the affect.

Letter to the fairies

A few weeks ago, my daughter Zohar told me with excitement that she wrote a wishing-note to the fairies and threw it out of the window (we live on the third floor of an apartment block). I am embarrassed to say that my first response was getting upset with her for throwing things out of the window and cluttering our neighbourhood, but I quickly managed to get my bearings together and shared her excitement. "What did you ask for?" I enquired, and Zohar, who is five and a half years old, whispered in my ears, "To have wings, so that I could fly." It really moved and excited me.

I guess that being a good father and trying to be a good father are sometimes oppositional forces. I was deeply touched by Zohar's initiative, and wanted to be a good dad, and so went downstairs to the garden to look for the note. It was there, between the blades of grass, a shiny note with hearts drawn on it and my daughter's beautiful and naïve handwriting asking the fairies to give her a pair of her very own fairy wings to fly. Wanting to make her happy, I took a piece of paper, glitter, stickers and a flowery envelope and sat with my wife to write down a note.

We wrote: "Dear Zohar, thank you very much for your letter which is attached here. We were very touched to hear your request. While little girls in the world of humans cannot have wings like we do, we want you to know that we are keeping a pair of fairy wings here just for you. Every time you visit us in your dreams or your journeys to the fairy world, these wings will be yours to use as much as you want. With love, Tinkerbell, Ellie, and Ruby." Both my wife and I were aching for the sweet hope and dream and were hoping Zohar would be satisfied with this letter.

We brought home the letter and Zohar opened it and read it quickly, excitedly, jumping up and down with joy that the fairies answered her letter. Zohar asked me if I would take her to the land of the fairies that night. We often practised lucid dreaming together, using trance to open to those magical worlds which were still open for Zohar and that I have managed to reclaim with a lot of practice—worlds which were far more accessible for me in Zohar's company.

The evening approached and while hugging Zohar during our bedtime ritual she started crying. At first her tears were soft, barely noticeable, but then it became a heartbreaking sob. I knew what it was about and felt sad for her, discovering what Freud would probably call the tension between the pleasure principle and the reality principle. I also felt guilty.

"I think the fairies misunderstood me," said Zohar, "I don't want wings just for fairy-world; I want wings for this world, real flying wings, so that I can fly in the kindergarten and in the playground of our neighbourhood." I suggested she stayed in bed with us this night and held her while she cried herself to sleep. It felt like a deep grief over something she had lost. Shuy Grace, our eighteen-month-old daughter, woke up from Zohar's sobbing and got up. She sat on Zohar's belly and started jumping up and down; "Jumping," she said. "Jumping up and down." I guess it was hard for all of us to bear witness to Zohar's pain. It is hard to bear witness to the pain of somebody you love.

An internal tug to respond or narcissistic disturbance?

Relational psychoanalyst Stuart Pizer (2012) called it an "internal tug to respond", which constituted the analyst's "generous involvement". He discussed our internal pull towards responding to another person's suffering. I believe that a common characteristic of the psychotherapeutic profile was this very urge to respond, to feel this internal tug calling us to attempt to meet the other person, to attempt to alleviate their suffering.

In her seminal book, *The Drama of the Gifted Child*, Alice Miller (1981) referred to this phenomenon as a *narcissistic disturbance*. She wrote: "It is often said that psychoanalysts suffer from a narcissistic disturbance ... His sensibility, his empathy, his intense and differentiated emotional responsiveness, and his unusually powerful 'antennae' seem to predestine him as a child to be used—if not misused—by people with intense narcissistic needs" (p. 22).

Can you identify with Miller's statement and with Pizer's conceptualisation? Can you relate to the pain of witnessing my daughter's pain which led me to this regulatory attempt? That my internal tug to respond has narcissistic elements is clear. It is also more than just a narcissistic response, I hope, but the making of me as a father and as a therapist.

Let us ponder for a moment about the profile of a responsive psychotherapist—one who is able to respond. Following from Miller's understanding and Pizer's somewhat kinder take on this tug, I think about the balance between self and mutual regulation in the psychotherapeutic clinic, and, even more so, about the making of a psychotherapist.

To be good enough psychotherapists, we need to be sufficiently narcissistically wounded. The pain of the other has to move us, to mobilise us to want to "do something about it". Many of us share the basic predisposition for external attunement as well as hold the two following beliefs, even if unconsciously, that (a) it is my role and/or duty to do something about someone else's pain and (b) that it is possible for me to do something about somebody else's pain, that my attempts will make a difference. This predisposition and accompanied beliefs could be seen as narcissistic, as well as understood as empathetic. They are, of course, both. The therapeutic personality and the therapeutic act, I believe, require us to be sufficiently narcissistic to care and think that we can do something about it, while at the same time to have sufficiently worked through our narcissism in order for us to appropriately respond, allowing the other autonomy and self-direction. After all, everyone is entitled to their suffering. Somehow, this very internal tug is the source of the empathetic therapeutic act and at the same time it holds a potential for arresting or disturbing this very therapeutic act, by blocking natural regulatory processes.

I need you to let me help you, please

At the time, I thought that my note to Zohar was an attempt to regulate her distress—to support her in the journey of balancing reality and fantasy, in expanding her potential space. It was also that, and I do not wish to completely condemn my act, but I was also using Zohar as a selfobject—I was using her to regulate my own anxiety concerning her suffering: I needed to feel that I could do something to make her feel better, and that something could be done. I am pleased that Zohar was unwilling to serve (at least not fully) as my selfobject.

I propose that for the psychotherapeutic act to be effective, our clients are consciously and (more so) unconsciously required to meet some of our needs as psychotherapists. Mostly they do so simply by suffering and wanting us to help. It is not only we who regulate our clients but also (and sometimes more so) our clients who regulate us. By providing us with opportunities to help, our clients satisfy our "narcissistic disturbance". We receive meaning, we become; we build our sense of our worth. When my clients let me be meaningful for them, when they let me help them, they give my existence meaning, they regulate my characterological need for attunement. If we insist on adopting a pathological point of view, we might say that the practice of psychotherapy can be a repetition compulsion of our narcissistic disturbance. In other words, as the twelfth century philosopher Moshe Ben-Maimon (Maimonides) has allegedly suggested: if you have an aptitude for blood, go become a butcher.

Hence, the therapeutic act is not merely an altruistic voyage; it also stems, and deeply so, from unresolved and possibly unresolvable narcissistic pathologies whereupon my self-regulation and self-worth are dependent on the capacity to help. At the same time, being a psychotherapist is not simply sublimation of pathological disturbance, it is also about a true wish (not need) to love and be loved, to regulate and be regulated, to mutually meet and be met. One of the important enterprises of relational psychoanalysis (E. Balint, J. Mitchell, & Parsons, 1993; Greenberg & S. Mitchell, 1983; S. Mitchell & Aron, 1999) was to conceptualise human connectedness and mutual needs as important aspects of humanity which could not and should not be reduced simply to pathological sublimated drives.

How can we balance the pathological and generative aspects of our inner tug to respond? How can I take ownership of my utilitarian and narcissistic needs on the one hand, while on the other hand not shaming myself and acknowledging also the beautiful, empathetic, and loving aspects of my choices?

Bodied wings and somatic regulation

A few days ago, when I came home from work, Zohar approached me. "I've been thinking, daddy, and I don't think that the fairies wrote this letter. I think it was you who'd written it." I was taken by surprise. Unexpectedly, I felt relieved. "Yes, Zohar, it was me. I wrote the letter from the fairies." Zohar continued: "I know you just wanted to make me happy, but it didn't help at all." I apologised to Zohar. She has not let go of wanting to have wings, though, although she told me, yesterday, that "I don't want to have wings like birds—not to fly to the sky. I want to only fly so that my feet will be above mum's head, so that we can still touch each other, not higher than that."

Perhaps, when we allow ourselves to de-idealise the therapeutic act, and recognise the (sometimes deeply) pathological aspect of the psychotherapeutic profile, we can better appreciate what our clients do for us: they provide us with some of our deepest and oft-unmet needs for worth, acknowledgment, and with ample opportunities to matter, to make a difference. We have an opportunity to have some needs met on a daily basis thanks to our clients' generosity. I feel humbled when I can appreciate how much my clients are doing for me, mostly without me realising.

Perhaps, too, when we can celebrate our pathologies they become more than pathologies—without this internal tug to respond our world will be a sad, isolated, and lonely place.

Furthermore, what was made explicit by psychotherapist Gil Arad (Arad, Askarov, Gihon, Lieblich, & Medina, 2013) at the beginning of this section, and only realised in hindsight by me with Zohar, was that the tug to respond was a resonance phenomenon (Chapter Eleven is dedicated to discussing resonance). To reiterate, the pain of the other as well as the resources of the other were directly experienced by us as if these were our own, that the other was alive in me. Chapter Eleven clarifies and exemplifies my claim that resonance is primarily somatic, that our ache is first and foremost bodily. To experience resonance, we have to have an anatomy; a neurology—we experience the other through our bodies and in our bodies (I would furthermore argue that it is not strictly my body, but our shared, intersubjective body).

Perhaps, when we are attentive enough to our own bodies, we stand a greater chance of realising the extent of regulation that we require in our psychotherapeutic work and can find creative means of having those needs met (or at least addressing them) benevolently—some outside therapy and some within therapy. Simply said, we use our clients as much as they use us; we need our clients too. By cultivating embodied mindfulness of the ways I need my clients (and my daughters), I hope that I can become a better psychotherapist and a better father.

The morning after the sobbing night, Zohar came to me with body paint. "Can you draw a pair of wings on my back," she asked. I drew two pink wings on her back. "It's not what I really want," she made sure that I understood, "but it's OK for now." Shuy Grace, my young daughter and Zohar's young sister, was running in the playground, shouting with glee, "I am flying, I am flying, I am flying."

Exercise: peeling the onion

(In pairs)

This exercise is meant to deepen our familiarity with our most common bodymind organisations, and introducing the prospect of flexing these. We explore this through experimenting in peeling our public faces (our persona) through embodiment. This is a ritual, and it is therefore suggested that you keep to its simple structure. The ritual is particularly appropriate for workshops and training, but could also be used in therapy. It is an adaptation of an exercise I learned from Pamela Gawler-Wright.

The two participants "tune in" by closing their eyes, centring, and opening their eyes softly.

1. The therapist asks: "Who are you?"
2. Client answers with an identity statement: "I am X" (for example, "I am a man", "I am a mother", "I am a psychotherapist", "I am curious").
3. Therapist asks: "Show me the X that you are," and client adopts the bodily organisation which fits the identity statement and exaggerates it: the bodily posture, muscular holding. When she feels that she had embodied this aspect she says: "See the X that I am" (e.g., "See the woman that I am" or "See the mother that I am").
4. The psychotherapist validates the statement (after connecting with it): "I see the X that you are. And who else are you?"
5. The process is repeated (1–4) at least five times.
6. Process, share, and—if appropriate, swap.

Notes

1. The following vignette is an expansion of material previously published in the *USA Body Psychotherapy Journal* (Rolef Ben-Shahar, 2010b).
2. The quote is from "A Bond of Love, Emotional Risk, and Daring", by Ofra Eshel, published in *Psychoanalytic Dialogues* and is reprinted here by permission of Taylor & Francis Group (http://www.tandfonline.com).
3. This case material is an expansion of a vignette, which appeared in a paper published by the *USA Body Psychotherapy Journal* (Rolef Ben-Shahar, 2011b).
4. Parts of this section were previously published in *Somatic Psychotherapy Today* (Rolef Ben-Shahar, 2013c).

CHAPTER TEN

One tender touch: touch in body psychotherapy

The ultimate magic of attachment is touch. And this magic enters through the skin.

—*Daniel Stern* (1991, p. 99)[1]

Introduction

There are some pubs where any topic of conversation is allowed except for politics. The combination of alcohol and political discourse usually ends up with fists. In these pubs you may speak and fight over football, rugby, or the royal family; naturally, you can talk about the weather. But politics? This is too hot. There are some topics in the psychotherapeutic "pubs" (discussions, conferences, workshops, and trainings) which hold a promise for elevating the energy in the room, requiring the mature and responsible eye of a bartender, to observe the atmosphere and, if necessary, keep the place from falling apart: sex, money, and touch are the holy trinity.

For the majority of clinicians who encounter body psychotherapy for the first time, the issue of touch is the one to draw interest and cause apprehension, to attract and repel. The body psychotherapist is often perceived as a priori threatening, as if she carries some infectious curse by her mere clinical orientation. Alongside this demonisation, body psychotherapy has also been idealised, particularly concerning the use of touch: the body psychotherapist apparently manages to "touch the core of the issues", or meet the client "where nobody ever managed to meet her before" and other such sweeping declarations.

Today there is a general societal consensus, not least in psychology research, concerning the developmental need for touch, both in our infancy and in our adulthood. Considering this consensus, the taboo against touch in psychotherapy is more bewildering still. On the one hand, we emphatically declare the importance of tactile communication for establishing security and attachment, for supporting socialisation processes, and for identity formation. As psychotherapists, we offer a secure relationship, an opportunity to form an attachment which would foster self-regulation and self-organisation. On the other hand, our actions and avoidance of touch present touch as holding uncontainable and unmanageable danger; we declare our distrust in the very same human connection which we hail as crucial. The vote of distrust in touch, opposed with the recognition of our human need for contact, nonverbal validation, and physical connection creates a dissociating and confusing experience for our clients; possibly for us as well.

In the opening chapter of the important book *Bodies in Treatment*, psychoanalyst Frances Sommer Anderson (2008) shares with the readers her experience as a client of bodywork alongside her psychoanalytic work: "In the world of moving and breathing—the sensory, motoric, and visceral domain—I made contact with what Winnicott (1960a) referred to as the true self" (p. 22). Anderson continues: "Bodywork, combined with traditional analysis, helped me discover developmental trauma at a visceral and affective level, through transferences to my bodyworkers and analysts and through imagery in dreams" (p. 23).

At its best, body psychotherapy suggests that these two complex and complementary processes of which Anderson wrote, could be experienced within a single therapeutic framework, and with one psychotherapist. The body psychotherapist working with touch is trained to work with both the verbal and symbolic, and with the subsymbolic, with the language of touch. To use this language appropriately and professionally requires training, and different approaches in body psychotherapy offer training and practice in the different dialects of the language of touch.

A touching distance

> Touch can be healing, and although it is unfashionable to say so, psychoanalysis is also very much about healing, and I wonder what kind of disservice we do by *not* touching.
>
> —Susie Orbach (2004a, p. 40)

In the introduction to his excellent co-edited (with Frances Sommer Anderson) volume *Relational Perspectives on the Body*, Lewis Aron (1998) declared: "It is the intention of this book to bring the focus of psychoanalysis back to the body, to the bodily rooted self, to bodily based communication, to bodily and affective experience, and to somatic and psychosomatic phenomena, now all viewed in a relational context" (p. xxvii). It is my belief that psychoanalysts, as well as psychotherapists from other modalities, would benefit by training in touch, thus enriching their clinical repertoire and translating contemporary understandings into clinical applications of touch. It is the intention of this chapter to introduce the reader to the breadth and depth of working with touch in psychotherapy, in the hope that some readers would be curious enough to gain practical training and experience in touch skills.

Before delving into technical, ethical, clinical, and theoretical questions regarding touch in psychotherapy, I wish to stress that not all body psychotherapists use touch in their work. Body psychotherapy does not *require* touch; a touching distance could be observed; but in many cases it is not. Incorporating touch in psychotherapy may increase the potential for affective, regressive, aggressive, and erotic amplifications in the transference dynamics, but it may also offer immediate and unmediated mutual human connection. Psychoanalyst John Bowlby (1988) argued that: "There are occasions when it would be inhuman not to allow a distressed patient to make some form of physical contact" (p. 154).

As illustrated in Chapter One, therapeutic touch was an essential part of the early days of psychoanalysis and psychotherapy (Kertay & Reviere, 1993). After all, psychoanalysis developed both from medicine and hypnosis—and therapeutic touch was central to both, as the first chapter demonstrated. Certainly, touch as an encouraging agent for expressing emotion was not invented by psychoanalysis: every parent knows that when you hold a sad child, tears would more easily surface, followed by calming down; that kissing a wounded knee eases the pain.

Nor was Freud the only psychoanalyst who used touch. However, while Freud abandoned touch and no longer viewed it as legitimate for psychoanalytic use, analysts like Sándor Ferenczi and Wilhelm Reich not only continued to work with touch, but furthermore encouraged touch and developed therapeutic techniques for working with touch, as Chapter Two illustrated. Hungarian psychoanalyst Michael Balint (1952), who was highly influenced by Ferenczi (and introduced his work to the object relations founders when he moved to the UK), described the patients' wish for touch during the later stages of therapy as the expression of fondness, mutuality, and deeper connection. He suggested that in such cases touch was a powerful form of connection which led to deeper intimacy and a "tranquil quiet sense of well-being" (p. 231).

The taboo against touch in psychotherapy was also instrumental in differentiating the psychoanalyst from the medical practitioner and the doctor-patient relationship from the analyst-analysand and it is still in place in mainstream psychoanalytic theory and practice. Some psychoanalysts would decline a hand extended for shaking even at the end of many years of analysis. In Chapter One I mentioned psychiatrist Karl Menninger (1958), who made his position clear by exclaiming: "Transgression of the rule against physical contact constitutes evidence of the incompetence or criminal ruthlessness of the analyst" (p. 40). Analysts and psychotherapists like Winnicott, who touched their clients, were forced to either do it secretly or make themselves subject of scrutinising criticism and attack.

With contemporary developments in psychoanalytic thinking, primarily relational psychoanalysis, the last three decades saw a new spirit of willingness to re-examine the justifications for and against the use of touch in therapy. Is avoiding touch in therapy always justifiable? Could a dogmatic inner position concerning touch (for or against, it does not matter) be of service to the therapeutic process, the therapist, the client?

Body psychotherapy does not occupy a polarised position to psychoanalysis. While orthodox psychoanalysis religiously maintains a touching distance, touch in body psychotherapy is not conducted without discrimination. Just as the psychodynamic or psychoanalytic practitioner examines the appropriateness and relevance of an interpretive intervention, so does the body psychotherapist examine the appropriateness and relevance of intervention with touch. Body psychotherapist Arnt Halsen (1995) importantly claimed that: "Knowing when to touch and when not to, and how to touch, needs just as much insight and training as knowing when and how to interpret" (p. 103). Notwithstanding the complexities and risks of using touch in psychotherapy, when therapist and client consent to consciously work with touch, there sometimes emerges a magical, fertile, human, and mutual therapeutic meeting of bodyminds which is second to none.

The developmental importance of touch

> We are brought to vibrant life through touch and in its absence we wilt and shrivel.
>
> —Valerie Sinason (2006, p. 50)

The 1950s, 1960s, and 1970s were a fertile period for significant yet horrid psychological research and experiments, where animals and people were put through emotional and physical torture in order to acquire theoretical and clinical knowledge about love, hate, obedience, and attachment. Many of these experiments would not have been approved today by ethical committees (for example, the Stanley Milgram's (1974) infamous *obedience to authority* experiment, in which subjects believed they administered lethal electrical shocks to other subjects). One of the most painful experiments of the time, at least in my view, which is still studied by every psychology student today, was Harry Harlow and Robert Zimmermann's (1959) experiment, which studied attachment and maternal bonding. In the experiment, infant rhesus monkeys were separated from their mothers, and were given a choice between two wire-based monkey models: a naked-wire surrogate mother holding a milk bottle, and a soft and cuddly (cloth-covered) wire-based mum, who did not offer food. Time and again, those poor baby monkeys chose the pleasant-to-touch mum, despite the fact she offered them no food, only comforting touch. Harlow's monkeys have since become a synonym for the deep and primary need we have for touch.

Touch is our earliest form of communication, and the infant is highly dependent on its tactile sensitivity and sense of touch. The Winnicottian concept of *the psyche indwelling in the body* (1960b, p. 44) is an invitation to connect to the basic embodiment of our human experience, as well as to our need for touch. In her review of the developmental importance of touch, psychodynamic psychotherapist Maggie Turp (1999) elaborated on Winnicott's position concerning touch: "In relation to this extreme dependency, Winnicott focuses on the infant's non-negotiable need for 'holding', which includes both the holding of the baby in mind and empathic identification with his state of mind, and physical holding" (p. 24).

The baby's physical proximity to the mother (or main attachment figure) allows him to learn how to self-regulate, providing the gradual transition from a primarily dyadic identity into the formation of an individual self. Thus, touch provides the baby with his body—helping the child embody himself within it. Safe touch with an attachment figure facilitates the internalisation of a good enough relationship between inside and outside, body and mind (i.e., the creation of potential space). The physically supported and touched baby learns, through touch, to balance the somatic expressions of self with the emotional and mental ones.

It is with touch that the baby becomes a person: moving from an *I–it* relationship with his body and selfhood (Buber, 1958) to developing the self as relating and embodied: the baby organises himself (together with the mother) as a body-centred self. The influential neuropsychologist Allan Schore (2003) portrayed the therapeutic process as paralleling attachment processes during infancy: "The intuitive empathic therapist attunes to and resonates with the patient's shifting affective state, thereby co-creating with the patient a context in which the clinician can act as a regulator of the patient's physiology" (p. 48).

Ethics of touch: boundaries and touch in psychotherapy

> Touch is a lifesaver and a life giver. However, as with any basic human need, it has its traumatic side.
>
> —Valerie Sinason (2006, p. 50)

The issue of touch in psychotherapy is a hot cauldron of discussions, disagreements, fears and anger, unending ethical questions, and heated arguments—both outside the field of psychotherapy and within it. Ethical positions concerning touch cause many psychotherapists to lose their curious politeness and openness to differentness and variety: conclusive positions are frequently made around touch, unquestionable and unchallengeable truths tend to form, and absolutes characterise the thinking around touch in psychotherapy. Indeed, touch can ignite our vitality and inner fire, and at the same time set on fire dialogues between psychotherapists from different modalities. Few are the discussions around touch in psychotherapy which are held without dogmatic exchanges and conclusive arguments for or against.

To touch or not to touch? What might touch bring to the client, the therapist, or the culture within which both live? What are we avoiding and escaping by not touching? What are we avoiding and escaping by touching? All these are heated topics in the body psychotherapeutic dialogue.

Perhaps we should start by acknowledging that touch in psychotherapy is indeed a complex matter. The therapeutic relationship is highly complicated as it is, with a priori bias towards inequality and complex transference dynamics which include, among others, erotic transference and imbalanced power dynamics. *Working with touch in psychotherapy should not be done lightly, and requires appropriate professional training*. The decision whether to touch or not (and how to touch) requires understanding of the context within which the relationship takes places, and the meanings carried with and through touch (Kertay & Reviere, 1998). These meanings include cultural, therapeutic, biographical, gender, racial, and other aspects. As a side point, transgression of boundaries in psychotherapy into sexual relations between clients and therapists occur across the therapeutic modalities, whether these incorporate touch or not (Gabbard & Lester, 1995; Sinason, 2006).

Many of the psychoanalytic papers concerning touch (for instance, Patrick Casement's (1982, 2000) seminal papers on the subject) primarily indicate for me the need for (and lack of) appropriate therapeutic training, and not necessarily an established position against touch in psychotherapy. A psychotherapist, experienced as she might be, who was not trained to work with touch but chose to touch her clients, will be more exposed to the dangers and risks in touch than a body psychotherapist who was trained to use touch in psychotherapy. When I emphasise the need for training, it is not merely techniques I am referring to, but primarily practice and training in learning to recognise what is conveyed with touch and how to "speak" it, how to converse and communicate with contact as well as with words, which includes substantial training in recognising and working with somatic countertransference.

In cultures where touch was not the norm—and psychotherapy is one such culture—touch is frequently perceived as an active technique done by the therapist on the relatively passive client, preventing the client from developing symbolic capacities. Body psychotherapist Bernd Eiden (1998) refers to this argument thus: "The rationale that touch inhibits the process of symbolising implies that the body is related to the concrete literal level and the mind to the symbolic level only—an outdated dualistic concept" (p. 2).

Touch in psychotherapy is often understood as if the therapist operates *on* the client in order to mobilise something, to do something, or get somewhere. Touch is frequently seen as an active intervention, as doing. This perception is very far from the depth of connection and communication which could be conveyed with contact. First and foremost, touch could be a *being* movement—expanding our mutual presence, telling the other (and myself) that "I am with you." Touch could validate and affirm depths of connections, deepen attachment, and flex rigid or stuck emotional, mental, and cognitive organisations. Touch could in fact assist in the organisation of symbolic thinking and subsymbolic processes. In my experience, touching a client may facilitate the creation of intersubjective spaces in psychotherapy without compromising the therapeutic dialogue.

Another common argument against the use of touch concerns the belief that touch serves the needs of the id and the pleasure principle, and is unfaithful to the reality principle. Drive theory holds that the baby arrives in the world full of drives and urges, and is motivated by the desire to satisfy those needs—the pleasure principle. Only gradually does he learn to adapt and adjust to his surroundings, sublimating his needs and accepting the burden of the reality principle (Freud, 1920g). Object relations theory, attachment theory, and the relational approach already presented another attitude, according to which the baby was object seeking from infancy, and this active seeking for connection was a powerful motivational force, as much as the desire to regulate pain and hunger (D. N. Stern, 1985; Summers, 2002).

The body psychotherapist may add three answers to this argument. First—the capacity to surrender to pleasure without losing contact with myself or the surroundings (and the other) was the main Reichian indication for mental health (Lowen, 1965; Reich, 1942): touch may help to foster surrender into the bodily orgiastic flow, which was not the same as narcissistic egocentricity, but the opposite—it contributed to functional object relations. The second answer concerned the quality of touch: there are methods of touch which could actually strengthen the boundaries of self, support individuality, and in so doing contribute to a healthier relationship between the pleasure principle and the reality principle. The third answer relates to psychotherapeutic relationship as a potential space. When clients internalised secure attachment, their organism naturally aspired to growth and independence: this answer presupposed that in our core, our human organism aspired to full expression of its potential, and given the sufficient conditions we shall not choose to remain in the regressive symbiotic uterine-touch. The vignette on the oral character structure in Chapter Six exemplified this argument. Despite Gina's concern that her son Robert would never cease from sucking if she continued to breastfeed him, as soon as the dyad was regulated and calm Robert stopped when he was full.

The family therapist Virgina Satir (1988) wrote: "Touch remains the most trusted connection between people. I will believe your touch before I believe your words" (p. 61). Later in this chapter we shall examine different types of touch interventions, including touch as facilitative of establishing rapport and building trust. True, physical touch holds highly affective, emotional, erotic, and aggressive potential, but this is also true for transference, love, and human life. Ethically speaking, categorical avoidance of touch is a deep declaration concerning the innate danger of touch—we convey to our clients that there is something principally and a priori dangerous, unsafe, and uncontainable in our touching (in us). Psychologist Bertram Forer (1969) challenged us to consider how the taboo against touch in psychotherapy perpetuated "the patient's own conviction that words are good and touch is always erotic or destructive and bad" (p. 101). Such attitude might turn the transitional space to dangerous and annihilating (i.e., collapsing the transitional space), and thus the categorical avoidance of touch might in fact, at times, communicate therapeutic dangerousness and lack of security (Lawry, 1998).

When clients come to see a body psychotherapist, they usually expect and seek the *possibility* of working with touch, and the therapeutic contract surrounding such possibility and the nature of touch is usually done explicitly and transparently with the adult client (while continuously checking with younger self-states).

Within body psychotherapy there are many legitimate fields for using touch. Psychotherapy, as I hope to demonstrate, could incorporate touch which is clearly therapeutic, holds clear and transparent boundaries, while exercising a sensitive and declarative dialogue. The US Association for Body Psychotherapy (2007) offers guidelines for the ethical work with touch in psychotherapy: "Because use of touch may make clients especially vulnerable, body-oriented therapists pay particular attention to potential for dependent, infantile or erotic transference and seek healthy containment rather than therapeutically inappropriate accentuation of these states" (pp. 7–8).

When dialogues about touch arrive in the psychotherapeutic arena, the most common immediate question arising is *to touch or not to touch*. Discussions pertaining to this question are indeed fascinating, and the answers to this question are many, but it can easily invite a binary answer of "either/or". Relational body psychotherapist Shoshi Asheri (2009) wisely identifies the seduction in a dichotomous answer to this question. On the one hand, she argues, we can find the orthodox psychoanalytic position according to which touch satisfies the client's infantile needs, turning the symbolic into concrete. Touch in therapy is prone to encourage power struggle, and moreover, touch might cause transgression of sexual boundaries since it encourages sexual arousal for therapist and client alike. On the other hand, Asheri continues, we can find the orthodox body psychotherapeutic position, according to which touch is life-giving, strengthens self-boundaries and self-perception; touch can melt rigid bodymind organisation and encourage affective regulation. "Through the lens of this framework," writes Asheri, "we are led to conclude that touch is not only appropriate, it is the 'answer'" (ibid., p. 108).

Immanent to the wider mind, or intersubjective encounter, is a tension (explored in Chapter Five) between validating and recognising the other as an other-than-me subject and the willingness to surrender to connection—and denying the separateness of the other through transference, projection, and our inner fantasy space (in which we insist on viewing the other as an extension of ourselves) (Benjamin, 1990). The challenge we are facing, through the issue of touch as well, is to maintain the tension between those two movements. Indeed, a narrowing and possibly collapsing of this tension into one position or another is inevitable, but our attempt to reclaim the "both/and" (and mind our "either/or") is part of the relational endeavour.

Asheri claims that the decision about touch needs to consider the therapeutic encounter as an intersubjective and embodied dialogue. "In this sense," writes Asheri (2009), "having an unquestionable rule that touch is always 'right', or appropriate, will contribute to the collapse of the paradoxical tension of the intersubjective engagement as much as will the notion that touch is always 'wrong' or inappropriate" (p. 108). Asheri continues:

> When I wonder if it is appropriate to touch my client I cannot help but consider the fact that I'm negotiating the tension between internal and external realities. On the one hand there is an intrapsychic reality of both my client's and my own past relationship with touch (which may be associated with anything on the spectrum from love, care and nurturing to deprivation, exploitation and abuse). On the other hand there is the interpersonal reality of here and now, me and you and the concrete experience of possible physical contact between us. (pp. 107–108)

The psychoanalyst Hyman Spotnitz (1972) echoed a similar voice in saying: "Not touching is as objectionable as touching the client when this might foreclose therapeutic progress" (p. 462). In other words: satisfying needs or frustrating these, consenting to touch or refusing touch—these are neither appropriate nor inappropriate, good or bad, right or wrong, but instead require therapeutic dialogue and contextual examination.

Even if we lobby for the possibility of using touch in psychotherapy, we should acknowledge the challenges which arise when touch enters the clinic. Touch might intensify regressive transference and erotic charge in both client and therapist. Relational body psychotherapist Nick Totton (2006) boldly writes:

> Working with touch enables us to reach back into this infant world in very powerfully effective ways. At the same time, though, the passage through the Oedipal field takes up and transforms infant eroticism into adult sexuality; we can never wholly or permanently have one without the other. (pp. 159–160)

To examine the complexity Totton speaks about, we can consider Philip Bromberg's concept of multiple self-states (1998). According to Bromberg, there is an immanent multiplicity at the core of ourselves, and we constantly move between different self-states (e.g., a child, a toddler, and adult). We can enter and exit different self-states, sometimes consciously and at other times unconsciously. When we work with an adult client, younger self-states as well as adult self-states are always present, and therefore different facets of sexuality are present in the room—infantile (pre-oedipal) sexuality, child (oedipal) sexuality, and teenage and adult (post-oedipal) sexuality. When we are touching a client, it is important to ask who is touching whom, and recognise the other's self-state as well as our own. However, even the regressive client, as Totton illustrated, is not merely a "toddler" but also an adult, and the touch will reach both places. We are therefore called to exercise choice while understanding the complexity of touch, a choice which gives up dogmatism on the one hand, and naïvety on the other. We can be mindful of "who is touching whom" in terms of self-states, and use it as a clinical guide, yet nonetheless appreciate that other parts of us are engaged too and other parts of the clients are touched, which may come to the foreground and require our different attention.

The pros and cons for using touch in psychotherapy are but the beginning of our dialogue. My clinical interest rests elsewhere. For me, the question whether to touch or not is less interesting than how touch arrives or not in therapy—the manner of the psychotherapist's positioning of herself both inside herself and in relation to her client around touch. *How we touch or not touch* are not technical questions at all.

What do I do when I touch, what kind of touch do I use? These too are separate questions. Later this chapter we shall examine types of touch which the body psychotherapist may use, and demonstrate their application. The *what* is a pragmatic issue—both practical and clinical: did I take the client's hand? Did I hold him in a regressive space? Did I apply deep tissue bodywork to loosen muscular holding in the back? All these are possibilities relating to the praxis and therapeutic technique. Similar to these are questions regarding the context—the gender of the client and therapist, whether touch was in a group setting or in the clinic, whether the work was on a mattress, massage table, or while seated in "the client's chair". The potential types of touch are very interesting to explore and body psychotherapy offers a rich repertoire of interventions with touch.

However, I wish to return and examine the question of "how to touch", which is connected with therapeutic stance and positioning, and is therefore an ethical question as well. A psychotherapist may, for example, use deep bodywork directly on the body of the client (hence, involving some nakedness) out of deeply respectful psychotherapeutic dialogue. At the same time, a simple handshake could be a completely technical intervention, external to the therapeutic relationship and transgressing therapeutic boundaries. The choice not to touch could similarly express such tension. For instance, the psychotherapist may choose to acknowledge the client's need for touch but refuse such touch in order to confront the mourning for the asymmetrical and non-real aspects of therapy, and in so doing deepen the therapeutic relationship and support the client. The psychotherapist may also refuse a request for touch simply out of adopting a theoretical position and dogmatically applying it without inner or shared dialogue. The question of *how* requires the psychotherapist to examine her readiness and willingness to maintain connection with the other and with the processes which emerge from this relationship. This type of dialogue is a place where touch in psychotherapy becomes highly relevant to therapists and analysts from non-bodily modalities.

The following sections examine transferential issues with touch, types of psychotherapeutic touch, and questions regarding the therapist's position when touch enters into the clinic.

Touch and transference

> Playing is always liable to become frightening. Games and their organization must be looked at as part of an attempt to forestall the frightening aspect of playing.
>
> —Donald Winnicott (1971a, p. 67)[2]

During an NLP course I participated in, four of us were having lunch together. To our surprise, we discovered that all four of us worked with touch. The first person was a medical general practitioner (GP). The second man was a voice coach and voice teacher in an important theatre company in London. The third person was an Alexander technique teacher, and there was me—a body psychotherapist. We asked Robert, a lovely psychotherapist from Glasgow whether he would agree to be our touching guineapig, and he willingly obliged. We explained to him that each of us worked with touch in a different way, and that each of us in turn will touch him exactly in the same area (the chest) with the same type of touch (an open hand) for two minutes; we asked him to notice similarities or differences in the touch. For two minutes, each of us came to Robert and placed his hand on Robert's chest. After the four of us finished, Robert shared his experience.

"When Dan touched me, I knew that he knew exactly what was happening inside me, and that he made sure everything was OK. I felt that I wanted to let go; I felt that I was in good hands, I wanted to let him know how I was and for him to tell me what he felt." Dan was the GP.

"When Alex touched me, I felt myself growing taller, as if I was pulled upwards and stretched, my spine becoming more erect—I felt tall, capable, and full of power." Alex was the Alexander technique teacher.

"When Darren touched me I was mainly aware of my breathing. I felt it becoming fuller, and I wanted to draw a deeper breath, from inside, I breathed more easily, and my breath was richer—it was very pleasant." Darren was the voice teacher and voice coach.

"Your touch, Asaf, was the weirdest. On the one hand it was very pleasant, but on the other—a bit awkward. I felt that you wanted to get to know me, that you don't know things about me or understand how I am, but instead you wanted to get to know me and to meet with me—I couldn't just focus on my sensations; suddenly there was you and the touch between us." Robert identified a crucial aspect of relational body psychotherapy, which placed an emphasis on the therapeutic relationship. Unlike his response to the touch of the other three experts, his attention here was not only intrapsychic but also interpersonal and Robert was already mindful of our transference dynamics.

The different intentions behind each of our approaches to touch, and not only the technical skills, contributed to Robert's experience. A significant part of the training in body psychotherapy focuses on the ability to translate therapeutic intent and attunement into touch, and learning to gauge the meaning and intention given to this touch by the client.

Despite my love for touch, including its psychotherapeutic applications, it is important to recognise the cultural context within which we live and operate before we attempt to offer such interventions. In modern Western culture, there are few person-to-person relationships where touch is perceived as legitimate. There are three major categories of relationships where touch is understood as appropriate, and therefore three common transferential systems which are likely to appear when touch is applied in psychotherapy: touch between parents and a pre-oedipal child, erotic touch between partners, and professional touch between a doctor and patient (expert touch). Indeed, during the last years we have seen flickers of legitimising other types of touch—such as touch between girlfriends (who are not erotically involved), or professional touch in complementary therapies (like Darren the voice coach and Alex, the Alexander technique teacher); yet since we all live in a culture saturated for decades by these three transferential fields, they are likely to arrive in the clinic of the psychotherapist who uses touch. When Freud used touch in his work, his intent was instrumental. Touch was a therapeutic technique aimed at facilitating the hypnotic process—and he related to it as supporting the doctor-patient relationship. As is evident from the autobiographical note quoted in Chapter One, where Freud described a patient who unfortunately hugged him upon her awakening from hypnosis, the erotic transference which accompanied the technique was perceived as inappropriate and threatening (even when it was regressive and expressed infantile sexuality, as the above case was—at least to my understanding).

In the early days of body psychotherapy, therapeutic touch was indeed reliant on the convenience of medical transference. The therapist in the white robe, a skilled professional who knew the client's body and its secrets better than the client, approached the client like Dan, the GP. These types of transference are important, they allow working through authority issues, yet they also limit the client's sense of agency, autonomy, and self-direction; after all—the doctor knows best and does things *to* the client. The body psychotherapist could often find herself in professional medical transference dynamics, and it is worthwhile picking the elements which cultivated such transference. There are some times where the white robe positioning could be actively chosen (or at least consented to) as part of building trust.

As body psychotherapy softened, alongside its adoption by the humanistic psychology milieu, two complementary motives contributed to transferential shifts. Body psychotherapists wished to shake off the omnipotent white robe transference on the one hand yet wanted to avoid erotic transference dynamics on the other. During this time, many touch techniques developed which emphasised regressive, supportive, and loving touch. By and large, our culture is highly invested in preserving the psychotherapist as "good" and "clean", and if not an expert, at least paternal or maternal. Influenced by humanistic psychology, some touch techniques were developed which used this cultural bias towards parental transferences. This type of touch, parallel to *touch as comfort* (the next section expands on different types of touch), carries with it many advantages. Parental touch could facilitate deep reparative regression. It may remove the erotic threat from touch in psychotherapy, thus protecting the younger parts of the client, deepening therapeutic relationship, and supporting mutual attunement and rapport between client and therapist; all these serve to strengthen the intersubjective body.

However, this transferential stance also bears some dangers, such as delaying or inhibiting symbolisation, temptation to collusion, preserving regressive states, and ignoring erotic undercurrents in the therapeutic relationship. It is far more comfortable for most of us to remain in the position of the good parent with our clients than admitting our pleasure from the erotic intimacy, from being objects of erotic transference, from being attributed with so much power. The narcissistic and perverted motives, which go side by side with many psychotherapeutic acts, alongside altruistic, loving, and generative motives, are less pleasant to own. All-positive parental transferences are predisposed to saving fantasies and grandiosity in a subtler way, but not less dangerous than the expert position. Precisely for this reason, even if the body psychotherapist chooses to cultivate parental transference with touch (or without), it is important for her to note elements of mutual choice. Is the parent–child position vital for the therapeutic process, or is it inessential?

Psychologist David Bannay (2010) boldly spoke about sexuality in the therapeutic encounter. He described the core of erotic transference as deep desire for connection, relations, and sharing of the self. The third type of common transferences with touch, the erotic one, reaches most psychotherapeutic relationships, certainly those which intensify and emphasise emotional intimacy and provide space for expressing emotions (affect-friendly).

Shoshi Asheri (2004) examined erotic desire in the therapy room in general, and particularly in the body psychotherapeutic clinic. She divided the work with erotic material into different developmental stages: pre-oedipal, oedipal, and post-oedipal. Working with touch with a pre-oedipal client tended to create parental transference dynamics, and the subsequent quality of eroticism will therefore be pre-oedipal, infantile. The issue of touch with oedipal and post-oedipal clients was more complex, requiring skill, clear therapeutic position (some psychotherapists will touch a pre-oedipal client but not an oedipal client), and clear boundaries. But dealing with touch and eroticism was not limited to the act of touching in psychotherapy, but was an important aspect of the therapeutic processes in most modalities of psychotherapy.

When touch, and the material it stirs in the client and therapist, becomes a legitimate field for discussion and mutual examination, then the erotic aspects which may accompany touch could be appropriate, suited, and central to the therapeutic process. Asheri (ibid.) begins her paper with a question of a terrified supervisee, wondering if he "is allowed" to feel erotic desire as a psychotherapist. After an analytic, bodily, and transferential examination of the various dimensions of erotic transference, Asheri bravely seals her paper writing:

> To my supervisee's question, "Am I allowed to feel my erotic desire when working as a therapist?" I would go as far as to say that it is our responsibility to do so! The explosive material is in the therapy room anyway. I would rather learn to play with it, touch it, consciously and artfully and, by doing so, risk the chance of therapeutic transformation.

Psychotherapists who choose to touch their clients need to be sensitive to the transferential potential which is intensified in touch—for the clients and psychotherapists alike, and be willing to cautiously and consciously step into these transferential fields, play within them and expand them into further enquiry. These are not merely body psychotherapeutic skills; these are psychoanalytic and psychodynamic skills. To provide space for the complexities which arise from touch, the psychotherapist should be skilful in identifying transference and countertransference phenomena, as well as be skillful in working with these. When touch interventions are supported by psychodynamic grounding, the work becomes a potent field of Winnicottian transitional space, dangerous—yet full of potential. When therapeutic touch is applied without bodily training or skills on the one hand, or without being informed by psychodynamic understanding on the other hand, the danger ceases to be Winnicottian, and becomes concrete.

Encounters of the touching kind: types of touch in body psychotherapy

Touch in psychotherapy has variegated uses and expressions. Psychologists Morris Goodman and Arthur Teicher (1988) divided touch in psychotherapy into holding touch and provoking touch. According to Goodman and Teicher, holding touch was aimed at communicating therapeutic security and containment, while provoking touch attempted to create a response—to facilitate the surfacing of therapeutic material and to make it accessible for the therapeutic dyad. Nick Totton (2006) offered five categories of touch in psychotherapy, and this section will make use of Totton's division as a base for exploring types of touch in psychotherapy. The categories offered by Totton were: touch as comfort, touch to explore contact, touch as amplification, touch as provocation, and touch as skilled professional intervention. To these five categories I added another type of touch: touch as relational affirmation. Each category will now be explained and demonstrated with a short clinical vignette.

Touch as comfort

Similar to Goodman and Teicher's understanding of holding touch, comforting touch could at times provide a safe space even amid the most painful and frightening experiences (Rolef Ben-Shahar, 2009). Touch as comfort is highly valuable when working with fearful or regressive clients (or clients in fearful or regressive states), whose self-perception is indistinct or incomplete, and touch may answer their developmental need for holding.

The main type of touch offered by Winnicott was touch as comfort within regressive ego states (Totton, 2006). This is also the main use of touch exercised by Sándor Ferenczi, who supported his clients in regressive states as part of his work with developmental traumas (Keith-Spiegel & Koocher, 1985; Raubolt, 1985). Ferenczi believed that integrating touch in psychotherapy, as part of the transferential work, could be possible and appropriate: he believed that the therapist needed, at times, to provide the clients' (regressive) love needs by holding or cradling them (A. Kaplan, 1975). Freud's biographer and former analysand of Ferenczi, the psychoanalyst Ernest Jones (Jones, Trilling, & Marcus, 1961), portrayed Ferenczi (with such force and impetus that it felt like character murder) as encouraging bodily contact out of his own personal striving for emotional and sexual satisfaction. Jones argued that Ferenczi's therapeutic style stemmed from Ferenczi's sickly and insatiable craving for fatherly love, thus putting Ferenczi's entire enterprise under a question mark. It is interesting to note that it was Jones who did receive the very fatherly love that Ferenczi allegedly sought, and from the very same father (Freud). Psychoanalyst Patrick Casement (1982) also argued against the use of comforting touch in psychotherapy, which might lead to insoluble complexities in therapy, particularly to collusion.

I wish to support Shoshi Asheri's call to psychotherapists from different modalities to reconsider the place of the body in therapy and the possibility of including touch; notwithstanding this call, and as Asheri herself (2009) as well as Totton (2006) and others emphasised—body psychotherapists too ought to examine the clinical and contextual appropriateness of intervening with touch, and familiarise themselves with the arguments against it. There are some cases in which avoiding touch is a kinder, more benevolent, and clinically appropriate intervention.

Touch as comfort is particularly appropriate for clients expressing fragmented or oral character positions (expanded upon in Chapter Six), or when these developmental stages are at the forefront of the clinical encounter. The psychotherapist may offer a hand, hold, or cradle the client. One of the clearest (and most human) examples for this type of touch is contact as a response to crying. Many psychotherapists struggle to hold back from reaching out a hand to support the sobbing client, who seems unable to take comfort in the untouching presence of the psychotherapist alone. The momentary "inadvertent" touch which may accompany the handing of the tissue box (a sin which many psychotherapists have shared) is an almost comical substitute for the comforting hand—after all, the tissue box is as concrete as the touching hand.

But touch as comfort is not only relevant in regressive contexts; it can offer a human connection to the client, momentary dyadic regulation which allows the containment of what might otherwise be too painful. In these cases, touch could release the client from retraumatisation or regressive freezing in fragmented self-states. The following vignette will demonstrate such an intervention:

Dave speaks of a dream he had this week and tears are in his eyes. Suddenly he swallows some air, his neck becomes tight and red and the pulse in his neck is more visible. A childhood memory emerges and Dave starts relaying it. His eyes no longer seem alive, there is no affect in his voice, and Dave speaks quickly with an almost robotic monotony.

"What's happening now, Dave?"
"Nothing."
"What are you feeling now?"
"Nothing."

I reach my hand out to Dave, offering it to him. He receives it wordlessly. The hand holding mine is sweating, holding me tight. Dave's breathing seems heavy and distressed, and I can feel my own heart pounding strongly. After a while, Dave's eyes rise to finally meet mine with a questioning gaze. I strengthen our physical connection, we are here together. Dave carries on with his memory, this time much slower. "I'm back," he says.

Touch as a means to explore connection

Touch can be a language. In fact, some of the clients who come to body psychotherapy are far more fluent in touch and movement than they are in words and sentences, and the psychotherapist's willingness to converse in these languages too actually enables the therapeutic process. Expecting someone to speak psychological language when their native tongue is nonverbal in the name of symbolic superiority is as arrogant as insisting on speaking English with a non-English-speaking immigrant, qualifying it by saying—"This is England!" With time, the therapeutic dyad might learn to expand its vocabulary and also speak in the verbal tongue. We can ask questions with touch, or make offers with touch. The body psychotherapist may offer a spontaneous intervention or an exercise to explore the therapeutic relationship. This exploration may deepen trust and security, and support the surfacing of unconscious material.

It is one of our first sessions together, and I offer Jolene my hand as a way of exploring contact.[3] Jolene is an experienced client, with many years of psychodynamic work behind her. And yet, the field of body psychotherapy in general and working therapeutically with touch in particular is a completely foreign land for her. She came to see me specifically to explore her anxiety in relation to others through therapeutic touch. I sense caution in both of us alongside curiosity and willingness to engage. Jolene accepts my offer and touches my hand. Our first contact is apprehensive; Jolene lowers her eyes—like a wild animal testing the safety of contact. I can sense the potential for both danger and comfort in this first hand-to-hand connection. I feel that my hand is being tested—that I am being tested, and it comforts me, as well as slightly unnerves me.

Soon, Jolene makes eye contact and breathes. She seems bewildered. "What's going on, Jolene?" I check. "I'm surprised how quickly I feel safe with this touch. It's like my body knows that it is safe, but my head tells me I shouldn't trust so quickly," she says. The tango of checking for safety continues on; Jolene lets go of my hand and resumes touch, each time surprised to discover this discrepancy between her bodily felt sense and her cognitive schemas. Who shall we listen to? We use this exploration to later draw on the body as a compass, not just a source of anxiety.

Jolene and I could have had this dialogue in many other ways, with touch or without it. Nevertheless, I believe that when Jolene touched my hand she knew me in a visceral way, which allowed her to feel safe enough, and that it would have taken much longer to establish this kind of safety with words. I also know that, as a client, I need touch to establish safety; that in order to feel my psychotherapist and be able to trust her or him I need my body to sense them first.

Exercise: dancing the relationship

(In pairs)

The next exercise is drawn from the martial arts (I first encountered it with Silke Ziehl) and it forms a lovely dialogue through touch and movement. This is one of the most potent exercises I know and I use it extensively in training and workshop situations, and sometimes in therapy too (with couples and individuals)

1. Take off shoes, stand facing one another, unlock knees, and loosen your jaws. This exercise is done without speaking.
2. Find a safe way to establish hand-to-hand contact and notice what sensations accompany such touch.
3. Decide (nonverbally) who leads first, and begin to explore movement, touch, and flow without completely letting go of the contact (for example, you may only touch the fingertips—but keep contact). The leader leads the movement and the follower follows the movement. You may move with your eyes open or closed, or play with both.
4. As a leader, allow the follower to learn about your rhythms. Let yourself be daring, creative, curious, and playful.
5. After about four or five minutes exchange roles: the leader now follows and the follower now leads.
6. After five more minutes, maintain contact. Now that you are slightly more familiar with one another's rhythms, let movement take over—without leading or following, or while the two of you lead and follow at the same time. Submit to the movement which wishes to emerge out of your relationship. Allow for at least five minutes of shared exploration.
7. Thank one another, process and share.

Touch as amplification

The psychotherapist draws the client's attention to feelings and thoughts, slips of the tongue and dreams, fears and hopes, behaviours and expressions. Drawing attention creates movement; it amplifies affect in the corner which is illuminated by attention.

Touch invites paying attention, and touch as a way to draw attention is a basic human gesture. Tapping a shoulder for "Excuse me, can you tell me how I get to …" or placing our hand against the heart which accompanies a "You wouldn't believe what happened to me yesterday" are common examples of touch as amplification.

Many modalities in body psychotherapy use touch to help the client focus on her body and pay attention to bodily responses and their associated cognitive and emotional material. This could be self-touch ("What's happening in your stomach when you are speaking? Is it OK to place your hand on your tummy when you talk, breathe into it and see what comes up?") or touch by the psychotherapist. Touch as amplification (mainly self-touch) is highly common in process-oriented modalities like Gestalt therapy and focusing. The bodily attention could illuminate unconscious processes in unmediated ways, and the body psychotherapist may therefore use these to assist her clients in exploring bodily arenas en route to better knowing themselves.

A supervisee tells me of a strong, diaphragmatic stomach-ache that started shortly after a particularly good session with a client; so strong was the pain that it prevented my supervisee from sleeping at night. She describes the session as pleasurable. For the first time in their work together, her client was willing to engage in a relationship with her and to enjoy this connection. After two laborious regressive years, oedipal material began to emerge and therapy was now deeper and more "fleshy". I invite my supervisee to lie down and touch her diaphragm. After a few moments of deep breathing and self-touch something loosens: "You shouldn't feel pleasure," says my supervisee. "Inside the session it was OK, but in the real world my client is forbidden from feeling pleasure."

Touch as provocation

Deep bodywork can assist in softening the *muscular armour* (which was discussed in Chapters Two and Four), inviting inner vitality to express itself more freely. Touch as provocation relies on the Reichian tradition of touch as energetically charging (Lowen, 1975). Commonly, the psychotherapist will exercise skilled bodily pressure on body tissues, allowing for a release (discharge) of pent-up emotional and bodily energy. The release might be accompanied by emotional expressions, thoughts, images, and beliefs connected with this chronic muscular tension (these would occur spontaneously or with the encouragement of the therapist). Provocative touch involves changing bodymind organisations and therefore requires great therapeutic skill, as well as a stable and supportive therapeutic relationship, which can "speak itself", that is—material which may surface in the client and therapist ought to be given space before touch, during touch, and following the touch—openly and while assuming shared and respective responsibility.

Tickling touch or even poking could be considered as provocation, and sometimes the psychotherapist may use these types of touch. For example, in my work with Kate, a highly dissociative client, I used to annoy her quite frequently with slightly poking but non-threatening touch. Kate tended to enter, easily and spontaneously, dissociative states of terror and dread where she shook, contorted, and uncontrollably sobbed for long minutes, unable to recognise me as Asaf. I turned into a dangerous and threatening figure in ongoing loops of retraumatisation.

When I annoyed her (for example, with small, playful pokes in her shoulder), Kate would get irritated but not frightened—she remained present and we could hold a dialogue without her being swept into what she called "my black holes". These provocative irritations were, at the beginning of our work, interventions which were a central part of trauma work.

The following vignette describes one part of the therapeutic process with Grace,[4] herself a psychotherapist, who came to see me following nine years of Jungian analysis. She being an experienced client, we were able to rely on her previous psychotherapeutic experience, deepening where her analysis stopped. The following session was about a year into psychotherapy.

> Grace writes: "As Asaf's hand works its way down my rigid neck muscle, pressure increasing, I want to hold my breath and fight the urge to swear—I never swear. Asaf is urging me to release my breath 'with noise.' I feel totally disoriented, lost; it is the scariest feeling of my life as every nerve in my body feels like it's jangling. There is nothing beneath me and I am falling, falling into an abyss. Somewhere through the fog I am aware of Asaf's soothing voice ... I cry like a baby as he strokes my hair while I lie curled up in foetal position within his protective embrace. Things gradually settle and I become calmer ... yet in some ways, more hypersensitive than before. Strange as it may sound, it's like there is more substance to me. I know that my body's always been there but I haven't really given it that much consideration/regard before. Now, well ... it's there!" (Rolef Ben-Shahar & MacDonald, 2011, p. 57)

When somatic organisation is characterised by rigidity, very little emotional motility is possible. Grace was always softly spoken, but when we approached painful material in her biography she became almost muted, and her voice disappeared into a whisper. We loosened the fascia associated with voice, using deep bodywork techniques from postural integration (Painter, 1984). I worked with the trapezius, the sternocleidomastoid, the scalene muscles, and the diaphragm, and we temporarily removed the habitual muscular obstruction of Grace's voice: around the cervical segment. It seems that during the bodywork Grace experienced deep regression and was able to liberate her voice and feelings in new ways—the voice which could not have been heard before came out: animalistic, raw, and uncensored. Following this session Grace managed, more than before, to speak her mind in uncensored and vital ways: both in therapy and outside it. Grace and I processed this session for long weeks thereafter.

Touch as skilful professional intervention

Body psychotherapists train in a variety of bodywork skills: massage, rocking, pulsing, joint mobilisation or adjustments, and other soft or deep tissue techniques. Body psychotherapists may offer bodywork as part of the therapeutic process, when it is perceived as advancing the therapeutic work, goals, and the therapeutic relationship.

Touch as skilful professional intervention poses complex requirements for the psychotherapist: on the one hand, the capacity to be an expert, to know what he is doing, how, and why he is doing so (including a completely different set of expertise to the psychotherapeutic ones, regarding anatomy, physiology, and pathology). On the other hand, the professional positioning also bears complicated transferential potential, and the psychotherapist should be mindful of the complexities such intervention may introduce to therapy. It is seductive, but mostly undesirable, to become the "white-robed doctor" narrowing the relationship with the client to authoritative transference dynamics between a doctor and her patient.

Nevertheless, when the client knows his therapist is also professionally skilful in touch, new material will arrive in therapy which may not come into solely "talking therapy". Clients may bring bodily experiences, pains, and somatic symptoms, hence expanding the field of work in psychotherapy. More of the persons (client and therapist) may enter the clinic. Moreover, the pains and symptoms could arrive in therapy earlier, telling and showing what the client cannot yet conceptualise verbally. Thus, skilled professional interventions in touch could expand the therapeutic enquiry (allowing entrance of material that would not have arrived in other therapeutic modalities) but might narrow it down too (cultivating authoritative and doctor-patient transference dynamics).

The previous vignette described touch as provocation, which was also skilled professional intervention. Another example, from my work with Jacob, will demonstrate the complexity of dialogue between transferential and intersubjective encounters and skilled professional touch. I chose to illustrate this type of touch with a complex example since bodywork as skilled intervention was in the past frequently practised while maintaining an oblivious attitude to transference dynamics, and was therefore prone, at least in my opinion, to abuse, retraumatisation, or perpetuating doctor-patient dynamics. I find it important to demonstrate the integration between an expert consciously working with muscular organisation and the psychodynamic practice.

Jacob, a forty-year-old psychologist and father of two, sought therapy to deepen his bodily exploration. He "warned" me in the beginning that one of the issues he wanted to work with was his bisexual orientation. Jacob and I quickly dived into an exciting analytic examination of his relationship with his father. I really was looking forward to our sessions together. Psychotherapy with Jacob was moving, without threats to the therapeutic frame or challenging of boundaries, without resistances or acting out; he really came to work. Even though our shared positioning was comfortable for both of us, it also became too convenient—somehow it prevented regressive processes. At the same time, our mutual positioning kept a safe distance from erotic material. What was comfortable at first became limiting as soon as we wished to deepen our work. And then, eight months after commencing treatment, Jacob's back started to hurt.

We both loved integrating deep bodywork in our psychotherapy, and we decided to meet the pain directly through the body. For a number of sessions we worked with deep tissue bodywork techniques, integrated with postural integration strokes. Parallel to this, Jacob started showing more vulnerability in our sessions, and at times brought younger self-states in. One day, following a deep tissue release of his lower back, I felt a wave of sexual arousal surging inside me. At first I was apprehensive and withdrew internally. I looked at this man, who dared to explore his sexuality more than my private homophobia had allowed me to. Jacob noticed the qualitative change in my presence; he reached out and took my hand. "What's going on, Jacob?" I asked, having recomposed my position (with defensive effort, I must add). "You know, Asaf," he replied, "I think you are trying to ease your embarrassment from this shared moment we just had." He was right of course. This shared moment was not the erotic arousal (this was fine), but the moment afterwards, where our transferential structure lost its habitual organisation and for a moment we experienced mutuality and potential symmetry—more than I was comfortable to admit. Following this session we had an important conversation concerning the ways Jacob protected me and himself from this homoerotic tension, and we were able to process and work with his sexuality (and our sexuality) in therapy in more honest and authentic ways. The bodywork we have done loosened a transferential impasse between us.

Touch as relational affirmation

> If touch is to be considered psychotherapeutically, then the psychotherapist needs to have a theoretical basis for the touch, a means of evaluating the touch and the possibility of discussing it in process in the consulting room. Otherwise, how do you know what your touch has communicated? I believe that the key elements of touch as relational affirmation are presence, intention, and the ongoing relationship between client and therapist.
>
> —Angela King (2011, p. 121)

By and large, touch in therapy requires sufficient establishment of the therapeutic relationship before applying bodily interventions. The categories of touch covered in the last sections presume a certain degree of connection which forms the basis for the therapeutic intervention. The more provocative and evocative the intervention, the more stable the therapeutic relationship and the dyad's capacity to process need to be. However, touch could also be a part of the process of establishing therapeutic relationship in general, and the formation of the intersubjective body in particular. Touch could be (and is in many ways) a part of how I make contact with the other; it can be an extension of my presence rather than a therapeutic intervention. While exploring new and unfamiliar therapeutic territories, when the client and therapist are both required to let go of the separated individual identity, touch could become an important anchor to the ground, while at the same time a bridge into the therapeutic connection. In some cases, as I shall soon illustrate, touch can serve as the legs and the strings which strongly connect to earth, allowing our dyadic kite to soar to impressive heights.

In her beautiful paper on touch as relational affirmation, body psychotherapist Angela King (ibid.) argued that touch interventions could at times be what psychoanalyst Beatrice Beebe (2004) conceptualised as an *action-dialogue*. King portrayed this orientation to touch as a bodily translation of Martin Buber's (1958) I–thou, a human connection holding within it the transferential tension without ignoring objective or intersubjective realities.

Touch as relational affirmation is an excellent communication agent when verbal conversation is too complex or impossible. We can get to know one another *also* through touch; you can tell me about yourself and listen to me through touch. You could learn to feel safe, to enquire and ask, check and converse—through bodily communication. In this sense, the person for whom touch is not a basic and fluent communication channel would not be able to offer this kind of intervention. In order to offer this basic type of touch I need to be a touching person, not just a therapist who attained training in touch.

For example, when Susan, a sixty-five-year-old musician came to therapy, she opened with a long and fast-paced monologue, the first of many, where she counted all the different reasons which brought her into therapy. I asked to put my feet next to hers and she consented. Once in a while, as she spoke, I moved my foot closer to her. I wanted to be by her side, but without contact I could not listen to the flood of words or be with her—I found myself needing to choose: staying with the narrative, or staying with Susan. Touch allowed me to remain present. To this extent, the physical contact helped me at least as it was there for her. Even if this type of touch could be seen as erotic, we had no erotic charge at all (at this stage); this has come at a much later stage in therapy.

Our sessions continued with my foot making its way to meet Susan's, who did not seem to notice this or demonstrate insights concerning our therapy. After about three months, Susan came one day and started her usual monologue, when suddenly she stopped. "Where is your foot?" she asked. "I miss it." "I didn't notice," I admitted. "But when you don't touch me you cannot listen to me," said Susan, "and I tend to talk at you and not with you as well. When we have contact you are with me and I am with you." And with this Susan managed to conceptualise what I was unable to fully grasp for three months.

A cup, grasping my fingers: musing on touch[5]

> A cup can be grasped only if our arm is long enough to reach it, and only if our fingers are strong enough to lift it.
>
> —Yann Coello and Yvonne Delevoye-Turrell (2007, p. 667)

My fingers, grasping a cup

My fingers are clicking on the keyboard. I particularly like the letters F and J, since they have little bumps on them to assist in touch-typing finger positioning. There are many ways to type, some better than others. I am an OK typist, not great, but OK. We can talk of the many ways to type on a keyboard; there are plenty of disciplines and not one discipline fits all. From a phenomenological point of view, a keyboard has no meaning without typing. It becomes a keyboard in our making it a keyboard—in my typing on it I help it become a keyboard.

Typing is like holding a cup. The grasping of the cup (the comprehending of its physical meaning) depends on the physical activity of reaching it and letting our fingers grasp it. The object *cup*—the cup which is in front of me, in the here-and-now, cannot be grasped by mere intellectual gymnastics, it will be the idea or concept of the cup (the "cup-ness") that I will understand, not the cup itself.

Since we are embodied beings, since relationships are not merely soul-to-soul relationships but also body-to-body ones, I wish to propose that in order to grasp another human being we need to touch them, that to be a human being means to have a body and bodies can only be fully realised in a relationship. We can understand the idea (concept) of someone else, but to grasp them, to truly know another, I will need to reach out and touch. Should you accept my reasoning, this may present a clear and compelling argument for the power of touch in body psychotherapy.

Let us think about this in three stages: first, we become in relationships (Buber, 1958); second, our bodies become in relationships (Orbach, 2003a), and third, we need touch to be bodies and be known as embodied beings.

a. Martin Buber (1958) phrased this argument poetically: "The person becomes conscious of himself as sharing in being, as co-existing, and thus as being" (p. 63). Buber therefore conceptualised our being (or rather, our becoming) as dependent on the interrelations with another—with the subjective thou. It is in the action of acknowledging the other that the other becomes thou (a subject).
b. Relational psychoanalyst Susie Orbach (2003a) brought the body into this relational-Buberian equation. Once more, let me repeat her argument: "To paraphrase Winnicott's famous and oft-repeated phrase, there is no such thing as a baby, there is also, I suggest, no such thing as a body, there is only a body in relationship with another body" (p. 11). Reiterating her position, a body was not only a thing (object), it was also a person; therefore, our "self" could not be grasped outside an embodied relationship, and our bodies were dependent on other bodies interacting with them.
c. But how can bodies be grasped if not physically? Can true grasping (not theoretical understanding, but unmediated knowing) of another person take place without physical contact? Although it is not fashionable to say this, particularly in our transference-laden era where we are continuously cautioned against touch in psychotherapy (even body psychotherapists), I personally do not believe that we can. I believe that in order to know another person I need to touch him or her.

This, of course, is a relational argument. If the individual-separated self is first and foremost for and by itself, then my argument is refuted altogether. But I propose an understanding of the self as not only (albeit also) separated—a self for itself but also dependent on relationship. Relational body psychotherapy conceptualises the self as partaking in a dance between two (or more) part-selves which only become selves in their connection. I am both a separate bodymind and a part-bodymind which becomes in connection with another part-bodymind. From this point of view, embodiment and relationality condition one another—we need other bodies and other people to become bodies and to become people. To grasp a cup, my hand needs to reach it. Now comes the interesting bit because cups do not grasp the hands that grasp them.

Cups do not grasp me

Cups, unlike people, do not return the favour. Cups do not grasp the hand that grasps them—people do. We are not only affirming the other when we acknowledge them and touch them, it is not only thou that is created in the act of relating. We are also created in this dance, or in Buber's (1958) words: "I become through my relation to the Thou; as I become I, I say Thou" (p. 11).

The idea that our clients may hold the power to create us, to help us in becoming (and so that, on the soul level, there is a true equality of relationship) is both exciting and scary for me, perhaps equally so. Consider the following example: a woman attending a seminar told feminist leader and psychologist Carol Gilligan (2004) how she "… was sitting in the living room one day when her four-year-old son came up to her and asked: 'Mommy, why are you sad?' Wanting to be a good mother, she thought she should not burden her son with her sadness. 'No, I'm not sad,' she said. 'Mommy,' he said, 'I know you. I was inside you'" (p. 113).

If we consider this when talking about touch, then, when we touch a person (and in this context, a client), they get to know us too, and deeply so. True, this knowing is also tainted by transference dynamics, by cultural conditioning, and therapeutic positioning, and so forth. But also, and at the same time, we serve ourselves to be known by the other, to be created by the other as subjectivity, and in return, they allow us to create them and know them.

Just like the boy who knows his mother from inside, in touching we allow our clients to feel us from inside and know us, whether we want it or not: imperfect as we are, sexual and vulnerable, power-seeking and faulty, shamed and scared, loving and hating, lusting and joyous, bored and jealous. I deeply believe that all touching therefore involves a relational event and ignoring the relational aspect of it is a counter-therapeutic act, naïve, and potentially dangerous. I propose here that for true knowledge of a fellow human being, which would allow him or her to become, we need to touch, and when we touch, we grant the other a similar opportunity (even if they lack the conceptual tools we might have) to know us, to facilitate us in our becoming.

If what I propose rings true to you, then it makes the practice of touch in psychotherapy a stance rather than a technique—a declaration of connection. It is not just something we do, it is a way for us to become. I would like to demonstrate what I mean with a short clinical vignette:

Eliot sits with me, shrunk and contracted. He is a young-looking twenty year old, who sought therapy because his amorphous gender identity (and gender-amorphous appearance) has attracted much violence since his childhood. It is our fourth session, and Eliot is unable to make eye contact. "Your room is far too scary and much too bright," he says in almost a whisper. "Please don't come near me, and don't look at me." I draw the curtains to darken the room.

I reach out and extend my hand to him. "You are welcome to take my hand or refrain from taking it. If you take my hand you can stay for a moment or for a long while, and you can refuse my hand altogether. I'm here."

Despite his lack of eye contact, I notice Eliot is rolling his eyeballs. "You must be joking. You'll hurt me, and once you feel me you'll be disgusted by me. Touch is always painful." In my countertransference, I feel so old—tired, weary, and old. "I'm closing my eyes now, Eliot, and want to invite you to imagine that you reach out to touch my hand and that you can feel it." I shut my eyes, and think, what a relief, then imagine the way Eliot is testing me now to see if I am cheating. To my surprise, I feel his hand touching me, tender and tentative like a wild animal approaching the hand of a person.

"Hello hand," I say, and Eliot replies with utter seriousness. "Hello." I offer Eliot the possibility of withdrawing his touch and coming back as many times as he likes and to choose whether he prefers to continue with or without touch.

Many minutes pass in silence during which Eliot comes and goes—touching and leaving. I delight in getting to know him and also in the times I get to be on my own; there is a gentle satisfaction noting the developing trust between us and Eliot's pro-activity in securing such trust. After a few moments his hand finally lands inside my own hand. "You can open your eyes now; I don't think I'm afraid of you anymore." We look at each other and burst out laughing. "How did you reach this diagnosis?" I ask. "Dunno. You feel safe," he replies.

I have to admit that I hate being known by my clients almost as much as I crave it. When training to become a psychotherapist, I was comfortable being out of the central stage, having the attention directed at my clients. I believe this feeling is shared by many people who choose to give their lives to others. With time, I realised that I also deeply wanted—more so, I needed, to be acknowledged as a person, not just an extension of the client or a function in their development (part object or object), but also as me. The tension between those needs (to serve as an object for the other and to be a subjectivity for them) is, I believe, at the heart of our profession. Furthermore, it became clearer to me that in order to help another become a subject and appreciate himself or herself as a subject, I needed to do the same, that while many aspects of psychotherapy may remain asymmetrical, the human recognition of another was not one of these.

Liking myself does not come easy. And I have learnt from Eliot, later in therapy, that through our touch (which was touch to explore contact, as well as touch as relational affirmation) he noticed many aspects of me which I was trying to conceal: some aspects of myself that I was not proud of, and others which I was trying to protect him from. This visibility was at times intolerable, but it was also a de-shaming act as Eliot must have decided I was still a decent enough human being to trust and so he allowed me to make him safe. And in this act he did much more: he made me (although he was not the first, I was also made by others) a decent enough man, a trustworthy human being. He was a cup that reached out to hold the fingers that grasped it.

Therapeutic positioning and touch: touch as relational engagement

> I can touch somebody in such a way that my touch says: "You can take your time; I am interested to meet you; where are you? Is this OK for you? Will you meet me here?" I can touch in such a way that each finger has eyes and ears as I make contact with the other person. When I touch in this manner, I am more likely to be receptive to who the other person is, and what they want, and what they are saying with their body at the moment. From this somatic dialogue, we get to know each other more deeply.
>
> —Silke Ziehl (2005)

Touch in psychotherapy is ever so complicated and complex, confusing, misleading, and holding an explosive potential. At the same time, touch in psychotherapy is simple and clear, organised and organising, and holding a calming potential, strengthening attachment and security. Touch is not confusing *or* simple, misleading *or* clear—it is both. How does the client interpret touch? What meaning does this particular touch receive in the therapeutic context—and later, in the non-therapeutic world of the client (and the therapist)? How is touch processed and in what ways? Like many other therapeutic elements, these are all questions which are shaped and created throughout the therapeutic relationship and long after it had finished. Considering the answer to those questions we can establish whether the touch intervention was appropriate or not.

When touch stems from curiosity and desire to be co-created in an intersubjective space, it is second to none as a tool for fostering surrender to flow and to connection. With touch I can demonstrate that I am here, with you; that I am sharing each human experience, thought, or emotion which you may have, pleasant or unpleasant. Additionally, touch can express desire for intimate sharing which is both safe (boundary-wise) and dangerous: we are standing on the edge, facing the intersubjective tension of validating the other and negating the other. With touch I invite you to create intimacy along with me—intimacy which may change me as well, not only you.

Touch can be a powerful agent in dispelling the myth of our isolation, by visiting the world of the other or penetrating the world of the other and bringing our "discriminatory and meaning-giving" (N. Diamond, 2006, p. 89) subjectivity to the fore; thus, it is actually from this connection and meeting we may discover our subjective separateness. When the skilled body psychotherapist touches with enquiring and safe yet not-knowing hands (the skill is in the curiosity and the willingness to not know, as discussed in the section on touch and transference), she demonstrates in her own body the courage and capacity to surrender to the wider mind. At the same time, this type of touch is but an invitation to the client to act similarly: we cannot force the other into an intersubjective space, but we can certainly be there if the other chooses to join in.

This therapeutic position, which views touch as a bridge between inside and outside, between what is mine and what is yours, between the desire to merge with the other and the wish to separate from the other and individuate, is highly relevant to all psychotherapists, regardless of whether they use touch or not.

The question of the therapist's positioning concerning touch is not another type of touch, but an issue of how we approach touching, the "how" and not the "whether" or "what". By being willing to hold the potential space for touch—by allowing the possibility for touch—we already create a change. Relational psychoanalyst and poet Barbara Pizer (2002) phrased it like this: "In my view, whether or not we believe in or feel comfortable with any sort of physical contact in the psychoanalytic setting, if we arbitrarily split it off on theoretical grounds as a viable possibility in all circumstances, we invite dissociation" (p. 841).

Psychotherapists who wish to offer interventions with touch should, in my opinion, receive appropriate training, particularly in learning to regulate and monitor their somatic countertransference, and learning to calibrate their somatic attention and listening. Just as the psychoanalyst learns to use her ears, her language, her mind, and her feelings accurately and sensitively, so does the body psychotherapist learn to additionally listen to and communicate with her fingers, hands, and body, and continuously and methodically observe body language. The psychotherapist learns to examine the ways her intentions are translated into interventions, and the meanings her clients attribute to these interventions. Listening with touch requires the therapist to notice resonance, including countertransference, imagery, and sensations. For instance, when one day I touched Jeremy on his shoulder I was suddenly scared that he might leave therapy. Checking with him, he confirmed his fears of surrendering to both the therapeutic process and to his fiancée, out of worry that we might leave him or die. The next chapter will discuss resonance skills which are complementary to touch skills.

Beyond training and the capacities which developed therein, such positioning towards touch in psychotherapy requires us to carefully examine our prejudices and racist beliefs, as well as our willingness to mutually examine these and other sensations and feelings with our clients, since touch as a relational event is not merely technical even when it involves technical mastery. When we position ourselves as potentially touching we expose ourselves to our clients as they might see us as much as we might see them—both in the here-and-now, and in presenting our transference and projective reality, which are also expressed in the inhibitions, fears, and yearnings we express when we connect.

Touch as a relational event carries with it large doses of mutuality, even if we are still asked to maintain the asymmetrical nature of psychotherapy. When I touch you I declare my willingness to be known by you, I proclaim my desire to know you and my willingness to risk the possibility that you, too, might get to know me.

To touch or not to touch? And if we touch, how do we touch?

Shoshi Asheri (2009) suggested eight guiding principles in supporting the decision when to touch. These are explored here alongside some explanation:

- **When the client knows that touch is a possibility but not an inevitability**: Touch does not have to happen. Touch as a possibility allows the therapeutic dyad to remain working in the transitional space of fantasy, expectation, wish, and fear. Both extreme positions for and against touch may collapse the uncertainty.
- **When touch is guided by the client's material and not the therapist's needs or therapeutic agenda**: The therapist is attentive to the therapeutic relevance of intervention with touch. The therapist's needs and agenda will unavoidably influence the therapeutic direction and the client, yet I believe Asheri points to increasing awareness of these and encouraging conscious choice regarding the intervention.
- **When the nature of the touch is varied and unpredictable and not dictated by a technique (although technique may be involved) but by the therapeutic encounter**: That is, that touch would not be dictated by a procedure, but will mainly be attentive to the quality of the therapeutic relationship. "Last week we worked on your feet so today we need to work on your calves" is an extreme example for touch dictated by technique.
- **When the nature of the touch corresponds to the client's presented self-state and can appropriately and fluidly change according to the therapeutic needs**: Touching a regressive client who wishes to be cradled in the arms of the therapist ought to change when the same client expresses oedipal desire to possess the therapist. Psychotherapists are called to relate to multiple self-states in the clients and themselves and check their positioning in the interaction (who is touching whom). Touch should be in accord with this enquiry.
- **When touch is aimed at deepening dialogue with unconscious material and not used to avoid uncomfortable issues or uncomfortable dynamics**: Explorative and open touch maintains potential space. Any choice of intervention may result from a (conscious or unconscious) wish to avoid an uncomfortable issue of dynamics. If, for example, I find it difficult to stay with the client's suffering, I might offer physical support. While we cannot (and should not) obliterate such defensive positioning, Asheri recommends a conscious inner dialogue, to examine our motivation for intervention.
- **When there is an indication that the symbolic needs a concrete manifestation, but not when the concrete manifestation limits the possibilities which the symbolic could open**: Once, during a workshop I taught about touch, one psychotherapist got up and started shouting,

"I don't have to touch my clients in order to reach them." She was, of course (at least partly), right. This guideline checks the extent to which touch serves the potential space allowing the client to explore her needs and material, and the extent to which touch (or not touching) may obstruct such exploration.

- **When the therapeutic relationship and the nature or touch are congruent and aligned**: Like any other therapeutic intervention, this guideline concerns both timing and relevance within the therapeutic relationship. Choosing touch could be paralleled to providing an interpretation: the therapist who considers whether to offer an interpretation will examine the readiness of the client, the stage of therapy, and possible contingencies and consequences. The capacity to take risks and tolerate ruptures in the therapeutic relationships (necessary for deepening attachment) also depends on the therapeutic dynamics. Deep Reichian touch in a well-established relationship may be processed and serve as a transformative point in therapy, while the same touch in an unstable relationship may be experienced as traumatic re-enactment or as abusive.
- **When the ethical boundary of sexual abstinence is held as an essential and clear foundation of the therapeutic relationship**: This boundary is essential for the client, but it also protects the therapist and the therapeutic dyad, allowing both parties to explore freely. I invite the reader to revisit the section on boundaries in Chapter Seven, which will assist in understanding the body psychotherapist's complex reasoning when offering touch. The "clear cut" boundaries in body psychotherapy regarding touch concern touching genitals, genital-to-genital contact, and any type of penetration. Some early Reichian body psychotherapy involved touch which was aimed at sexually arousing the client, but today it is consensually agreed that touch which is aimed at sexual arousal of the client or therapist is unethical and should be prohibited.

Nonetheless, the therapeutic relationship could be erotic and sexual even when these guidelines are kept to (as noted by psychologist Efrat Even Tzur in Rolef Ben-Shahar, 2013a, p. 361). I see the dangerous erotic zones less in the "red" areas mentioned above and more in the grey ones, such as unspoken flirtations which turn the therapeutic field into a collusive and potentially abusive space. I doubt that it is possible to draw a finite and clear boundary here, but I can share my feeling that touch which ignores transferential complexities (and the fact that clients bring with them *also* younger parts—as do therapists), and which is done for the purpose of satisfying the client's or therapist's erotic needs is unethical.

These important questions could not and should not be examined by introspection alone. The therapeutic relationship takes place, as Asheri formulated so well, in spaces which are also erotic—and a good thing that they are! As long as these are spoken and not enacted, clearly explored and not hidden, processed in the psychotherapist's personal therapy and supervision. We cannot identify all the currents and undercurrents which activate us, and we need external support to better conduct ourselves in therapy—in the shape of supervision or therapy. Notwithstanding all the above arguments, the therapeutic relationship could be unethically erotic even when no touch is used at all.

To Asheri's clear guidelines I would like to add a few more points (Rolef Ben-Shahar, 2003):

When to touch:

- When we are clear about what we communicate with our touch, and yet willing to check it with the client and change it appropriately.
- When there is a clear contract regarding touch, defining boundaries and exercising the right of both parties to say no.
- When we are ready for the possibility that our client will touch us and get to know us through the physical contact.
- When we have sufficient touch in our personal life, when we are not deprived of touch.
- When we believe that touch is a valuable therapeutic intervention.

When not to touch:

- When we are uncertain, not ready, when we do not want to touch.
- When we are unsure whether we can offer safe touch.
- When we are deprived of or desperately crave loving touch or sexual touch.
- When we are incapable of sufficient self-regulation.
- When the client's boundaries are amorphous or too weak (although skilled and trained body psychotherapists could actually use touch here to support boundaries).
- When there is incongruity between the request (or consent) for touch and the client's nonverbal language.

Exercise: two initial types of touch

(In pairs)

This exercise is suitable for training and workshop contexts, and sometimes for therapy too. The psychotherapist and client decide on a static touch which could be a safe base for exploration—a shared position without movement, such as hand-to-hand or foot-to-foot contact.

1. Both parties centre themselves (please see Chapter Seven for centring skills).
2. The first type of touch is a present touch. Before the therapist touches, she prepares for the intent of contact, as if she says with her touch "I am here" and nothing more. This is neither diagnostic nor supportive touch, neither challenging nor curious—simply declaring and ratifying the therapist's presence. The psychotherapist checks if it is OK to touch and then establishes this touch which says: "Hello, I am here." Both client and therapist notice sensations, thoughts, and feelings.
3. After a moment or two, the therapist lets go and both sides centre themselves.
4. The second type of touch is slightly different from the first one, and attunes to the client. This type of touch says: "Hello, I am here—with you." This touch too is not supportive, diagnostic, or challenging. We declare our wish to meet the other with our touch. The addition rests in relating to the other, and unlike the first type, where we were simply "there", here the therapist attunes to the other with her touch. The therapist checks whether touch is

acceptable, and then establishes this touch which says: "Hello, I am here—with you." Both client and therapist notice sensations, thoughts, and feelings.

5. After a moment or two the therapist lets go and both parties centre themselves again.
6. Share experience, process together, and if appropriate—swap.

Exercise: touch and intention

(In pairs)

This exercise is suitable for training and workshop contexts and sometimes could be used within therapy as well. It helps in establishing skills of intention in touch, which is highly important for psychotherapists who are willing to touch their clients.

1. Client and therapist decide on a static touch which could feel safe enough to explore.
2. Both parties centre themselves.
3. The therapist checks if it is safe to touch and if it establishes touch. This touch will be there for the entire exploration; from now on all changes will reflect the psychotherapist's inner positioning—shifting of intent.
4. The psychotherapist sends his intent to the touch, as if all of him is in the contact. Therapist and client notice sensations, feelings, and thoughts.
5. Without letting go of the physical touch, the therapist withdraws his intent from the touch, gently leaving the client and coming back to himself. Is it possible to withdraw without abandoning? Therapist and client notice sensations, emotions, and feelings.
6. Steps 4–5 could be repeated a number of times to notice differences.
7. Client and therapist share experiences and possibly swap.

Notes

1. Excerpt from *Diary of a Baby* by Daniel Stern (1991). Reprinted by permission of Basic Books.
2. Reprinted from *Playing and Reality* by Donald W. Winnicott copyright © 1971. Used by permission of Basic Books.
3. An earlier version of this vignette was published in *Somatic Psychotherapy Today* (Rolef Ben-Shahar, 2012a).
4. The vignette is part of a paper, co-written with Grace, which was published in *Attachment* (Rolef Ben-Shahar & MacDonald, 2011). I would like to thank Karnac for permission to reprint parts of it here.
5. Previously published in *Somatic Psychotherapy Today* (Rolef Ben-Shahar, 2013b). Reprinted with kind permission. I wish to thank Will Davis for his stimulating dialogue which led to writing this section.

CHAPTER ELEVEN

Gliding on the strings that connect us: resonance in body psychotherapy*

Could my daughter be Chinese?

> The mission ahead of you requires a surrender of the attempts both to be still and to be shaken. We must patiently wait to be caught by the medicine. We cannot take this medicine. The medicine waits to take us.
>
> —*Bradford Keeney* (2007, p. 14)[1]

Last night, as I put my eldest daughter Zohar to bed she asked if we could play the make-believe game. In this game, we should both close our eyes (tightly) and invite the other to join our world of imagination. Throughout the day she had been a bee, buzzing from flower to flower, drinking nectar, and collecting pollen. So, as we lie I ask her to close her eyes and suddenly we are gliding over petals and playing on the flowerbeds, preparing nectar cakes made of roses, daffodils, and hibiscus flowers. These cakes are yummy!

"Can you hold me really tight until I fall asleep?" Zohar asks, and I partly delight in the opportunity to spend some quality time with her, but another part of me wishes to have some time for myself, or be with Tom or Shuy Grace, our baby daughter, whom I have barely seen during the day. "Sure," I tell Zohar and stay. I firmly hold her small body for a few minutes. At first our contact is all that I can feel, and it is the most precious gift I can think of. But then my thoughts take over and I find myself preoccupied with the many things I need and want to do later that night, after Zohar falls asleep, and tomorrow. Between my arms, Zohar irritates

---

*The chapter is partially based on a paper previously published in, and is published here with the kind permission of the *International Body Psychotherapy Journal* (Rolef Ben-Shahar, 2012d).

me, she wriggles and turns—I am waiting for her to fall asleep, but she is annoyingly restless, tossing and moving and not letting go: "I cannot fall asleep like that, daddy," she says. "You are not sleepy at all; your thoughts wake me up." And she is right, of course. I take a deep breath, allowing myself to feel more comfortable, letting my body sink ever so gently into the bed; then I close my eyes and slow down; the things I have to do can wait till tomorrow. Thoughts are still coming and going, this is their nature after all, but they too give way to quietness and slow down their pace. I can feel Zohar's little body softening, her breathing is a bit deeper, as well as my own.

The mind is drifting and floating as the body surrenders, yet I am not fully asleep. Zohar has fallen asleep, smiling, and I can imagine her little bee-wings as she travels from one flower bed to the next and the sense of freedom envelopes me, both soothing and exciting at the same time. And now, the choice is clear—I can either join her, letting go into sleep, or get up.

The capacity to sense the other through our own bodies can sound, as I hope this description does, as a most natural and innate human ability. At the same time, when skilfully honed, it can establish and contribute to highly complex communication processes, ranging from the therapeutic (noticing the unspoken), to the forensic (detecting lies, appraising threat), or even some so-called paranormal phenomena (mind-reading or channelling, for example). Therapeutic resonance can serve as a superb diagnostic tool, allowing us to feel into the relational field, picking up shown yet unspoken fragments of communication. And Zohar, in her highly attuned nature, easily sensed my energetic activity and was unable to sleep.

Moreover, there is another side to resonance. If affective fields indeed open wider selves in which we partake, then surely changes we personally make in ourselves (or rather, in "our side of the field") could contribute to the entire system. The principle according to which a change in a subsystem leads to changing the entirety of a system is a basic premise in systemic thinking (Keeney, 1983). Calming myself down and submitting into the rhythms of sleep affected Zohar and eased her falling asleep. This is an intersubjective crossroads where body psychotherapy, relational psychoanalysis, and shamanism meet.

When cultivated, resonance can prove a highly potent therapeutic intervention. The famous parable of the rainmaker, which Carl Jung allegedly told in every possible seminar (Jung & Douglas, 1931–1935), can nicely demonstrate the value of resonance as a therapeutic intervention. Once upon a time, goes the parable, there was Chinese village suffering a great drought. In their despair, the people of the village sent for the rainmaker, who lived in the farthest corner of China. As we all know, prophets frequently come from afar, or in the words of Jesus: "A prophet is not without honour except in his own country and in his own house" (Matthew 13:57). As the man arrived, the village elders gathered around him pleadingly. "What shall we offer you?" they enquired, yet the rainmaker asked for nothing but a place to rest in solitude. He was promptly provided with a small hut, where he sat and meditated while the entire village people impatiently awaited him outside. Two days and nights he stayed in the hut and the villagers' impatience grew bigger, and on the third day the rain started to come, and the rainmaker left the hut.

Excited and grateful, the village elders gathered around the rainmaker full of awe and curiosity. "How did you bring us the rain?" they asked. "What have you done?" The rainmaker shrugged his shoulders. "I have done nothing," he replied. "Nevertheless," the villagers insisted, "you have brought the rain after so many months of drought." "I don't know anything about that," answered the rainmaker, "but in the village I come from people live according to the ways of the Tao. We maintain the dynamic balance of Tao: people are sad and people are happy; babies are born, and people die; the sun shines and the rain comes. When I first set foot in your village, my stomach was aching; I felt completely off-balance, I couldn't think straight or calm down. It had taken me three whole days to retrieve my inner balance."

Jung's concept of synchronicity describes the interdependency between objective events, both among themselves as well as with the subjective observer. In his preface to Richard Wilhelm's canonical English translation of the *I Ching*, the Chinese Book of Changes, Jung (1949) wrote:

> The ancient Chinese mind contemplates the cosmos in a way comparable to that of the modern physicist, who cannot deny that his model of the world is a decidedly psychophysical structure. The microphysical event includes the observer just as much as the reality underlying the I Ching comprises subjective, i.e., psychic conditions in the totality of the momentary situation. Just as causality describes the sequence of events, so synchronicity to the Chinese mind deals with the coincidence of events. (p. 6)

The traditional Chinese perception of interconnectivity seems to fit the relational understanding of self, which was expanded on in Chapter Five. Adopting such a point-of-view will allow us to relate to resonance as an organic and natural phenomenon. Could synchronicity be a more appropriate logical construct to explain resonance than causal attempts?

Elle and the quest for a selfobject

I felt nauseated even before Elle stepped into the clinic room. Coming downstairs to meet her in the waiting room, we greeted each other and I walked upstairs, Elle following behind. I was extremely preoccupied and self-conscious about my weight and body, and felt threatened by her scrutinising glance as I climbed the stairs. I tried to walk as quickly as I could to prevent Elle from concentrating on my body; I wanted to hide. We sat in our chairs and a good proportion of my attention, throughout the session, strayed from what Elle was bringing and was instead directed at my body: I felt fat, ugly, and awkward. While these feelings are not completely foreign to me, their magnitude and timing felt too peculiar to simply ignore.

During our second session, I attempted to trust my instincts and asked Elle whether she was bulimic. She shook her head vigorously: "No, I just hate my body and hate being fat, but I don't throw up." When I asked her again, six weeks later, Elle responded with the same answer, but this time she was angry at me: "You're talking about building trust," she said, "but you don't believe me." In hindsight, I can recognise that my questions were premature. Elle was referred to me by a colleague whom I thought very highly of and whom I wanted to impress. Moreover, I just wanted to rid myself of these horrid sensations and feelings and hand these over to Elle (after all, they were "hers"). I felt embarrassed and ashamed of my body, and wanted her to take it away from me; to assume responsibility over her feelings and liberate me from my own intolerable feelings. I spent a long time being (internally) angry with her for not taking responsibility for her feelings and difficulties.

Elle was a stunning thirty-year-old woman, and during the initial stages of therapy, regardless of what she spoke about, I felt that everything went smoothly and easily for her in her life. During the first two months of therapy, and although Elle was clearly very distressed, my main feelings towards her were envy, jealousy, and resentment. I wanted to have what she had, I wanted to be more like her; and for the life of me I could not understand what such a beautiful, charming, and intelligent woman had anything to be sad about. In fact, I felt irritated at her "insistence" to remain unhappy and her difficulty made me angry: how spoiled and ungrateful could she be! Elle was financially stable. She studied something she was very passionate about and was doing brilliantly at. She had a loving boyfriend who was ten years older than her, and Elle said he was "everything my mother would have liked in my husband to be". During the first year of therapy we discovered that her mother, whom Elle first considered as "my best friend, my soul mate, my true twin sister", always used Elle to regulate her own unstable emotional life. Elle was the one expected to comfort her mother from a very early age, to perform perfectly in order "to make mum happy", to fulfil the spoken expectations and moreover to guess and deliver home the expected goods of mum's implicit and unspoken expectations, lest her mother would slip, yet again, down her depressive slopes.

Elle therefore never attained appropriate differentiation from her mother; she continued to exist as a partial-system, unable to self-regulate, too frightened to leave mother behind. Unsurprisingly, time and again Elle entered relationships where she felt disconnected and distanced, feeling betrayed and lonely. In this context, Israeli psychologist Eytan Bachar (2001) explored bulimia through the lenses of self-psychology in terms of the difficulty to occupy space. Bachar claimed that the role-reversal, commonly observed between the bulimic client and her attachment figures (primarily her mother), represented a parental tendency to excessively use the child as selfobject. Interestingly, during the early stages of psychotherapy with Elle, I found myself doing the same and using Elle. For example, my insistent questions regarding her bulimia were directed at regulating my own needs. The empathic failure I experienced with Elle was similar to that of her mother, and this powerful and complex transferential dynamic was, as my supervisor helped me to realise, an expected re-enactment of Elle's attachment dynamics.

With the help of my supervisor and my own psychotherapy, I realised that in order to help Elle I had to survive myself, to regulate myself in her presence. For many weeks, as soon as Elle entered the room I would feel "bombarded" with physical discomfort, self-loathing internal dialogues, an urge to cover myself or hide, and debilitating nausea. Going back to basics, I kept practising conscious breathing techniques (G. Hendricks, 1995) and a lot of inner-child work. This practice, influenced by the work of Silke Ziehl, was a type of self-hypnosis where I directed kind attention to my younger self-states, relating to them as holding precious transferential potential, as well as assisting me in processing some unresolved personal issues. Gradually, I felt a little bit more stable in Elle's company, and the need to push her into speaking about her difficulty and admit her negative feelings subsided. Her suffering and distress became more apparent to me, and it was relieving to feel my therapeutic empathy returning and therapeutic positioning regained. About that time, Elle admitted to having been bulimic for the last five years: "It's just that your questions seemed invasive at first. I didn't even know you," she said.

When I was blindly drowning in the countertransference dynamics, I was too deeply ashamed to share any of my processes with Elle; but self-disclosure at that stage would have been easily understood by her (and rightfully so) as being used, again. It was only when I was able to self-regulate more successfully and recognise my maternal countertransference, that sharing my countertransference and resonance with her became valuable. When the mother (or therapist) was able to acknowledge her (my) needs and sufficiently differentiate herself from her daughter, Elle stood a chance of acknowledging her needs and take her own space. As psychoanalysts Arnold Rachman and Velleda Ceccoli (1996) argued, therapist self-disclosure should occur within the context of empathic attunement and responsiveness, and in the psychotherapeutic process with Elle, it accompanied the growing differentiation, as well as connection, between us.

It took two further years of therapy for Elle to stop her bingeing and purging behaviour. During these two years, a significant part of our therapeutic work was my own regulation of the invasive resonance (or somatic countertransference) I experienced in her company. Slowly I learned to tolerate and even like my body with her, and it felt as if we were both recovering from a prolonged and painful addictive process. Elle stopped speaking with her mother a few times a day and was even willing for her mother to suffer without her feeling directly responsible for "making her better". The changes manifested in many facets of Elle's life—as well as within the therapeutic space. While the beginning of our therapeutic work was characterised with a lot of physical holding (like a baby), during the last year we spent most of our sessions facing each other. Touch was no longer *necessary* for Elle, but instead became a possibility that was gauged according to the wish and need, and to our shared unravelling dialogue.

In the beginning of this chapter I described Zohar's bedtime rituals. These two processes—with Zohar and Elle—share a contextual resemblance, even though the content was very different. With both Zohar and Elle—my attempts to "do something to" them miserably failed. With both I had to closely monitor my narcissistic needs and attend to these myself before attempting to attend to Zohar and Elle and respectively support them. Perhaps the rainmaker was right, and retrieving our own balance, inasmuch as we were part of the village, was the best that we could do?

Relational psychoanalyst Susie Orbach (2003b) wrote: "Our patients are already using our bodies just as they use our psyches" (p. 31). But could we consciously and electively present our bodies to our clients? The therapeutic work with Elle continued for three more years, and resonance experiences continued to be central to our work, even though the magnitude of resonance decreased. It was as if the relational field slowed down; our wider mind (or intersubjective self) held us close together, encouraging us both to be apart from one another, and a part of each other, and both at the same time.

Non-cerebral consciousness: sensing the field

> The brain is the seat of the ideal consciousness. And ideal consciousness is only the dead end of consciousness, the spun silk. The vast bulk of consciousness is non-cerebral. It is the sap of our life, of all life.
>
> —D. H. Lawrence (1928, p. 47)

That a great deal of communication between people occurs nonverbally is both common sense and broadly agreed upon (e.g., Benjamin, 2000; Klein, 1960; Knoblauch, 2000; Ramberg, 2006; S. Shapiro, 1996). "Considering that words account for as little as 7% of the perceived message," wrote Jungian body psychotherapist Gottfried Heuer (2005), "a cure exclusively relying on talking is an impossible endeavour indeed" (p. 108).

Resonance is a central therapeutic skill in body psychotherapy and constitutes a significant aspect of relational work. Resonance, as the term will be used here, describes a primarily nonverbal and affective response to what is happening in the other. It is a conversation taking place in an unmediated fashion between bodies and between unconscious processes; where the experiences of the other move and live through us and are sensed through *our own bodies*. Freud (1915e) was deeply curious about this phenomenon: "It is a very remarkable thing that the unconscious can react upon another, without passing through consciousness," he wrote (p. 126). However, if we recall the arguments of the intersubjective approach (discussed in Chapter Five), which saw the self as primarily dyadic—whereupon the *us* preceded the *I*, then this would be slightly less peculiar (Rolef Ben-Shahar, 2008b).

When a depressed client enters the room and the therapist immediately feels tired and struggles to concentrate, or when we are able to complete the sentence which the other began with an inner, bodily, knowledge that we experience (not simply know about) the other as part of us, we enter resonant fields. A more analytic term for this specific form of resonance is body-countertransference (which was discussed and exemplified in Chapter Nine), noting that our bodies serve as amplifiers of the system (which includes ourselves and the other). Later in this chapter I shall offer some distinctions between somatic countertransference and resonance.

It was Freud (1912e) who recommended that the analyst "must turn his own unconscious like a receptive organ towards the transmitting unconscious of the patient" (p. 115). This opening of our unconscious towards the other is attained through sensory channels—it is a bodily receptivity. Somatic resonance allows us to connect to the shared field in an attuned manner, responding to a showing that is not yet a telling (Schafer, 1992; Turp, 2000). Relational body psychotherapist Ronen Levy (2013) similarly related to the connection between Bion's reverie and resonance, claiming both were transpersonal phenomena requiring surrender to the relationship and willingness to speak this surrender and process it together.

We may perceive resonance as a sociobiological skill, which is necessary for survival, since it allows for communication within systems and between them, like the neural network of a large village, and corresponding to the entrainment theory of the biophysicist James Oschman (2000), which was mentioned in Chapter Seven. When a cheetah approaches a herd of antelopes, it ignites a resonant response: as soon as one antelope senses the predator's presence, a wave of fear passes through the herd almost instantly. An expression from the other (mostly non-conscious, frequently belonging to the autonomic nervous system) is making an impression on us, registering first and foremost through somatic processes. An antelope insisting on maintaining its individualist consciousness, and shutting off interconnected messages, which are communicated resonantly, will probably end up as dinner.

The phenomenon of resonance receives poetic meaning when we consider it a marker of surrender to a greater self, a wider mind. When the personal self expands to partake in a larger, communal self, sensing the other (resonating) ceases to be an interpersonal act, but instead becomes a process taking place within the same system and between its parts. Inasmuch as we partake in this expansive self, this wider mind is within us (Bateson, 1974). Resonance could be considered the epitome of relationality: we are asked to surrender our narcissistic-solipsistic fantasy, namely, letting go of solely holding the self as an independent object which belongs to us (Stolorow & Atwood, 1992).

A basic working premise for therapeutic use of resonance is that as soon as we enter an affective field with another, nothing simply *belongs to us* any more: no thought, feeling, image, no sensation is fully disconnected from the other and the relational field. It is therefore not "the other person's processes", which we sense either. Instead, it means that once we have entered an affect-laden relationship, we partake in a larger system, and are both a part of as well as apart from the other. Whatever event and experience emerges through us and our sensory, emotional, and cognitive systems during the interaction, is also a manifestation of this shared wider mind.

According to traditional shamanic philosophy, assuming otherwise is considered purely illogical: perceiving the individual person as disconnected from her surrounding can seem completely nonsensical to the shaman, since we are primarily seen as a part of the whole (Capra, 1982; Castaneda, 1971; Jung, 1920; Keeney, 2005; Sheldrake, 1987). This worldview will be expanded later on in this chapter.

Even though our resonant sensory experiences are valid and often self-evident, it does not mean that we are able to accurately interpret them. We acquire resonant information inasmuch as we partake in a dyad. Therefore, we cannot successfully and methodically (without feedback) interpret the other, since what we sense is not the personal *other* but the emergent *us*, a dynamic self, which is different from *you* and *I*. For example, if my client speaks of a new relationship she entered and my stomach begins to ache, my bodily response indeed indicates a movement (a dissonance of sorts) in the shared field, but it does not provide me (or us) with a linear causal explanation for the event (e.g., this relationship must be a mistake). Instead, I rather relate to resonant information as a compass for curiosity and wonderment about synchronised contexts. We are seeking connections, rather than cause and effect. I might say for example: "As you were telling me about your new boyfriend, my stomach began to hurt. Does it have any meaning for you?" The client may respond to this with: "Yes! This is just how it feels, it's been so long since I was so excited by somebody; and I have butterflies in my stomach every time we meet, just like I used to when I was a teenager."

Thus, when I enter an affective connection and am washed by thoughts, images, or sensations which emerge in me, I presume these are inevitably relevant to our shared relational field, and that these cannot but be relevant to our dyadic self and should not be disconnected from this intersubjective context. At the same time, however, I relate with suspicion to my interpretations of those resonant experiences, and endeavour to appropriately process them with the client. Could individual events be at all considered as meaningful outside their relational context? Could private experiences and personal thoughts be meaningful and possible when we are in a relationship? Thoughts, sensations, emotions, and memories all belong to the tension between private and public: their very domain changes. The relational dynamic is one of pulsating tensions and dialogues between negotiating systems: a process taking place within us (intrapsychic aspect), between us (interpersonal aspect), and within the system which emerges from our connection (intersubjective aspect) (S. Pizer, 1992). In this regard, the relational self is a transitional phenomenon. That is, a phenomenon belonging to the potential space—between fantasy and reality, between inside and outside, between the intrapsychic space (mine and yours) and our intersubjective connection (ours) (Winnicott, 1971b).

Relational psychoanalyst Steven Knoblauch (1999) described resonant minding, a model of mind where "the analyst continually inquires of herself, 'To what am I attending, and to what am I not attending?'" (p. 44), thus used herself as a source of information about the other, and moreover, the unravelling relationship between the two. The analyst's subjectivity became a significant marker of the dyad, and deciphering the therapeutic engagement therefore necessitated analysing and attending to the analyst's experience.

In her seminal and controversial paper "Love in the Afternoon", psychoanalyst Jody Messler-Davies (1994) shared her erotic countertransference with her patient. "I don't think that there's anything sick and disgusting about the sexual feelings that either of us have had in here," she told her patient (p. 166). Despite her prolific writing, this paper received great attention, both positive and critical, and to an extent shook the psychoanalytic community. Almost twenty years later, relational psychoanalyst Jonathan Slavin (2013) addressed Davies's decision to share her sexual feelings with her patient. He wrote:

> In my view, what Davies did was not a self-disclosure at all. She did not say anything that was not known to her patient. It was there, filling and poisoning the air between them, as it had with his mother … But it was a moment of truth, in the sense that all her work, and the therapy itself, was at stake. When she spoke to her patient, Davies punctured the perverse scenario and made what was undeniable something that could be said, for the first time. The moment of truth was speaking the truth, not disclosing it. (p. 145)

In a similar vein, I would like to suggest that sharing resonance material with clients is mostly not self-disclosure, but instead—as Slavin conceptualised it—moments of truth. When resonance material appears in the therapeutic field it has a felt presence, an event which is enlivened in the field. Sharing it is naming the experience, not disclosing it, and while it is undeniably risky, it also has the potential for therapeutic transformation when appropriately and sensitively conducted.

The psychotherapist's appropriate sharing of resonance experiences is among the most powerful tools in the therapeutic encounter. Traditionally, analysts noted their countertransference reactions and kept them to themselves, or, if sharing, found a way to de-personify the event and minimise the relevance to themselves as subjects. Today, primarily thanks to the relational turn in psychoanalysis, sharing countertransferential material and resonance material sometimes takes a different form—of bringing the therapist's person more into the dyadic relationship (Aron, 1997, 1999; Aron & Starr, 2013; Messler-Davies, 1994; Renik, 1993; Searles, 1979), and of furthermore recognising the therapeutic dyad as the affective, analysable unit.

In fact, we may look at self-disclosure as an intervention which fosters integration (Ziv-Beiman, 2013), perhaps in its essential validation of the resonant context—the multiplicity of client, therapist, and the intersubjective field. The therapist's disclosure of his resonance (or countertransference) could be powerful in mobilising the client's resources, in deepening relational aspects and trust, and in focusing on the undercurrent occurrences in therapy (B. Pizer, 2006; Rachman, 2001). Sharing resonance may further validate and shed light on the client's unspoken experience, and foster a better differentiation between fantasy and true occurrence. Notwithstanding its potential therapeutic use, when prematurely shared or insensitively executed, sharing resonance material may also prove a disruptive force that imposes pace, direction, or otherwise interferes with the client's natural rhythms and the therapeutic process. Clinical decisions regarding the appropriateness of sharing resonance, and the amount of disclosure involved, require a responsible clinical position, experience, and practice (and willingness to get it wrong).

Gliding on the strings that connect us: shamanism

> The rope is the most important thing we know.
>
> —Cgunta I Kace (in Keeney, 2007, p. 62)[2]

The shamanic body of knowledge may express a different terminology to the one characterising body psychotherapy, which was presented thus far, yet it portrays similar phenomena to resonance, and might therefore support our understanding of resonance, particularly in its clinical applications. The shamanic worldview speaks in the language of symbols, magic, energy, and faith—and you are invited to relate to the following section as a metaphoric and symbolic structure.

Shamanism emphasises the unity of all that is alive and the aliveness of nature. Shamans believe they can attain direct contact with the spirit world, but also with other people (Capra, 1982). Through focused attention, the shaman can surrender to oneness with minerals, plants, animals, people, and God—partaking in their identity.

These connections are made possible and conducted through energetic strings or ropes (which were mentioned in Chapter Seven, in the section on *grounding*). These strings, which are independently discussed and mentioned in various shamanic cultures, are connecting agents. There are strings which connect different geographical places (horizontal), strings which connect one person to another and to all living beings, and strings that connect us to other realms of realities (vertical) (Keeney, 2005). These strings are found cross-culturally in many shamanic traditions. For example, the strings have been described in the Bushman shamanic tradition, but are also found in the Polynesian (Hawaiian) religion of Huna, where connection between selves is visualised as a cord, which prayer can activate and vibrate its flow (Boadella, 1988). Don Juan's "men of knowledge", who followed the tradition of the Yaqui shaman Don Juan Matus, are experts in travelling along the fibres, which radiate from their stomachs (Castaneda, 1974; Mindell, 1982). The physical body (form) is understood as secondary to the principle of energetic organisation—connection and relationship, the organisation between forms.

When we surrender to a wider mind, or to the big spirit, explained Don Juan to Carlos Castaneda (1971), we sense the other through those strings which connect us to become one. He elaborated: "Every man is in touch with everything else, not through his hands, though, but through a bunch of long fibres that shoot out from the centre of his abdomen. Those fibres join a man to his surroundings; they keep his balance; they give him stability" (p. 33). One of Freud's major intellectual assets concerned a similar insight: our behaviour was predominately dominated by unconscious pulls and reactions; we kept responding without awareness to pressures and movements which were invisible to us (S. Mitchell, 2005). The shaman described such pressures and influences in terms of vibrating energetic strings.

Since the individual in shamanic cultures was perceived as woven within the cultural and social contextual lattice, illness too was understood as connected to the sociocultural balance. When a person suffered an illness in her body or mind, she actually expressed a systemic imbalance: it was the village which lost its dynamic balance and she had generously taken upon herself to manifest this imbalance within her. Consequently, it became the responsibility of the entire social-communal structure (the village) to retrieve the balance, not merely the personal responsibility of the "ill" or "diseased" person (Rolef Ben-Shahar, 2013d). Shamans took the shape of the animals and plants they knew to be medicinal (Jung, von Franz, Henderson, Jacobi, & Jaffé, 1964) and were therefore able to administer these medicines from within, through sharing in their psychic identity. Shamanic medicine was therefore a process of re-establishing lost connections between different parts of an individual, between one person and another, and between those two and the lower and upper spiritual realms. The shaman performed a similar act to the rainmaker, expanding and transcending her personal identity, allowing herself to be deeply shaken and destabilised, and making appropriate rituals to regain inner balance. Adopting Bromberg's (1998) notion of multiple self-states for a moment, imagine that the community itself is those multiple self-states, and in its coming together it represents an organism which is kaleidoscopic and multiple in nature.

The shaman glides on the strings which connect us by mobilising the centre of self from the skin-bound individual self to the pulsating field self (wider mind). Could my daughter have done the same when she used me to fall asleep, as described in the beginning of this chapter? The shamanic worldview sits well with attachment theory and relational perspectives. In fact, most people who have experienced a deep sense of empathy and felt an experiential bond with another could probably relate to this description intuitively. I believe that empathy in general, and skilled therapeutic resonance in particular, involves a very similar act, as I shall later demonstrate. To smoothly and effectively glide on the strings we require a highly attuned and calibrated sensory organ, one which can move between the private and the public, between the individual self and the wider mind. Such an organ is bodily in its nature, requiring both body-awareness and embodiment to be appropriately, skilfully, and consciously used in therapy, and in life.

Transference dynamics and resonance

Transference is an unavoidable psychological phenomenon. In short, our early experiences of relating and interacting, particularly those relationships we formed with our attachment figures during the first five years of our lives, seriously influence and impact the way in which we relate to (and with) others as adults. Our early relationships provide us with lenses through which we look at later relationships in our lives. Developmental psychologist Inge Bretherton (1992, 1995) developed the concept of "internal working model", which described how internalising attachment figures later shaped the way we ascribed meaning to events and to the world, and the way we responded to the world and others.

Principally, I believe it is impossible for us to relate to others except through those early relational matrices. We use these transferential patterns to show ourselves to the other, in the deepest possible sense. When client and therapist meet, they both bring their biographical lenses and together attempt to relate to one another not merely as actors on the stage of their historical dynamics, but also as here-and-now subjectivities. The polishing of our attachment lenses is the heart of the psychodynamic endeavour: an attempt to retrieve subjectivity. This quest is therefore two-fold, resulting from the tension between our need to use the other as an object (part of our deep need for lenses in the story of our lives)—and our need for the other as an other-than-myself person, where the other is the centre of his or her own universe, a separate subject.

This complex dynamic becomes even more complicated since we are not only bringing our own biographical relationship-matrices (our own lenses), but we also, naturally and unconsciously, respond to the other through her or his life story, re-enacting their historical relational dynamics (and they re-enact ours). These two facets of transference were distinguished as reactive countertransference and responsive countertransference (Racker, 1968).

Reactive transference dynamics is easy to understand. However much we have processed our history with many years of analysis or therapy, we nevertheless bring our past ways of relating into new relationships, including the therapeutic relationship. We therefore tend to, at times, respond to the other (and as therapists, to our clients) through the beliefs, generalisations, limitations, and distortions of our past relating.

For example: Don came into the session uncharacteristically proactive. After many weeks of severe depression, accompanied by suicidal ideation and very little motivation to change, Don sat in the clinic and enthusiastically described different job interviews he had applied for that week. More than focusing on his news, I noted how Don was actively choosing to reintegrate himself in social structures; how he was choosing life again, and it made me smile with gladness. Don continued to speak, but as he spoke he seemed to be losing patience and getting increasingly agitated. "What's going on, Don?" I asked. "Why are you mocking me, Asaf, is it not enough for you?" he replied. "Whenever I make a real effort to do something for myself I am mocked." Don was shocked to hear that I smiled because I enjoyed seeing him so vital and proactive. As his history was interspersed with his parents and family mocking and belittling him, it was easy for Don to interpret my response as belittling.

To exemplify the parallel transference response in the therapist (reactive countertransference) we can look at Roger, with whom I found myself, time and again, frozen and rigid. Every time Roger spoke enthusiastically or wanted to emphasise an important point, he would wave his finger at me. It took me a while to realise that, for me, the waving finger was registered as a threat from my own early childhood. Awaiting punishment, I became quieter and quieter, moving very little to avoid taking too much space. My response was, in turn, perceived by Roger as indifferent, so he amplified his finger-waving motion and spoke louder still. Our two life stories interwove into a paralysing and highly frustrating bond.

Traditional psychoanalysis considered reactive countertransference as an evidence of insufficient processing of the analyst's biographical material. If the analyst continuously failed to avoid reactive countertransference experiencing, he or she would be advised to return to analysis and deepen their personal work. In contrast, relational psychotherapy related to countertransference (including reactive countertransference) not only as inevitable, but also as invaluable and meaningful for the therapeutic process, and holding a genuine therapeutic potential (Loewald, 1986; S. Mitchell, 1998, 2005).

Whereas reactive transference involved our own biographical buttons being "triggered" or activated, responsive transference described a more complicated communication dynamics, which was more interesting to our exploration of resonance. Responsive transference and responsive countertransference describe how we respond to the other person's biographical patterns and become a part of their repeated and re-enacted story; and how the other, on the other hand, returns the same favour. The way I responded to Elle in the vignette presented earlier in this chapter exemplified responsive countertransference: without knowing it, I felt like her mother and responded like her mother. Another simple example could be the tendency to be late for an appointment with the one client you really did not want to be late for, since everybody in her life always forgot her. Projective identification (Klein, 1975) was indeed based on responsive transference dynamics. It meant that, while we submitted and opened into an affective field, we also accepted (not by choice) a role in the other person's continuously repeating and unfolding life story. With introspection and curiosity, we might stand a chance to unravel, understand, and (hopefully) transform these roles.

Even though reactive transference is a highly fascinating phenomenon, at the moment I wish to wonder about the means through which we become actors in someone else's life theatre: what makes responsive transference possible at all? Many theoreticians and clinicians attempted to explain projective identification. Heinz Kohut (1959), for instance, believed that the therapist provided the client with missing functioning, projected on her by the client until the client was able to internalise the therapist's functioning and self-regulate. In other words, the therapist served as selfobject en route to enabling the client to internalise these qualities and attaining sufficient self-regulatory capacities. Wilfred Bion (1989) proposed that the origin of the phenomenon rested in the mother's containment of her baby's negative feelings. However, both clinicians explained *why* projective identification occurred but not *how* such body-to-body and unconscious-to-unconscious communication was possible.

Body psychotherapist Babette Rothschild (Rothschild & Rand, 2006) views projective identification as the psychobiological foundation of empathy. This brings us closer to looking at the mechanisms which enable transference. As I shall later suggest, I believe these mechanisms are based on resonance, or if we use the shamanic metaphor—these mechanisms are based on the strings which connect us.

While transference dynamics is a psychological phenomenon, resonance is a sociobiological one. As social organisms, we are highly sensitive and attuned to our environment. We may, for a moment, adopt a biological terminology and speak of Antonio Damasio's (1994) somatic markers theory, which proposes that emotional experiences begin with a gut feeling which appears as a response to various internal and external stimuli. When we attempt to understand how a client might feel, for instance, we tend to assume her affective and physical gestures, which in return create a gut feeling inside our own body, letting us know her from inside. As Chapter Five illustrated, research into mirror neurons (Gallese, Fadiga, Fogassi, & Rizzolatti, 1996; Preston & de Waal, 2002; Wolf, Gales, Shane, & Shane, 2001) also provides interesting arguments for the physiological nature of empathy, and thus of transference and resonance.

I shall now attempt to present a clear distinction between these three synergetic phenomena: empathy, resonance, and transference. We can begin by recognising the similar characteristics of the three: in all three phenomena, there is a transition (primarily unconscious) of sensations, emotions, images, and thoughts from one person to another. Psychotherapist Robin Balbernie (2007) wrote: "We are inherently 'designed' to have visceral reactions to each other's actions, mishaps and feelings" (p. 309). And indeed, all three phenomena manifest a similar intersubjective movement.

Transferential fields: The concept of resonance, as astutely noted by body psychotherapist Oded Avigdori (2010), is broader than the concept of transference. In transference, an inner conflict concerning *a different past relationship* is projected by the client onto the here-and-now of the therapeutic relationship. Transference and countertransference involve adopting roles of the "historical theatres" of both client and therapist and their interaction. The therapeutic relationship serves as a (hopefully) safe platform for exploring and examining those forces, which pull us towards re-enactment, and thanks to this dyadic scrutiny, a novel dynamics is made possible. Transferential fields therefore represent the unavoidable interaction with our history, and the complex biographical intertwining of therapist and client. That is, the therapist and client, inasmuch as they are human beings partaking in an affect-laden relationship, tell each other about their past in their behaviour, by responding to one another through their own historical and biographical buffers. Time and again, the subjects in the room become blurred due to the powerful forces of their past relating; time and again both parties attempt to disentangle these past relationships and retrieve their subjectivity. Somatic transference and somatic countertransference are the first channels through which transference dynamics occur: transferential emotions, thoughts, images, and ideas all appear later on.

Empathy: In the spirit of Heinz Kohut, Zehava Osterville (1995) defined empathy as "an accurate and specific recognition of the complex subjective point of view of the other, and the ability to express it in such a way that the other feels understood" (p. 58). Kohut himself (1982) related to empathy as vicarious introspection: a process where the listener attempted to find in himself a similar experience to that of the speaker. Here too, we can notice a transition from the depth of an intrapsychic experience to an interpersonal experience. Empathy, however, was not limited to transference of past experiences or past relationships. In a co-written paper, Elad Hadad and I (2012) considered empathy as one of the most powerful therapeutic tools and suggested that:

> Empathy is the basis for human connection in general and the therapeutic act in particular, and is arguably essential for the survival of the human species. [...] When empathy is conscious and mindful, we may be able to translate our humanity and demonstrate it and, therefore, act compassionately. The basis upon which therapeutic intersubjectivity is created, one that permits us to say 'I know that you know that I know' or 'I feel that you feel that I feel' (D. N. Stern, 2004, p. 75), rests upon empathic capabilities. (pp. 55–56)

Resonance: I see resonance as a sociobiological phenomenon expressing the deep interlinks between two organisms who are in physical, emotional, or affective proximity to each other.

When we are in contact with another person, particularly when meaningful intersubjective dimensions open between us, the other moves through us and we share sensations, feelings, and thoughts. The resonance phenomenon illustrates a move from personal sensing to public sensing, and subsequently from our personal body to the intersubjective body. Resonance stems from our deep and primordial familiarity with intersubjectivity—from the fact that the wider mind is where we developed from. Resonance occurs spontaneously within affective fields, but it is also a skill which one can consciously cultivate or narrow. To simplify the concept, we might describe resonance as *the sensory and bodily apparatus of the wider mind*; resonance could be understood as *the communication system of the collective, the intersubjective body*. Resonance takes place when, once in a relationship, a sensation which belongs to the field emerges in us, and we sense it through our intersubjective body: through the place within us that belongs to us and at the same time marks a broader and wider body (the wider mind) to which we belong.

I propose here that both empathy and transference dynamics are made possible through resonance phenomena. To reiterate: the mechanism of resonance allows for empathy and for transference—our dyadic body is expressed in empathy and transference via the dyadic sense apparatus: resonance.

Important theories in brain research and neuroscience attempt to provide explanations for the mechanisms behind empathy and transference; however, when explaining social and psychological phenomena, the biological-causal explanations are insufficient for the psychotherapist. Of course, mirror neurons demonstrate how we express empathy, but are we really resonating and feeling empathy *because of* mirror neurons? Are our unconscious adoptions of another person's postures and the subsequent registration of these postures in our gut *the cause of* empathy? As I hope to have demonstrated in Chapter Five, attempting to explain social phenomena using biological language is based on erroneous use of metaphors (Bateson, 1974; Capra, 2002). However, if we reject the biological explanation as the cause for transference phenomena, how are we then to explain it? How can we justify and explain intersubjective experiences?

Chapter Five illustrated Gregory Bateson's theory of mind, which related to mind not as an object but rather as a process taking place in the field of relating. Therefore, when therapist and client sit together, affectively relating to one another, mind is not merely the two separate individuals but is instead the two people together, their implicit and explicit background, their multifaceted relationship, and the context in which they connect. Within an affect-laden relationship our individual identity is but a partial identity: I am separate, yet I also take place within a broader wider mind.

The strong Western inclination (and need) to maintain the belief that the self (and therefore the mind) is a personal object—that our thoughts, feelings, and sensations are ours, and ours alone—is understandable. During the process of identity-formation and organisation, it would have been too big a challenge (and a frightening one as well) to tolerate the paradox that the self was both a personal, and at the same time an interpersonal process. If we truly choose to adopt the relational (or shamanic and Jungian) perspective, then intersubjective phenomena, including resonance, become the clearest example of communication. *We resonate because we are a part of an organic system, and the nature of organic systems is to communicate*; it is what they do! We resonate through our whole bodymind—our nervous system, our affective system, and our energetic system: we glide on the strings because this is what we are made of and what we are made for. As argued in Chapter Five, resonance is an emergent phenomenon; hence biological explanations belonging to the biology of the separated body, even if these are useful, aesthetic, and successful metaphors, they still miss and limit the logical level and the broad horizons of the wider mind.

To summarise, I have claimed here that transference is a psychological phenomenon, which is expressed through the wider sociobiological phenomenon of resonance. Transference dynamics is a form of resonance, but not all resonance is transferential. Personally speaking, I am more comfortable with explaining resonance (and therefore transference phenomena) through the Chinese concept of synchronicity, as offered by Jung (mentioned above), than through causal logic (biological or otherwise); and through the shamanic notion of the strings that connect us, rather than through mirror neurons. But this preference is clearly a matter of personal taste in metaphors.

Resonance protocol

Relational body psychotherapy offers practical ways of cultivating resonance skills. Sensory attentiveness and embodiment, centring and working with somatic countertransference (skills which were described in Chapters Seven and Nine)—all these enable the body psychotherapist to use his or her body as an amplifier, strengthening the capacity to surrender into the intersubjective body and work inside it.

The following suggested protocol is one of many ways of cultivating resonance skills, and was created from numerous resonance workshops for therapists which I had taught in the last ten years. The process described (accompanied by a clinical vignette) is an experiential exercise. Once the skill is better honed, you can develop your own personal resonance style.

1. **Centring and strengthening somatic awareness and embodiment**
   Establishing the separate self and familiarising with our body will allow us to better identify bodily changes when we cease from being separated and partake in the wider, intersubjective body. Without self-awareness, and particularly body awareness, we would struggle to distinguish individual sensations from those belonging to the shared field. The following exercises are useful in strengthening centring, body awareness, and embodiment skill: the embodiment exercise at the end of Chapter One, the tracking down our breathing exercise at the end of Chapter Two, and the grounding and centring exercises in Chapter Seven.

   For example: before Lexie arrives in therapy I take some time to compose and centre myself. As I breathe deeply, I notice some contracting in my diaphragm and pleasant sensations in my lower back. My thoughts are active and I sense readiness in my body without much stress.
2. **Opening to a wider mind**
   Before inviting our clients to submit to connection and therapy, we are called to demonstrate and role model both attention towards and attunement into the creation of a wider field of connection, the surrender into a wider mind. In fact, this stage involves an expansion of identity into an intersubjective self. To use shamanic terminology, we begin to glide on the strings. Skills of working with alternative states of consciousness and trance, particularly

dyadic states of consciousness (Tronick, 2004), energetic work, and unmediated bodily connection (such as touch) increase the probability of creating a wider mind. This notion could help us understand the words of psychoanalyst Michael Diamond (1984), who presented the hypnotic relationship as a combination of Winnicott's (1958a) "alone in the presence of the other", which was a balancing act between individuality and sharing, and Martin Buber's (1958) "I–thou", which presented a spiritual stance of unity. Similarly, psychoanalyst Jessica Benjamin (2006) described the intersubjective encounter as a "dyadic dance that is mutual and co-created though not symmetrical" (p. 387).

The exercise suggested at the end of Chapter Five is appropriate for cultivating skills for opening to wider mind.

Lexie enters the clinic, she sits and starts talking. I listen to her, but at the same time notice that the rhythms of our respective breaths slows down. I allow my eyes to become softly focused, a type of reverie, and I open to peripheral vision. In myself, I imagine the bubble that is wrapping us both. Our physical proximity becomes more easily sensed and I can feel my own centre moving from my own body to the space between us.

3. **Resonance—inner searches and tracking changes**
Once we open to the intersubjective body we are in fact called to introspect while looking for changes. I ask myself: "Now that I am in an affective relationship with you, how did I change? What sensations, emotions, images, and thoughts emerge in me now?" My working premise is that whatever experience we have from the moment we entered a relationship (and sometimes before) is relevant to the therapeutic dyad. To cultivate this skill, I propose staying with body sensations to begin with: how are these different now to the way I experienced my body earlier, when I focused on my separateness? Some exercises for sharpening resonance skills are offered at the end of this chapter.

Lexie is speaking about her previous week and a painful telephone conversation with her mother. I notice my tense diaphragm, and remember it was there before. A dull pain begins to pound behind my eyes, mainly behind my left eye. The pain makes it more difficult to concentrate. At first, I disregard it, considering it irrelevant to our conversation, yet it keeps grabbing my attention.

4. **Reflection and mindful disclosure**
At this stage the therapist shares his resonant experiences with his client, in a monitored fashion and appropriately to the therapeutic stage, the client, and his own clinical style. I strongly suggest avoiding therapeutic interpretations of the nature of experience, and instead sharing unprocessed feelings or sensations, without an accompanied psychological explanation. The observation and resonance exercise at the end of this chapter can help cultivate skills of process-sharing (sharing sensory-based countertransference).

I address Lexie, saying: "You know, as soon as you started speaking about this phone conversation I notice a dull pain behind my left eye. Does it have any meaning for you?"

5. **Feedback and recalibration**
Assuming that resonance experiences belong to the intersubjective body, then the therapeutic conversation which accompanies them (self-disclosure) is an attempt to bridge and integrate between the wider mind and the individual selves included within it. When the therapist makes a conscious choice to share material which is not fully processed with the client, she

does so with the aim of co-processing the emergent experiences and calibrating resonance. This stage is not accompanied by an exercise because working with feedback and calibrating involves psychotherapeutic dialogical skills, not resonance skills. Additionally, these skills depend on emergent material and are hard to procedurally create.

Lexie replies: "It is interesting, because in the last couple of months I developed a migraine every time I spoke with my mum on the phone, and then her voice sounded far too loud but I wouldn't hang up, it's as if I needed to stay and check how much of her I can take." My own headache subsides. "How curious, Lexie, for me this headache felt like extreme neediness." Lexie smiles, "It doesn't feel like that for me, Asaf. I actually feel angry with her and her lack of sensitivity to me—so yes, of course there is also neediness there, but this is not the main component for me."

6. **Coming home—centring, strengthening somatic awareness and separated embodiment** Following the dyadic intervention, the therapist "withdraws" to her separate self, once more by practising embodiment, centring, or grounding and cultivating her body awareness. To resonate well we need a pulsating movement: between the distinguished self and the intersubjective us.

   I ask Lexie to take a moment to myself, and breathe. Inside me, I pull back from Lexie and breathe. I remember my separate self—I centre, and in my mind's eye I call upon some personal memories and significant relationships. I feel my own hands—this is me, this is my body. Once more, I open my eyes towards Lexie. "You've come back to me," she says. "I am back," I reply.

Exercises for establishing and developing resonance skills

Exercise: co-listening: presence without intervention

(In pairs)

This is a preliminary exercise preparing for work with resonance. It helps partners to focus on their bodily listening and waiting. It is particularly suitable for workshops or training settings, but can also be applied in couple therapy.

1. Establish a static touch, without movement, which could be safe for both parties—for example, hands touching each other, or foot touching a foot. We use touch with the premise that body-to-body communication can help foster and accelerate the creation of wider mind.
2. Both partners close their eyes and centre themselves.
3. The first person speaks for about five minutes about a meaningful emotional experience (of any kind), which she is comfortable enough sharing with her partner. The other listens with dual focus: both to the words of her partner and to what is taking place inside her own body. The listener offers only her presence, without commenting or validating, no physical gestures or changing the touch: she is just there, with the other, noticing the ease or difficulty in being without doing.
4. After five minutes thank one another and swap roles—without sharing. I suggest that the exercise is done without any sharing regarding the spoken content. It is an exercise aimed

at developing bodily and conscious awakening to the way our bodies respond to another person.

Exercise: observing and resonating

(In pairs)

This exercise too is a preliminary process for focusing on sensations and minding the gap between observation and judgment and interpretation. The process is appropriate for training or workshop setting and, with minor adjustments, to therapy as well. It is an adaptation of a process I have learned from Silke Ziehl.

1. Sit in front of each other. For three or four minutes the first person reports sensory observations, while avoiding interpretations (it is not as easy as it sounds). I suggest using the following ritualistic form: "I notice X" or "I see Y". For example: "I notice that your lips are moving outwards and up" (instead of "I notice that you are happy").
2. Change roles.
3. Repeat the exercise, only this time—after the observation share your resonance—please note, this is not about the other but instead about sharing of your inner events: sensations, feelings, thoughts. What happens inside you when you notice the reported observation? I suggest using the following formula: "When I notice X in you, I notice Y in me." For example: "When I notice that your eyes are shutting down, I feel ashamed for boring you." This is an opportunity to extract our interpretive thinking, fantasies, and beliefs and assist in clarifying and distinguishing resonant material. Once more, allow three or four minutes for each round.
4. Swap over, and then share and process together.

Exercise: bla bla bla

(In pairs)

This is a classic resonance process, which I frequently use in my training and sometimes, if less often, in therapy as well.

1. Sit next to each other and centre yourself.
2. The client thinks of an affective/emotional experience (on a scale of one to ten, please avoid feelings lower than five and higher than seven)—happy, sad, painful, excited, or angry. The type of feeling is not so important but the presence of affect is. Choose an experience you could speak about for ten minutes.
3. The client speaks about his experience to the therapist, but instead of speaking in English, he speaks gibberish. I propose using the simple formula of "bla bla bla" to save you from thinking and focusing on this. For the process to work, the client enters the experience and speaks from within it (with feelings …). It might be funny or awkward to begin with, but after a short while it becomes clear and simple.

4. For the first two minutes the therapist sits, centred. He opens to sense the wider mind feelings and listens to his own body. Notice sensations, emotions, thoughts, images—assume that whatever is happening to you and inside you, however distracted it might seem, is relevant to the client's dialogue and to your relationship.
5. After about two minutes the therapist begins to speak with the client. The client continues to answer in bla bla, but every few sentences he allows the therapist to respond. The therapist responds by sharing his resonance in words. This is not an exercise in mind-reading or successful guessing. You are not examined here but instead invited to be honest. This part should take between five and eight minutes.

   For example, resonance sentences which the therapist could say:

   - "When I heard that last part, I found it difficult to focus, my thoughts kept wandering to dinner and I needed to make a real effort to reconnect."
   - "You speak and I feel that the earth swallows me and I become a shy little boy."
   - "I suddenly feel very close to you."
   - "I am so angry with my mother when I listen to you."

6. In both parts, the client need not relate directly to the therapist's resonance. He or she may continue their conversation as it were. However, accurate resonating will help the client in going deeper into the relational field and will be felt by both parties.
7. After about ten minutes, the gibberish conversation stops and the client may share his experiences: when did it feel accurate?, what was interesting?, etc.
8. If you wish, you may now do another round of resonance (the feedback round serving to calibrating resonance skills).
9. Swap, share, and process together.

Summary

> The Good Walkers are those who "step out" in altered states of consciousness to "fight for the fertility of the field."
>
> —Stephen Karcher (2007, p. 208)[3]

During a course I taught on resonance, musician and body psychotherapist Roy Friedman (2013) joined in to give a lecture about music and resonance, which we then connected to psychotherapy. The following paragraphs are excerpts of his talk.

> The field of music and acoustics can be used to nicely demonstrate the concept of resonance. One of the ways of getting the string of a musical instrument to vibrate (obviously, besides plucking or hitting it) is to play, in close proximity, a note whose frequency (what we conceive as "pitch") is similar or close to that of the string itself. For instance—if we bring our mouth close to the strings of a piano (while pressing the right pedal, thus allowing the strings to move freely), and sing a single note, we will hear the note we sung being "played back" to us. Although this may sound at first like an echo, it is in fact resonance, which is an entirely

> different phenomenon. What we hear is not our own voice reflected to us (what we know as "echo", or reverberation).
>
> In fact, our voice will have caused the strings whose frequencies are similar (or close) to the frequency we just sung to vibrate. We will notice that while the strings whose pitch is closest to the pitch we sung will sound the strongest, many other strings will vibrate too. This has to do with the series of overtones that every note has, and the balance between them (what we perceive as "timbre," or "tone"). The mathematics of overtones (first explored by Pythagoras) would be too complex to get into here, but the acoustic effect is beautiful—not only will we hear the note we sung being played back to us, it will also sound surprisingly like our own voice, and not like a piano—this is the result of the overtones in our own voice resonating with different strings (and their overtones) of the piano.
>
> Some musical instruments (like the sitar) have a set of strings which are not meant to be played at all—they are only there to resonate ("sympathetic strings"). The musician does not play those strings directly, but their resonating with the strings that are played creates the rich and unique sound of the instrument. The sitar player will tune the sympathetic strings according to the scale (or "*raga*") they are playing, to maximise the effect.
>
> We can notice this acoustic phenomenon even when "normal" objects, which are not musical instruments, are concerned. Most of us are familiar with the experience of listening to a song (or a speaker) on the radio, when every so often—when the song or speech reaches a certain frequency—we can suddenly hear the sound of a loose screw, or a glass seems to vibrate; we might in fact hear the noise of any object, which can freely vibrate or move. At that particular moment, the frequency of speech or song was identical (or close enough) to the self-frequency of the vibrating object. A shattering glass during highly pitched singing is an extreme example for the power of resonance.
>
> It is important to note that even on the mechanical level, *the force which is required to activate a string (or any other object) through resonance is significantly lower than the force needed to directly move or activate it* (by strumming or tapping the keyboard, for example).

Two things particularly excited me when listening to Roy Friedman's lecture. First, the simplicity with which acoustics and music related to the fact that each object has a frequency—and that, in certain moments, those frequencies could be tapped into, and continued to impact us and be impacted by us. Second, was the notion that resonance allowed for a much more ecological way of activating a string. It is my belief that, when appropriately used, resonance is a powerful therapeutic skill for doing exactly that: vibrating the song of the intersubjective body. Resonance can accelerate the creation of intersubjectivity and require far less energy, time, and efforts to do so than many other therapeutic methods.

Resonance is an organic and natural phenomenon, yet it is also a skill which could be honed and calibrated. By opening to a wider mind we drop into an expansive sharing space which is bigger than ourselves, a mind that includes us but is not limited to us or excluding the other from us. Resonance is not only an aesthetic and ecological therapeutic practice; it is also a skill which could be supported by, and deeply relevant to psychotherapists from other therapeutic modalities.

The dawn of psychoanalysis was characterised by an attempt to let go of the body and rely on the thinking head, as famously captured in Freud's (1933a) saying: "Where id was, ego shall be" (p. 79). The early days of body psychotherapy were symbolised by an opposite and rebellious declaration—to leave the head behind and open to the body, or, as Fritz Perls (1969), founder of Gestalt therapy wrote: "Lose your mind and come to your senses" (p. 39). Contemporary body psychotherapy is less binary (and greedier): we want it both, and we want more. We attempt to have both, to think deeply, and remain deeply connected to our bodies and senses. And indeed, for skilful practice of resonance we require both the embodied capacity to open to our senses (to tune in to the frequency of the strings), and at the same time, the analytic capacity to name these for ourselves and appropriately use this information therapeutically. When we are able to reconnect with other fields of knowledge, we stand a greater chance at growing and developing as a profession, and as people. No longer is it satisfying to be a disembodied mind or a mindless body.

The manner in which resonance is used in therapy depends on the psychotherapist's orientation. While resonance can offer a deep and often a quick sense of empathetic sharing, it is not about therapeutic fireworks. As Roy Friedman (2013) suggested, resonance requires astute listening to the frequencies of connection. The therapeutic task of naming those surfacing aspects, which are calling for recognition and validation, is a complex clinical practice. Premature disclosure of countertransference can be damaging for the client, the therapeutic process, and the therapist, who is also exposed in this disclosure.

How can we open and speak of that which has not yet been opened and spoken of without hastening the process prematurely? How can we do so without shaming the other person, or dangerously exposing ourselves? Relational psychotherapist Sharon Ziv-Beiman (2013) argues that self-disclosure is a significant integrative tool, required from the unavoidable presence of the therapist's subjectivity. As we saw earlier, Jonathan Slavin (2013) considered these types of sharing "moments of truth", of naming what was already present in the room, and of which both parties implicitly knew. However, I am still struggling to find answers to these questions. Perhaps one aspect of the answer can be found in the ongoing negotiation of and dialogue with these questions.

Surrender to the wider mind, the intersubjective field, allows the therapist great flexibility both diagnostically and in terms of therapeutic interventions. I may regulate aspects within "me" and by so doing impact the therapeutic dyad and (indirectly, by resonance) the client, assist in reducing levels of anxiety or step into unchartered territories together. But the surrender into connection which happens during successful resonance is much more than a potent therapeutic technique—it fosters mutual and unmediated knowing of one another. Our connection allows us to know each other (and ourselves); intersubjectivity is fruitful for both my client and me—but not without risks. When I am able to submit and surrender into this wider mind I may become a better therapist; but I risk the possibility of changing, as a person, in deep, significant, and unexpected ways. Wider mind is an emergent phenomenon and with it, the client and therapist are reorganised and recreated.

Dalia, a talented sculptress, used to bring flowers to therapy. She kept a vase in the clinic and was excited every week to present herself through the flower or flowers she brought. Despite her blossoming creativity, the flowers, which were left in the clinic during the nights, reminded me of the ceremonial flushing of the dead fish in my childhood, and it made me sad. I remember how, at five or six, I used to run every morning to the aquarium in the living room and my heart sank to see the floating fish, which were regally flushed down the drains.

One day, during a significant therapeutic session where Dalia made a crucial and risky life decision, we entered a particularly intimate space. Dalia was anxious and at that moment I could sense the chaotic anxiety in my breathing. "You can see, Asaf," she said, "it's frightening." We both knew that we knew what was happening at that moment. I felt that she felt that I felt her. I soothed my pounding heart with lateral breathing and Dalia relaxed as well: "Thank you."

And then, as if from nowhere, Dalia said: "You don't really like my flowers, do you?" I smiled apologetically. "I find it difficult that they die so quickly, Dalia." It seemed that the space between us became more condensed still when Dalia replied: "But everything dies in the end, the flowers, and the fish, and the birds, and us. You keep telling me that it is worth my while to open my heart and allow relationships space even if these will end one day." I did not need to know how she knew (or whether she did) about my fish. Dalia was right, and I have inadvertently allowed her to get to know me intimately. At that moment the child in me calmed down, felt supported and enlivened. From then onwards I could delight in Dalia's flowers, and moreover I could bring flowers home, a symbolic step which marked a much deeper change in my positioning against death, a reorganisation between my child-state connection to death and my man-state.

In the course of good therapy, the client undergoes transformative processes of growth and self-acceptance, alongside the reorganisation in relation to the suffering and pain she brought into therapy; perhaps the client is more able to maintain connection to herself and others. But for me, good therapy also involves transformation inside me: the client gets under my skin and into my body and heart, and I leave therapy a different person from the one who entered therapy. Few are the long-term therapeutic processes which have not changed me—and almost always the transformative moments occur in wider mind fields, deep within resonance.

Notes

1. Bradford Keeney's epigraph from *Shaking Medicine* (2007) is reprinted here with kind permission of Destiny Books.
2. Bradford Keeney's epigraph from *Shaking Medicine* (2007) is reprinted here by kind permission of Destiny Books.
3. Reprinted by permission of Stephen Karcher and the Carl Jung Institute of Los Angeles.

SUMMARY

The relational matrix—a suggested model*

Three dimensions of relationships and their therapeutic relevance

Every meaningful relationship is a matrix of dimensions. The interplay between these dimensions creates the rich tapestry of human relatedness. This summary is offered here as a possible model for explaining the various levels of relating, particularly as these manifest in psychotherapy. This simple structure may help the reader better orient herself or himself throughout the book.

The first relational dimension is that of utility (or function). We need to acknowledge that every relationship we have fulfils some needs: we want something from the other, be it material or emotional. Our engagement with other people includes a functional, utilitarian side to it.

The second dimension is transferential. It means that as we enter any relationship, we bring the wealth of our previous relating history and style with us, in particular attachment relationships, and the way we have internalised these. Any newness in relating is therefore partially coloured by our previous relating-models (forms).

The third dimension is the humanistic one. In this dimension, notwithstanding the transferential and utility relationships, I suggest that there exists a genuine meeting of people inasmuch as they are people. This meeting takes place beyond the roles and functions, beyond the history and future.

These three levels interact and are not mutually exclusive. Mature intimate relationships exist in a fourth dimension which is created by the dialectic and playful tension between these three fields, a matrix which includes both mutual and unilateral aspects, symmetrical and asymmetrical, utilitarian and humanistic, transferential and transcending transference.

---

*A previous version of this appendix appeared in the *USABP Journal* (Rolef Ben-Shahar, 2012c).

Many distinctions between different therapeutic approaches might be understood through this relational matrix model. The following subsections offer a closer look at these four dimensions as they manifest in psychotherapy, examining the multifaceted nature of relational organisation.

Utility/functional relationships

Whether one assumes a highly biological philosophy like Freud or a humanistic one like Maslow, we need to acknowledge that even though we might have noble and altruistic aspects to our behaviour, we are not all altruistic. To survive we need oxygen, nourishment, and company. As adults, we form deep and meaningful relationships *partly* because we need something from these relationships: we need connection and company; we need to disperse our sense of aloneness, to belong to a social structure to discover ourselves in, to have worth. Each relationship fulfils many functions or utilities for us, serving both to perpetuate our wounds (repetition compulsion) and to provide opportunities for healing. For example, each therapeutic relationship feeds my need to gain love through being at service. The part of me that does not believe that I deserve love unless I give first is potentially cultivated by my professional choice. At the same time, each of these relationships confronts me with myriad unresolved childhood needs, offering me an opportunity to work through these and find "other voices" be it through my own therapy, supervision, or within the therapeutic process with my clients.

In many relationships, the functional aspect is reciprocal. Friendships require a degree of mutuality: both parties *get something* from the relationship. While the child's needs from the parent are usually voiced much louder, parents need the child too. Children provide us with genetic continuation, with an opportunity to become parents, to occupy different social, interpersonal, and personal spaces which we would not have been able to otherwise. Children supply us with a love-object that may allow us to love parts of ourselves in a way we have not been able to before. But even when there is a seeming unilateral functional relationship, a degree of reciprocity is always there. The Buddhist sponsor receives an opportunity to advance his or her consciousness; plumbers get paid for their job; charity volunteers get to feel better about themselves.

When two people enter a relationship, however simple or complex it is, this functional relationship is frequently the first filter of connection, and a field of function opens between the two. This field of the utility/functional relationship is depicted in Figure 2.

This relational field has an intersubjective quality (i.e., it is a third), as it emerges from the function but is not equal to it; it has an "us-ness" quality to it. It would become clearer if we observe the utility field in psychotherapy. The therapeutic relationship is very clearly first and foremost a functional one. Our clients come to see us because they want something from us: they enter therapy because they hurt and they want this hurt to ease; they want us to help them, they want to hurt less or achieve more. Even though the therapeutic relationship may become a central axis for achieving their goals, we rarely seek psychotherapy simply because we want to "connect with the therapist and let this wider self change us".

On a very basic level, the utility relationship is the motivation for seeking therapy and all other relational dimensions are somewhat accountable for this relationship. By the end of therapy, if no shift occurred for the client, if none of her goals (or her orientation towards her goals) has changed, this would not seem like a good outcome. Our clients usually arrive to therapy hurting, and are willing to give us, in return, what we want. Psychotherapy is not a sacred profession; we do want things from our clients too. On the functional level, these are very clear: they pay us. We receive a socially accepted reward for our worth; we are paid for being willing to put our own utility needs aside when we enter a relationship with our clients and primarily attend to their needs. The payment is therefore a compensation for the inequality of the utility relationship, as well as acknowledgement of our expert *service*. We are, on this level, seen as psychological plumbers.

The functional field is an intricate relationship of service, interdependence, mutual needs, and utilitarian gain which develops between the therapist and client. Some relationships centre upon and are almost limited to the functional field. Service relationships, for example, could be an example. When I pay someone to paint my flat, we contract a functional relationship. Not only is our relationship focused on the function, but I may even limit the development of other relational dimensions lest it would obstruct the work. For example, I might leave the house and come back only when the work is done. The language of utility relationship is one of contracts.

The therapeutic contract is often seen as a rigid one. Possibly because so many other dimensions of relationship develop, we ensure and protect our needs and functions very early on: our

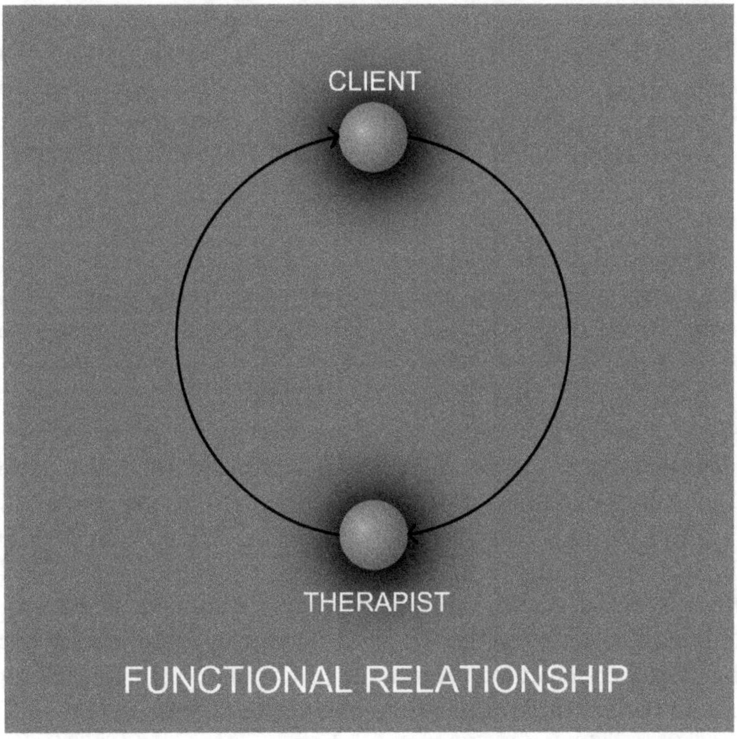

Figure 2. The utility/functional relationship.

meetings are fixed in time, there is a firm cancellation policy in place, and money is frequently paid without real place for negotiation.

The particular nature of the service we are giving (our function) and the exchange rate (money for help) turns the utility dimension into a power relationship. Both parties fulfil functions for the other, but our primary reward (money) is indirect and a compensation for the lack of reciprocity. Our client's utilities are placed at the centre of the relationship. They need, and we provide. The utility relationship of psychotherapy is clearly asymmetrical, one where both participants partake but unequally contribute to the functional field. The therapist here is mainly a service provider and the client the recipient of service—the customer. Within the utility relationship, the basic question we pose to the client is, "What can I do for you?" (or, to assume a psychotherapeutic jargon, "How can I help?") and the quality of the relationship is measured by our capacity to engage with their answer to this question satisfactorily.

Transferential relationships

Were humans simply machines, the relational complexity would have ended here, in the utility field. A huge web of utilitarian functions and interests would have created a complex enough world of needs and contracts, all driven by explicit and implicit agendas of functions. Thankfully, though, we are not merely machines. As relational psychoanalysis argues, we are first and foremost object-seeking, social creatures whose social needs cannot and should not be simply reduced into animalistic needs and drives. As soon as we enter a relationship, however simple it may be, we (both of us) inevitably position ourselves in the relationship in accordance with our previous relational forms (Boadella, 1992; Pulver, 1963). This projective process, which has been recognised in many shamanic and spiritual practices (Rinpoche, 1998; Ruiz, 1997), not just psychoanalysis, is the essence of *transference dynamics*. Consider Bateson's (1979) description of transference:

> *Transference* is a general phenomenon in human relations. It is a universal characteristic of all interactions between persons because, after all, the shape of what happened between you and me yesterday carries over to shape how we respond today. And shaping is, in principle, a *transference* from past learning. (p. 13)

Everything we know about relationships is with us from the onset of any new connection. We bring our mothers and fathers, siblings and teachers, heartbreaks and expectations. Harry Stack Sullivan (1954) illustrates this thus: "Even though only two people are actually in the room, the number of more or less imaginary people that get themselves involved in this two-group is sometimes really hair-raising" (pp. 8–9).

The psychotherapeutic relationship is from the outset an intimate relationship (we talk about our deepest pains and yearnings) on the one hand, and a very asymmetrical relationship on the other. Add to that the functional dimension of suffering and expecting the therapist to help, and an ideal *petri dish* for transferential dynamics is created, or as Sigmund Freud (1926e) famously noted, "Personal influence is our most powerful dynamic weapon" (p. 224). While all relationships carry transferential dimensions, the therapeutic relationship is special for a few reasons: it tends to create common transferential patterns (parental, authoritarian, erotic) and is moreover structured and characterised by its willingness to name these influences, work with them and do so (hopefully) without shaming. What signifies the therapeutic relationship is not the existence of transferences, but the commitment to work through these consciously. The transferential relationship is illustrated in Figure 3.

In classical psychoanalytic theory (as well as in traditional body psychotherapy), transference was seen as a unilateral event, where "the patient-therapist 'dyad' becomes a stage on which the patient re-enacts formative experiences and reactions, and so brings directly into the interactions between the patient and the therapist the very processes by which his personality developed" (Karle & Boys, 1987, p. 200). It was recognised that the patient transferred past experiences and expectations, primarily of attachment relationships, onto the therapeutic situations and an important goal of therapy was to help the patient disentangle the tainted projections of previous forms (Dozier & Bates, 2004; Klein, 1960). In this one-person psychology model of transference, the analyst was at most responding to the projections of the client.

Questions then started to arise regarding the realistic presentation of this unilateral dimension. Jung, for example, perceived the therapist as deeply and emotionally involved in the therapeutic process (Field, 1996) and Sándor Ferenczi (1930) recognised that the transferential dimension represented a bilateral relational field, where the analyst's personal biography and experiences (transferential history) played out as well in the therapeutic field. Hans Loewald (1986), whose

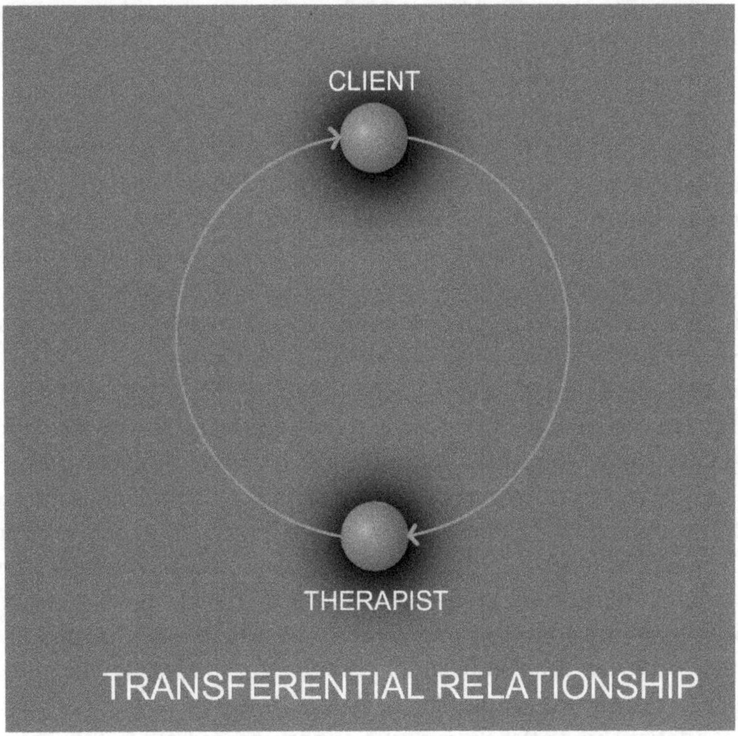

Figure 3. The transferential relationship.

work contributed to the forming of relational theory, exemplified the disenchantment of the therapist's neutrality:

> The resonance between the patient's and the analyst's unconscious underlies any genuine psychoanalytic understanding and forms the point of departure for eventually arriving at verbal interpretations of the material heard or otherwise perceived. The analyst, during that internal journey, in his effort to stay sane and rational is often apt to repress the very transference-countertransference resonances and responses, induced by the patient, that would give him the deepest but also most unsettling understanding of himself and the patient. (p. 283)

Loewald therefore understood the transferential dynamic as a bilateral field. The past histories of both psychotherapist and client affected the current therapeutic relationship, and both parties had to collaborate in order to realise genuine connection from this complicated biographical matrix. This entanglement was not merely verbal, though, it also manifested, and very much so, in the bodily attitudes of both therapist and client towards one another (Orbach, 2004c; Schneck, 1966).

Relational psychoanalysis represents the culmination of what Ferenczi and Loewald began arguing for. Relational psychoanalyst Steven Knoblauch (2000) illustrated it succinctly: "Affects are not *in* the person. An affective field is continuously constructed and shifting *between* persons who *affect each other.*" The psychotherapist's own biography, as it manifests in the therapeutic relationship was now not only seen as inevitable but was further understood as essential for the therapeutic relationship. Stephen Mitchell (2004) succinctly wrote: "There is no way to filter out the analyst's impact on the process" (p. 540).

The disentanglement of transferential dynamics thus became a joint voyage of seeking clarity in the faith of the possibility of, and for the purpose of real connection. Influential psychoanalyst Christopher Bollas (1987), for example, suggested that the analyst must become "lost" within his countertransference "for long periods of time" (p. 203) before the process of identifying, sharing, and disentangling could take place. Bollas encouraged therapists to surrender to flow before inviting their clients to do the same. In fact, as Stephen Mitchell (2005) emphasised, if the patient did not get "under the analyst's skin" (pp. 5–6), then the therapeutic process was limited in scope.

While the transferential dimension is mutual—both parties engage in past and current patterns of relating, like the functional dimension, therapist and client enter the transferential dimension asymmetrically. The distress and dependency which clients bring to psychotherapy mean that most therapeutic relationships also activate attachment forms (i.e., parent–child organisations). Through the transferential dimension, the therapeutic relationship is not an equal partnership and has many qualities of a power relationship. The transferential dimension is informed by and is in tension with the utility dimension. Beginning therapists often get angry that transference phenomena seem to prevent the natural course of treatment, and clients get frustrated that instead of focusing on what they wanted to achieve they seem to be preoccupied with the therapeutic relationship and with the therapist.

Transferential relationships offer therapeutic opportunities both within the particular transference field and outside it. Within the transferential field, the relationship can take many forms. The therapist and client are in essence asking, "Who are we to one another?" We may be father–daughter, mother–child, two lovers, abuser-victim etc.; each dyad is certain to be of deep relevance to both our lives. Awareness of boundaries and of these dynamics can help attain a reparative experience. If the enactment is that of father and son, a better fathering experience may help to reshape the internalised attachment model (Arden, 1993). When a good therapeutic alliance is created in the transferential dimension, a secure attachment can form between therapist and client. Such a relationship was shown to be a reliable predicator for positive therapeutic outcome (Farber, 2008; Holmes, 1996).

The second type of therapeutic opportunity involves a different question, "How did we find ourselves in this relationship?" This question requires a different order of introspection, as it invites both parties to participate in the transferential dynamics yet at the same time observe it from outside and learn from it. We can learn to become aware and recognise the transference dynamics that we operate from, the type of relationships we tend to create, and therefore have a clearer sense of our disposition. With time, we may therefore become less at the mercy of our relational forms. Together, these two psychotherapeutic opportunities provide us with a chance for deconstructing and reorganising our relational patterns.

I–thou relationships

The previous two dimensions presented quite a grim prospect for novelty in interpersonal relationships. We were depicted as flooded by explicit and more so unconscious and implicit interests and agendas which shaped our communication. We operated out of utilitarian calculations all the while doing so without properly seeing the person we were with. All we were able to engage with were mirror images of our previous relationships. Indeed, at times we might feel that Freud's perception of human relations ended here. Should this picture truthfully represent humankind, then all we have left to do is learn and acknowledge our dark, egocentric, and forever calculated relatedness, to destroy our naïvety in favour of open-eyed, if hopeless, realism.

But we are more than that. We are more than our uncultivated drives which, at best, could be sublimated, granting us a noble façade and entry rights into society. We are also capable of deep experiential connections to other persons—connections which transcend utility or transferential dimensions; we are capable of genuinely meeting as people, uniting in our human similarities. Martin Buber (1958) described I–thou relationship as a stance. We could not fully know it or even speak of it without losing this connection. Buber wrote:

> I do not experience the man to whom I say *Thou*. But I take my stand in relation to him, in the sanctity of the primary word. Only when I step out of it do I experience him once more. In the act of experience *Thou* is far away. (p. 9)

This transcendence was transcendence out of utilitarian and transferential dynamics, and was primary and self-validating. It parallels what this work describes as surrender to a wider mind. Within the wider mind, it is meaningless to speak of me and you as separate: "If *Thou* is said, the *I* of the combination *I–Thou* is said along with it" (ibid., p. 3). Buber's relational stance connoted to the third relational dimension—the humanistic (or I–thou) dimension, depicted in Figure 4.

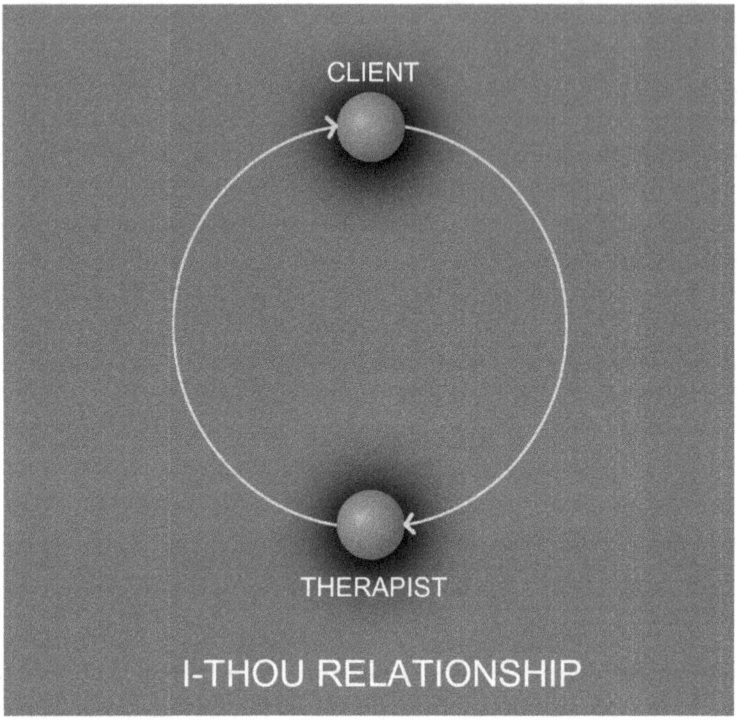

Figure 4. The I–thou relationship.

I take this to be our saving grace: genuine moments of connections occur despite all that was discussed here before. Regardless of our previous history and the involvement of our wounds in choosing our partners, friends, and professional direction; notwithstanding the truth of transferential trances and how tainted our connections are, real meetings of souls do take place in the world.

I–thou dynamics is a magical occurrence indeed. As Erich Fromm (1957) realised: "The desire for interpersonal fusion is the most powerful striving in man" (p. 14), and the momentary I–thou connections present a more hopeful prospect for humanity. The humanistic movement, considered the "third force" in psychology (positioned against psychoanalysis and behaviourism), insisted on the possibility of meeting. Relational body psychotherapist Robert Hilton (2012a) described this emerging relationship: "The therapist and client eventually create an I–thou relationship wherein each is taught and renewed as a whole person by the other" (p. 33).

It is easy to see that the I–thou dimension has a reciprocal symmetry at its heart: this is where we meet as one, regardless of our roles and gender, utility or function, history or age. This is where we meet as two people who share a self. There is something peculiar about I–thou connections in psychotherapy. While the previous two dimensions are asymmetrical and involve power imbalances, I–thou connection is a place of equality and symmetry. Amidst a highly unbalanced relationship, and mostly without intending to do so, a shared human place grows where we are nothing but the same.

In explaining Huna shamanism, Laura Yardley (1990) writes: "The bridge is the heart, the destroyer of the ego. It is the ego that separates the conscious and the unconscious" (p. 99). I–thou meetings are precious occurrences of intersubjectivity. They are effortless and deeply meaningful, mostly taking place in silence and often difficult to speak about even later on. These I–thou moments closely relate to Daniel Stern's (2004) *present moment* and Thomas Ogden's (1994a, 1995) analytic third. What happens in therapy when such a weird and uninvited dimension emerges? Is it totally irrelevant to the therapeutic endeavour? Certainly it challenges the previous two dimensions; but it can also be at service of both the functional and the transferential relationship. Humanistic psychology had put great emphasis on this dimension, believing that those moments of meeting could serve to promote health and humanity. Discussing heart-based ethics, Faith Kaufhold Ray (2001) suggests: "Openheartedness does not mean there is no direction in therapy, but rather that defining and categorising problems must never precede a kind, uncensored human connection" (p. 27).

The therapeutic question we pose in utility relationship is, "What can I do for you?" The positioning is that of a service provider (or at least servitude) and consumer. In transferential relationship we ask, "Who are we to one another, and how did we come to be so?" The positioning is multifaceted: parent–child, siblings, lovers: all the potential dyadic configurations live in such a relationship. Here, at the core of I–thou we declare, "I am here with you" and our declaration serves as an invitation to connect, an invitation with which we demonstrate our equal human longing for connection.

The fourth dimension: the relational matrix

Different therapeutic approaches organise themselves differently along these three described models. In coaching and outcome-oriented psychotherapy, for example, the transferential dimension is rarely addressed and if it does emerge, it is used at the service of the functional relationship. Similarly, I–thou connections may be seen as facilitative for the overall outcome but are not focused upon. Psychoanalysis, psychoanalytic psychotherapy, and psychodynamic approaches, on the other hand, may begin with the functional dimension but as soon as the transferential dimension emerges it becomes the central focus of therapy. The transferential relationship is understood therein as reflecting other areas in the client's life and as the axis for change. Humanistic—and subsequently some body-centred psychotherapies which developed within humanistic psychology (like Kurtz, 2007)—cultivate the I–thou dimension. In some cases, this was done at the expense of acknowledging the complexity of the transferential and utility dimensions of the therapeutic relationship.

The fourth dimension of relatedness is created by the kaleidoscopic multidimensionality of the previous fields, and is one of embracing paradox and withstanding tension (what Lewis Aron (Aron & Starr, 2013) called "undecidables"). I am suggesting that each and every significant human relationship exists in all three dimensions: the functional, the transferential, and the I–thou. The relationships we partake in are both reciprocal and asymmetrical, saturated with transferential projections yet holding potential for true meeting of souls, full of implicit unspoken agendas yet embedding transcendence of ego-centred utility. The tension between these three dimensions creates yet another order of connection: one where contradictory tendencies coexist in dynamic and co-created ways. Martin Buber (1958) described the awakening into relational complexity with one of the most beautiful phrases in modern philosophy: "But a moment comes, and it is near, when the shuddering man looks up and sees both pictures in a flash together. And a deeper shudder seizes him" (p. 72).

The therapeutic relational matrix is depicted in Figure 5 as a field of fields: it is the tension held between the three dimensions of utility, transference, and I–thou dynamics. This matrix includes symmetrical and asymmetrical aspects of relationship which cannot be reduced to either one or the other, transferential dimensions where no real subjectivity exists, alongside humanistic meeting. It is, as Stephen Mitchell (1988) writes, a "*multifaceted relational matrix* which takes into account self-organization, attachment to others ('objects'), interpersonal transactions, and the active role of the analysand in the continual re-creation of his subjective world" (p. 8).

What sustains the uniqueness and efficacy of the therapeutic relationship is the very tension between its dimensions. The relational matrix is an emergent third which connects not only client and therapist but also these various contradictory dimensions of relating. I view the essence of intersubjectivity as the tension between the wider mind and the subjectivities. Consider Thomas Ogden's (1994a) explanation of the analytic third: "The intersubjectivity of the analyst–analysand coexists in dynamic tension with the analyst and the analysand as separate individuals with their own thoughts, feelings, sensations, corporal reality, psychological identity and so on" (p. 4).

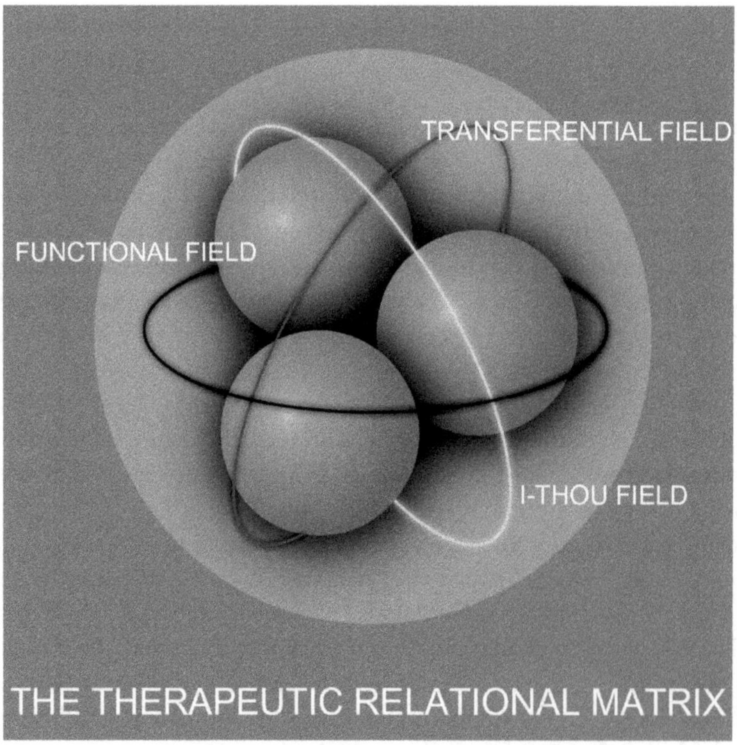

Figure 5. The relational matrix in psychotherapy.

One of the roles of the relational psychotherapist, as argued in this book, is to role-model mindful surrender to the unknown and to intersubjectivity, while communicating it to the client. This is potentially threatening not only to the client but also to the therapist's *person*. Relational psychoanalyst Barbara Pizer (1999) claimed that the analyst's fear of losing control may obstruct the patient's surrender. Relational body psychotherapist Shoshi Asheri (2009) complemented Pizer's stance by naming it the "danger zone" which took place "where both my client and I dare to flirt with a sense of aliveness that starts where habitual ways of relating end" (p. 119).

When the transferential and utility dimensions are positioned in tension with I–thou connection, the latter receives a deeper meaning. No longer is this a symbiotic union, but instead a connection which allows both for unity and individuality. Erich Fromm (1957) noted:

> *Love is an active power in man*; a power which breaks through the walls which separates man from his fellow men ... love makes him overcome isolation and separateness, yet it permits him to be himself, to retain his integrity. In love the paradox occurs that two beings become one and yet remain two. (p. 16)

By adopting the relational matrix of relationship we realise that the multidimensional intricacies of relationship will never fully be deciphered. As psychotherapists, we take upon ourselves to partly feel our way in the darkness of our client's psyche, as well as of our own. In Philip Bromberg's (1996) words, we enter a space "in which incompatible selves, each awake to its own 'truth' can 'dream' the reality of the other without the risk to its own integrity" (p. 519). Owen Renik (1993) suggested that the therapeutic metaphor should change from that of a reflecting mirror to a skier or surfer, "someone who allows himself or herself to be acted upon by powerful forces, knowing that they are to be managed and harnessed, rather than completely controlled" (p. 565). Steven Knoblauch (2011–2012) put forth a similar idea, according to which the analyst navigated emotional fluencies, to maintain rhythmic attunement to the unfolding relationship. These interweaving fields of relatedness form the relational matrix, which is at the heart of this book, of psychotherapy, and of relationships in general.

APPENDIX

The relational approach*

Relational psychoanalysis is a significant movement in contemporary psychoanalytic thinking, which includes a variety of theoretical and clinical schools. I have chosen to briefly review some of the origins of the relational approach due to their centrality to body psychotherapy. Contemporary body psychotherapy is indebted to relational developments. Additionally, the principles of relational body psychotherapy may be integrated in relational practices. Since this book presents relational body psychotherapy and makes use of relational terminology and conceptualisation, some familiarity with basic premises in relational thinking will support the reading of the main arguments in this book.

Introduction

In their brave scrutinising examination of the history of psychoanalysis, Lewis Aron and Karen Starr (2013) pointed to the historically dissociative context in which psychoanalysis was created. Oscillating between binary positions, psychoanalysis defined itself by exclusion, through limiting itself to the selected few (following the Jewish tradition which dominated its creation, and to this day characterises the psychoanalytic movement). Relational psychoanalysis, a current rebellious child in the psychoanalytic arena, wished to challenge some of the dichotomies adopted by orthodox psychoanalysis, while inevitably creating new ones. Like the somatic rhythms of pulsation, form and flow, construction and deconstruction, we were called to examine our oscillating polarities if we were to transcend them, all the while realising that these were also inevitable processes.

---

*Parts of this appendix were previously published in the *USA Body Psychotherapy Journal* (Rolef Ben-Shahar, 2010b).

The orthodox psychoanalytic framework aspired to cultivate an analytic position which refrained from influencing or directing the patient. The analyst was asked to adopt an attitude of an "evenly hovering attention" (Freud, 1912e, p. 111), in order to be a witnessing observer and allow the patient autonomy and self-direction (and, as psychoanalysis was defined against its hypnotic predecessor hypnosis, it was important to differentiate itself from hypnotic influence). This position, as noted by psychoanalytic psychotherapist Nathan Field (1996), also attempted to protect the analyst from the influence of transference which would later become the centre of the psychotherapeutic act, as well as strengthened the illusion that psychological treatment was a methodically organised science, fully comprehensible by cognitive means and capable of accurate operative control. This pseudo-scientific framework was possibly necessary at the dawn of psychoanalysis, since psychoanalysis was born as a science, not an art: an endeavour to create an accurate method for "the dance of connection" between two people, a dance where the rules were clear and the steps were planned.

Years later, Abraham Maslow, one of the founders and leaders of humanistic psychology, would principally argue against the attempt to provide scientific explanations to psychological phenomena (in Keeney, 1983); but at the dusk of nineteenth-century Europe, Freud's endeavours were not in vain: psychoanalysis received gradual support and validation as an established and esteemed professional field, and our unconscious lives became a legitimate arena for scientific and clinical examination. The grave prices we paid for choosing the scientific model included, among other binary splits, the split between body and mind which this book was dedicated to.

The relational approach challenges Freud's assumption that we could (or should) stay with a client without affecting him or be affected by him. It also challenges the Freudian exclusive emphasis on drives, and instead views humans as essentially object-seeking: aspiring to connect with others. People are understood as organisms who are born into connection and emerge from connection, thus require connections as part of our being. Relationalists believe that the self cannot fully exist, let alone be understood, outside relational contexts—independently of others (S. Mitchell, 1993).

Relational psychoanalysis was formed during the 1980s, bringing together different analytic voices which emphasised the importance of real (and imagined and internalised) relationships to our psychological health. According to this approach, the main human motivation was not merely biological, but socio-psychological. Relational psychoanalysis was influenced by post-modern theories, ethnological studies, and feminist approaches, and the concepts of context and emergence were central in it. The first book to present a cohesive relational model was Jay Greenberg and Stephen Mitchell's *Object Relations in Psychoanalytic Theory* (1983).

Greenberg and Mitchell used the term "relationality" to bridge between interpersonal therapeutic traditions, which emphasised the importance of real relationships in the external world, and the British object relations theory, which emphasised internalised relationships. While orthodox psychoanalysis presented the psyche as mainly comprised of animalistic drives and subsequent defences, thus portraying the person as an isolated animal fighting to control and restrain its wild sides so it may be accepted by society, Greenberg and Mitchell presented a transition to seeing the psyche as evolving from patterns of relationships and as existing, a priori, within relationships (S. Mitchell, 2004).

Relational psychoanalysis understood the tension between our internal world, the intrapsychic, with our external relationships (interpersonal), not as two contracting and polarising positions, but instead as complementary aspects of us which defined and created one another—this *and* that rather than this *or* that, both/and rather than either/or (Aron, 2003), which, incidentally, is another dichotomy. We cannot reduce ourselves or explain humanity through one aspect alone: we consist of both intrapsychic and interpersonal processes, the inside and outside, fantastic and real; the self emerges and becomes from the tension between these two fields. The formation of self and formation of object relations are therefore complementary and mutually dependable processes.

The next two sections will briefly review two of the fields from which relational psychoanalysis developed, because of their relevance to body psychotherapy: *attachment theory* and *object relations*. These two fields influenced the central stage relationality attributed to our real (attachment) and internalised (object relations) relationship, and to the dynamics between them. Heinz Kohut's self-psychology, which is also an important influence on relational thinking, is explored throughout the book and I have therefore chosen not to review it here.

Relationality and attachment

> The individual discovers himself within an interpersonal field of interactions in which he has participated long before the dawn of his own self-reflective consciousness. The mind of which he becomes self-aware is constituted by a stream of impulses, fantasies, bodily sensations, which have been patterned through interaction and mutual regulation with caregivers.
>
> —Stephen Mitchell (1993, p. 132)[1]

"Even if viewed from a purely biological point of view," wrote psychoanalysts Margaret Mahler and John McDevitt (1982) "the newborn infant is only a partial system: between the distress signal and the relief of need, there must be a mother" (p. 828). Attachment theory explains our freedom to engage with ourselves and others as largely dependent on the quality of our first relationships, particularly with our primary caregivers.

In contrast to Freud's developmental insights, which were constructed on his (albeit brilliant) philosophical and psychological conceptualisations, attachment theory was not created from deductive clinical thinking but began with infant observation, as the joint work of pioneering psychiatrist and psychoanalyst John Bowlby and psychologist Mary Ainsworth (Bretherton, 1992).

Bowlby (1951, 1965) studied the effect of maternal deprivation on children and noted how a benevolent relationship between the mother (or another significant figure) and child was crucial for the child's survival. Mary Ainsworth and her colleagues carried out elaborate studies through meticulous observation of babies and toddlers with their mothers, and characterised patterns of interactions which she termed "attachment styles" (Ainsworth, Blehar, Waters, & Wall, 1978). Ainsworth noticed that, upon separating from and then later reuniting with the attachment figure, children expressed clear patterns of behaviour: they were either capable of calming down and re-establishing connection with mother (secure attachment), or demonstrated myriad difficulties to re-establish good enough connection (insecure attachment).

Attachment theory provides us with one of the basic and most persistent organisational principles of development, and could deepen our understanding of bodymind character structure, which was presented in Chapter Six: while attachment theory points to the ways in which the quality of the parent–child relationship shapes the child and his relating patterns as an adult, bodymind character structure typology portrays the somatic and psychological organisations which accompany the relational form. These are complementary processes.

In attachment theory, the mother–baby dyad is seen as our primary identity, and is prior to our separate identity; it means that the intersubjective body (mother–baby) precedes the development of the individual body (separated self). In recognition of the primacy of this mother–baby dyad, Winnicott (1952) has famously stated that "There is no such thing as a baby" (p. 99) (without a mother). The wider unit of mother–baby relationship is in fact our first dialogic platform for forming connection, for separating, reconnecting, separating again, and so forth. A relationship which allows for good enough and safe attachment is a fertile playground for flexible identity formation, and therefore can indicate the measure of adaptability in the person's life. Secure attachment relationships provide the child with a solid "us" from which the "I" can emerge without paralysing fear from melting down or breaking apart—a safe ground from which it can leave and explore the world.

Prior to Bowlby, the common analytic perception held that the life of the infant and child was primarily determined by his drives and fantasies, that is—by his inner world. Bowlby insisted on the importance of our concrete early relationship, most significantly the maternal connection, which was a uniquely influential shaping agent of the psyche. In 1951 Bowlby wrote:

> If growth is to proceed smoothly, the tissues must be exposed to the influence of the appropriate organizer at certain critical periods. In the same way, if mental development is to proceed smoothly, it would appear to be necessary for the undifferentiated psyche to be exposed during certain critical periods to the influence of the psychic organizer—the mother. (p. 53)

Based on his empirical research, Bowlby concluded that healthy growth required that: "[T]he infant and young child should experience a warm, intimate, and continuous relationship with its mother (or permanent mother substitute) in which both parties find satisfaction and enjoyment" (ibid., p. 13). Bowlby believed that the role of the primary caregiver was to maintain an attuned and loving relationship with the child, providing the child with a sense of a secure base, a stable environment which met his basic needs and therefore allowed the child to explore the world. The quality, security, and stability of these attachment relationships were therefore deeply related to our emotional and mental health throughout life (Bowlby, 1980). The qualities of this primary relationship were mainly nonverbal, and were reliant on continuous, loving, and supporting touch (Turp, 1999; Winnicott, 1960b).

Influenced by attachment theory, relational psychoanalysis pays great attention to the clients' real connection in their lives (including the social support system), and examines their attachment styles in the past and present. Additionally, the relational willingness to relate to the therapeutic relationship as a connection which bears transferential and attachment facets alongside real and human connectedness was also influenced by attachment theory. We may say that attachment theory provided psychoanalysis with a sufficient theoretical grounding to adopt some principles of humanistic psychology.

Object relations theory

The object relations movement was pioneered during the 1940s and 1950s in the UK. While rooted in Freudian theory, it offered an alternative to Freud's central emphasis on biological drives. The term "object relations" was first coined by psychoanalyst Ronald Fairbairn, and among the important contributors to the field are Melanie Klein, Donald Winnicott, and Harry Guntrip. Instead of the focusing on drives, object relations theory considered the centrality of our relationships with the objects of our drives to the formation of our personality and for psychological health or ill health, positioning our relationships with those internalised objects "at the heart of what it is to be human" (Gomez, 1997, p. 1).

Psychoanalyst Melanie Klein, whose work is considered as the foundation of the object relations movement, believed that we were only able to experience the external world through our inner, subjective world. Ego strength and ego stability resulted from internalisation of good and safe objects (Klein, 1963). In other words, we needed a supportive external reality to internalise it and create a world with which we could maintain a connection. At the same time, we needed an inner psychic world to moderate between us and the other. The human experience was thus understood as the transitional space between inner world and external reality (Winnicott, 1971a)—a stance which was already in opposition to the orthodox Freudian theory. While the latter was conceptualised in biological language, object relations theory acknowledged the emergent qualities of the mind and offered a new, psychological language (Bloom, 2005), which has deeply influenced the way relational psychoanalysis conceptualises itself.

The self in object relations was perceived as a sphere which developed within a context of relationships (e.g., Greenberg & Mitchell, 1983; Sullivan, 1940). Freud's biological and physiological explanations were not completely abandoned but rather placed within social and cultural contexts. According to this view, the cultural, political, and interpersonal environment alongside the biological and somatic were two dimensions which conditioned each other, influenced one another, and together organised the person. In object relations theory, love was no longer simply perceived as the necessary but forced sublimation of sexual drive, but instead viewed as a basic human need for relatedness, which could not and should not be described in drive oriented language (Fromm, 1942).

If the caregivers were unable to tolerate and contain the child, the very organisation of self was shaken and threatened, since we would rather compromise our own integrity and cover our true self with a false self provided that we were accepted to be worthy of love (Winnicott, 1960a). Clients, who arrived with tight, dense, and contracted armouring, as if they have forever tried to look stronger and bigger, could be a good example of this phenomenon. Often, underneath the "I can do it all by myself" muscular organisation (a false self), we might discover a terrified and needy individual who did not trust in his right to need, or in the possibility to be loved with his neediness.

Object relations theory (like Kohut's self-psychology which offered further developments to object relations), placed an emphasis on the importance of internalised object relations, which formed significant portions of the person's inner world. In so doing, it provided a bridge between classical intrapsychic psychoanalytic perceptions and methods which emphasised the importance of our real, external relationship (interpersonal psychotherapy and attachment theory). It is upon this bridge, characterised by tension between inside and outside, between real and internalised connections, our drives and our inner world, that relational psychoanalysis was built and conceptualised.

But what happens to the therapeutic relationship?

While orthodox Freudian psychoanalysis sought to separate the subject of examination (the analysand) from the scientific observer (the analyst), relational psychoanalysis sought to link the two, arguing that the therapeutic relationship is an interactive process—similar to any other worldly relationship (S. Mitchell, 2005). "Therapeutic action requires mutuality," wrote Lewis Aron and Karen Starr (2013). "We can expect our patients to reorganize their identities only if we are open to revising our own" (p. 43). Under the relational paradigm, psychoanalytic interpretation was no longer directed towards the client alone, but was also directed at the therapeutic relationship and therapist herself or himself. As Aron and Starr recommended in the quote above, both parties opened themselves to one another mutually, deconstructing and reconstructing their mutual influence. This is why relational psychoanalysis was also called "two-person psychology" (in comparison with "one-person psychology" which solely focused on the world of the client).

As recommended decades ago by Sándor Ferenczi, a former analysand and student of Freud, who in his innovative approach conceptualised many of the relational arguments (Chapter Two expands the discussion on Ferenczi), the therapist became more active in therapy, and the place of the therapist within the relationship was no longer seen as obsolete but instead viewed as central to the therapeutic process. Appropriate self-disclosure, sharing mutual vulnerability, and focus on the therapist's own responses to the relationship (countertransference) became integral parts of the analytic-relational discourse (Benjamin, 1990). The meaning of mutuality in therapy was not a deconstruction and collapsing of therapeutic frame, but instead human involvement, albeit asymmetrical, in the process.

The relational therapist aspires to empathetically attune to the client, which is heavily reliant on nonverbal sensitivity. Such attunement supports the surrender into and creation of an intersubjective space, within which mutual regulation and mutual influence take place between client and therapist. Furthermore, gradually and appropriately to the stages of therapy, the relational psychotherapist maintains her own subjectivity in the therapeutic relationship, and aims at mutual validation and mutual recognition. It means that the therapist will not be satisfied with simply being an object for projections and transferences, and will endeavour to gradually extract herself—and the client—as two subjectivities: to find the *I–thou*, the *I* and the *thou* within the complex and ceaseless transferential matrix. Our humanity is also expressed in our capacity to maintain connection and identify the other-than-myself and myself as two subjects, both belonging to the intersubjective connectedness and separate from it at the same time.

This is a therapeutic position which converses with the spiritual-moral position of philosopher Emmanuel Levinas (1986), who asks us to recognise the infinite and divine in the face of the other (and therefore in ourselves too).

As a result of the increasing emphasis on the therapist's role in the therapeutic relationship, and on the mutual, authentic, and intimate aspects of the therapeutic interaction, the affective psychotherapeutic practice requires more improvisation, benevolent positioning, and creativity. Stephen Mitchell (2005) described the relational psychoanalytic focus: "The emphasis is now on interaction, enactment, spontaneity, mutuality, and authenticity" (p. ix). As Lewis Aron (Aron, 2013; Aron & Starr, 2013) argued, relationality positions the psychotherapist in a vulnerable place, expecting her to remain open to her own pains without dissociating these from the client, and further, to consider sharing unprocessed (or not fully processed) experiences with her clients, disclosing her own processes, and allowing herself to be deeply affected. Relational psychotherapy and psychoanalysis invites therapists to tread the same uncomfortable territory they invite their clients to walk, and this is an invitation to embark on a brave journey, which is at times risky and often human, vulnerable, and very moving (Ehrenberg, 1992; B. Pizer, 2003).

Interestingly, as relational psychoanalysis was advocating opening within the analytic and therapeutic relationships, it had also allowed for openness and mutual fertilisation with adjacent therapeutic fields, perhaps more than many other psychoanalytic disciplines. Relational psychoanalysis allowed itself to be permeable to humanistic influences, dialogic philosophy, transpersonal influences, and body psychotherapeutic ones, all of which have been explored through relational theoretical and clinical framework.

As expansively discussed in Chapter One, body psychotherapy was quickly exiled from psychoanalytic practice, since it did not fit with orthodox analytic principles. However, in the last three decades, following the popularisation of relational theory and practice in psychoanalysis, body psychotherapy could once more become relevant to the analytic discourse, be nourished by analytic developments, and reciprocate by contributing somatic skills and conceptualisation to the analytic field.

Note

1. Reprinted from *Hope and Dread in Psychoanalysis* by Stephen A. Mitchell copyright © 1993. Used by permission of Basic Books.

GLOSSARY

Affect: A concept relating to the subjective experience of emotional (affective) activation. *Flat affect* means a minimal emotional expression and experience; *full affect*—denotes a rich emotional expression and experience.

Attachment (attachment figures, attachment styles): The concept describes the quality of connection between people, which results from the quality of relationship between the toddler/baby and the main caregiver (usually a parent) in infancy and early childhood. Psychoanalyst John Bowlby discovered that good enough attachment between a baby and his mother was essential and central for psychological well-being later on in the person's life. Attachment figure is the person to whom the baby is attached, and *attachment styles* indicate the different patterns of connection between the child (and later adult) and his attachment figures (which are thereafter repeated with subsequent important, particularly romantic, relationships). These attachment styles were conceptualised by Mary Ainsworth and later expanded by Mary Main: secure attachment, ambivalent (anxious-preoccupied), avoidant (dismissive), disorganised.

Body armour/muscular armour: A term coined by Wilhelm Reich, father of body psychotherapy, describing patterns of chronic muscular tension, which unconsciously developed as a result of (inner and outer) environmental pressures against the child's spontaneous expression of feelings and sensations (e.g., "I mustn't be small, I shall inflate my chest and tense my buttocks"). When the muscles are tensed over a long period of time they become chronically held and organised as *character structure*. Alongside other interventions, body psychotherapy offers ways of directly working (physically as well) with the muscular armour. Chapter Two expands on the concept of muscular armour, and Chapter Six covers character structures.

Bodymind: A basic concept in body psychotherapy relating to the theory of mind in body psychotherapy, and illustrating the understanding of unity between mental, emotional, and somatic processes. Throughout the book I sometimes use the concept *body–mind* and at others *bodymind. Body–mind* denotes the inevitable affinity and complementary relationship between somatic and psychic processes. Body–mind still acknowledges the split between the two, resulting also from the cultural-historical context of Western civilisation (as discussed in Chapter One). On the other hand, *bodymind* signifies functional identity between the two. The choice to use one concept or the other in the book is contextual (when I relate to union I use bodymind; when touching on the split—body–mind). Chapter Five is dedicated to exploring the concept of bodymind.

Bodywork: A generic term for therapeutic methods which use skills of working with touch and movement. Many modalities in body psychotherapy incorporate a variety of bodywork techniques. Bodywork techniques are often used outside psychotherapy.

Catharsis: A central concept in early psychoanalysis, which relates to the discharge of emotional and physical energy (emotional and bodily charge). In some therapeutic modalities catharsis was abhorrently known as abreaction. Within therapy, catharsis may manifest in crying, expression of anger, laughter, bodily shaking, and more. Some body psychotherapy modalities encourage affective discharge, or catharsis. Chapter Seven discusses catharsis in some detail.

Centring: The skill of coming back home to the bodily-emotional centre. Centring is our capacity to connect to our core essence in a generative, calm, and relaxed manner. Chapter Seven explores and expands the discussion on centring.

Charge: The energetic building-up of *affect* in the body. To illustrate charge, think of pent-up anger, with its increasingly visible bodily expression. However, any emotional shade could express charge. This is a central Reichian concept and is expanded on in Chapter Seven.

Character structure: Bodily and emotional patterns representing different and characteristic ways with which we respond to the pressures that accompany our developmental processes. The developmental theory of body psychotherapy, which is explored in Chapter Six, relies on the theoretical concept of character structure and its clinical applications.

Collusion: A concept describing an enactment, where the therapist collaborates with unconscious wishes of the client in ways that may harm or be unhelpful for the client, the therapeutic relationship, or the therapeutic process (this is, of course, a simplification). For instance, an abused client may ask the therapist to "forcefully penetrate" his muscles with bodywork. In this example, the therapist's collusion may perpetuate the client's sense of abuse and retraumatisation.

Conversion: A central concept in the early psychoanalytic thinking, concerning body–mind interactions. Freud described conversion as the transition from an (intolerable) psychic pain to a symptomatic bodily expression. We may therefore say that psychosomatic pain could be an expression of conversion phenomenon.

Countertransference: (also see *transference*). In the therapeutic relationship, the therapist too is impacted and activated by the therapeutic relationship, and the concept of countertransference relates to the therapist's transference towards the client. The therapist's transferential responses could be activated as a response to the client's transference (responsive countertransference) or emerge from the therapist's personal biography (reactive countertransference). Mostly, both elements are present. Unlike orthodox psychoanalysis, which argued that the psychoanalyst needed to arrive as neutral blank slate to analysis, contemporary analytic theory understands that therapists could not (and should not) leave their subjectivity behind, including their biographic injuries and wishes as these were expressed in countertransference. Chapters Seven, Nine, and Eleven expand on different aspects of countertransference.

Dissociation: A psychological (or psychosomatic) phenomenon, whereby part of our experience is severed or split from the entirety of our experience. Dissociation could be normative and benign (e.g., we dissociate from the world when we are absorbed in reading or watching something interesting) and has a valuable survival function. Dissociation is also a defence mechanism (e.g., from traumatic flooding—an example of this could be found in Ruth Ben-Asher's vignette in Chapter Eight). In fact, many of the classical *defence mechanisms* involve a certain level of dissociation. Dissociation can also be part of an extreme reaction to traumatic events and may manifest in dissociative disorders, which are psychiatric conditions, such as dissociative identity disorder (DID, previously called multiple personality disorder). DID is characterised by splits between different aspects of the self, which may not know one another. Psychoanalyst Philip Bromberg claimed that we all manifested a certain degree of dissociation between self-states. He was among the main contributors to making the concept of dissociation central in relational psychoanalysis.

Ego states (self-states): A concept relating to familiar and repeated clusters of body-feeling-thought. These are clusters of experiences which characterise different aspects of ourselves at different times and contexts. For example the "me with my parents" ego state is usually different from "the unwell me" or the "me at work" or the "me with my daughters" self-states. Ego states could be made recognisable during therapy and we might work with these to introduce change. The concept is identified with attachment-based psychotherapy and intersubjective psychoanalysis, as well as systemic therapy, hypnosis, transactional analysis, and ego-state therapy.

Ego strength, ego stability: A Freudian concept which was further developed by ego psychology, describing the person's psychological stability and capacity to face the changing pressures of life. In the clinical setting, the psychotherapist considers her interventions also according to the client's capacities and stability—that is, according to his ego strength.

Embodiment: This concept relates both to the bodily shade of each and every one of our experiences (being in a body—being a body) and to the skill of connecting between our mental, emotional, and somatic dimensions. The concept is explained in Chapter Seven and demonstrated throughout the book in general and particularly in Chapter Eight.

Emergence: The principle of emergence describes a phenomenon of novelty. When certain organic processes reach a high level of complexity, new and novel characteristics which were not previously there emerge from the system (just like a symphony has qualitatively different characteristics, principally different to the notes from which it is comprised). The concept originated in philosophy and mathematics, and is used in this book to illustrate bodymind complexity, which is not merely causal. The principle of emergence is central in relational psychoanalytic approaches, as it points to the qualitative novelty of the space created from intersubjective interaction. The concept is expanded on in Chapter Five.

Emotional regulation (self-regulation, dyadic regulation): The capacity to tolerate and regulate various emotional experiences. *Self-regulation* relates to regulatory skills that the person can do alone. For example: I breathe deeply and calm myself before speaking to an audience. In *dyadic* (or mutual) *regulation*, it is the relationship that regulates the persons within it. For example, the mother kisses her child's knee to soothe the pain of injury. Chapter Seven discusses theoretical aspects of regulation and Chapter Nine exemplifies self- and dyadic regulation.

Empathic failure: A concept developed by Heinz Kohut and self-psychology, describing the failure of the psychotherapist (or parent) to be attentive and fully present to the client (or child), being completely attuned with the client's inner world. A possible clinical expression of empathic failure is the incapacity to feel empathy when the therapist "should have" felt empathic. Another, much more common, expression is when the therapist "doesn't get" the client, thus offering interpretations, interventions, or presence which are not compatible with the client's world and experience and perpetuate a feeling of not being understood or held. It is important to note here that empathic failure is not only inevitable (since we are all humans, even the therapists among us), but also that attachment-based and relational approaches consider empathic failure a crucial process of understanding the client and the therapy, essential for therapeutic (and relationship) progress.

Enactment: A concept describing our tendency to recreate patterns of older relationships in our current connections, by engaging in strong emotional and affective activities. When there is strong emotional intensity, the therapist too is activated (unconsciously), and so an inevitable repetition is created in the therapeutic relationship. Enactments are inescapable in affective relationships, yet early identification of these allows the therapeutic dyad to work in vivo with early patterns of relating in the here-and-now. Due to the impact of enactment on the therapeutic relationship and the therapist's involvement therein, the enactment has become a central concept in relational psychoanalysis.

Energy: This is a commonly used term in body psychotherapy, which began with the Reichian perception of the human being as a psychological-biological system. In Reichian approaches energetic and body appraisal are part of the therapeutic work. Today the clinical use of the term is mostly less biological, and is part metaphor, part concrete portrayal of the emotional-bodily-mental "snapshot" of the client (and therapist). Chapter Seven further discusses the concept of energy in body psychotherapy.

Felt sense: A term coined by the creator of focusing Eugene Gendlin, describing the preverbal sense of a bodily experience. Felt sense is a meta-sensation, a bodily awareness of sensation or feeling, but not a feeling in itself. Felt sense could be used as a compass for familiarising ourselves with ourselves and our behavioural, thinking, emotional, sensory, and relational patterns.

Form and flow: My term for describing the movement between bodymind organisations (like character structure) and the "in betwixt" spaces, where we are called to tolerate the unknown and the not-yet-realised (conditions which could be described as potential, or transitional, spaces). Chapter Four expands on these concepts which are clinically illustrated in Chapter Nine.

Gestalt: The literal meaning of this German word is "a whole pattern" or "a wholesome essence". In the book, the term usually relates to Gestalt therapy, which was developed by Fritz Perls and others in the 1940s. Gestalt therapy shares many theoretical and clinical principles with body psychotherapy, and pays great attention to processes taking place in the here-and-now and to bodily and nonverbal patterns. Gestalt therapy is described in Chapter Three.

Grounding: Is the skill of cultivating bodily and emotional relationship with gravity, our capacity to lean against, connect to the ground, live and act within the concrete and material world. The concept is theoretically explored in Chapter Seven and clinically expanded on in Chapter Eight, particularly in Shai Epstein's vignette.

Humanistic psychology: An important approach in psychology, which developed as an alternative to psychoanalysis on the one hand and behaviourism on the other. Wishing to focus on the human potential and viewing the therapeutic relationship first and foremost as meeting of two equal people, humanistic psychology is often known as the third force in psychology. Following its rejection from psychoanalytic circles, body psychotherapy was adopted and cultivated for many decades by humanistic psychology, and has been extensively influenced by humanistic philosophy.

I–thou, I–it: Martin Buber coined these terms, differentiating between a relationship where I only see the other and relate to the other as an object (I–it), and a relationship which blesses and is centralised upon the human encounter (I–thou), as an ethical and spiritual meeting between two subjectivities, who create one another and reflect their humanity in each other.

Intersubjectivity: A central concept in relational psychoanalysis, which developed also from Thomas Ogden's *psychoanalytic third*. In the clinical context, intersubjectivity describes the creation of a third entity (us) out of the affective therapeutic dialogue. This entity has its unique semi-autonomous characteristics and is in tension with the two subjectivities who created it (therapist and client), and is also a legitimate object of analysis and examination. There is a clinical approach in psychoanalysis, closely related to relational psychoanalysis, which is called the intersubjective approach. It is led, among others, by George Atwood, Robert Stolorow, and Donna Orange. The concept of intersubjectivity is discussed in Chapter Five.

Libido: One of the main concepts in classical psychoanalysis. Freud described libido as the sexual impulse, one of the main driving forces in our lives. Freud's developmental approach rested on the libidinal movement over the course of development and served as the platform from which Wilhelm Reich developed his own theoretical and clinical work. Reich expanded and deepened the libidinal theory, adding somatic elements to it and basing his bodymind character structure on this development of sexual energy.

Mindfulness: A concept describing the conscious drawing of attention inwardly, and outwardly. Mindfulness is a basic skill in many spiritual practices, particularly Buddhist meditation, which involves cultivating the conscious exercise of intention and attention, thus developing an inner (kind) witness, who can observe our experience while we are in it. Mindfulness practice was made popular in the West by Jon Kabat-Zinn who developed his adaptation of mindfulness practice called mindfulness based stress reduction (MBSR).

Mirror neurons: Neurons in the motor cortex, which were activated by proxy observation of another person's activity. Discovered in the 1990s by neuroscientists in Palma, Italy, mirror neurons made significant impact on relational theories and other therapeutic modalities. We may understand mirror neurons as the biological mechanism for *resonance*. You can further read about mirror neurons in Chapter Five.

Narcissism: One of the most complex concepts in psychoanalysis, carrying myriad meanings. In the therapeutic context, the term was developed by Freud following the Greek myth (and tragedy) of Narcissus. The concept points to a certain quality of self-love or self-centredness. According to Freud, narcissism described four phenomena: (1) a narcissistic disorder (and perversion), (2) a healthy and important narcissistic developmental stage, (3) narcissism as libidinal attachment to the ego (hence, I become the object of my love), and (4) narcissism as a kind of object-cathexis or choice (I love others inasmuch as they are a part of me, as long as they are "mine"). During the narcissistic developmental stage, the child perceives his entire world through his own existence. When the child is unable to successfully move on from this stage, it will be difficult for the child to see the needs of the other (or the existence of the other) as separated from his own needs and existence, and may become exploitative, lacking of empathy, self-centred, and sporting an inflated sense of entitlement. Narcissism is characteristic of the third developmental angle, which is expanded on in Chapter Six, where you can further discover how body psychotherapy relates to narcissism.

Object relations: A branch of psychoanalysis, which originated in the work of Melanie Klein, and described the person as object-seeking from infancy—seeking connections with real others and their internalised images. Object relations theory emphasises the importance of both real and internalised relationships for our psychological well-being and health.

Primary processes, secondary processes: According to Freud, primary processes were unconscious processes, experiences which have not been organised or symbolised. These processes also included bodily-affective phenomena which were unprocessed. Secondary processes were more "evolved" cognised processes, which were symbolically and cognitively processed, particularly through language.

Projective identification: A term coined by psychoanalyst Melanie Klein, describing an unconscious process whereby one person projected behaviours/wishes/fears on another person. As a response to the projection, the other person behaved in accordance with the projection thus ratifying for the first person the "truth" in the initial projection. The psychoanalyst Wilfred Bion, who furthered Klein's work, argued that projective identification was an unconscious and difficult-to-identify manipulation, which pulled the therapist into the client's fantasy. For example, a client believed that nobody remembered her and she was certain that her therapist did not remember her name. The therapist, without being conscious of it, began to "forget" important biographical details of this particular client (including the client's name) even if this was out of character for her, nor was it characteristic of her memory in therapy.

Regression: A return to a childlike self-state, either spontaneously or as a result of a therapeutic intervention. In the therapeutic context, in the early conceptualisation of hypnosis and psychoanalysis, Freud (and later Ferenczi) understood therapy as taking place also in regressive fields, and organised the therapeutic act around the parental-regressive transference relationship, which was weaved between client and therapist. Alongside Winnicott and other object relations psychoanalysts who worked with regressive states, regression was also explored and researched in the fields of hypnosis and body psychotherapy. Affective psychotherapy, including bodywork, tended to work with regressive self-states and many body psychotherapy modalities utilised regression techniques in working with clients. While holding great therapeutic potential, working with regression might lead to retraumatisation and requires skill, training, and sound ethical and theoretical grounding.

Resonance: A phenomenon describing the manner in which bodies (or people) can communicate without a cognitive interface. One person's body unconsciously and automatically receives (and is receptive to) changes, emotions, and sensations from another person, particularly when there is an affective relationship between the two. Chapter Eleven expands the clinical use and practice of resonance as a therapeutic skill.

Reverie: Reverie is "a daydream state of mind". The renowned psychoanalyst Wilfred Bion used the term to relate to the parent's (and later the analyst's) capacity to know what is going on inside the infant (or client), by surrendering to the free associations of the client and therapist, effortlessly drifting into the material. It is not a lazy position, but a disciplined practice of being present and letting go. Reverie could be thought of as a therapeutic skill for fostering resonance and the co-creation of intersubjectivity.

Selfobject: A concept from self-psychology and the psychoanalytic thinking of Heinz Kohut, portraying the maternal (and paternal) role at certain developmental stages as containing aspects of the infant which he cannot tolerate and contain for himself just yet. For example, I may feel fear when my daughters cannot fear at all, when feeling this fear might be too threatening for them—I am fearful *on their behalf*. Similarly, the psychotherapist may serve as selfobject for the client in certain stages of therapy.

Shamanism: A generic name for religions, philosophies, or cultures where sorcerers (shamans) use *trance* and other altered states of consciousness to heal and connect between the concrete and tangible and the spiritual dimensions. The philosophical theory of mind in shamanic societies is extremely relevant to the *intersubjective* theory of mind in relational psychoanalysis and contemporary approaches of body psychotherapy, and in particular to the concept of *wider mind*. Chapter Eleven expands on the shamanic worldview and its relevance to body psychotherapy.

Somatic transference: Transference is not merely a psychological phenomenon, but has somatic dimensions too. Somatic transference relates to the bodily aspects of transference. For example, a person who was hit as a child may respond to non-violent communication, which was accompanied by hand-waving, with contracting and physical defence, as if the speaker was about to hit him. Chapter Seven discusses the concept which is later clinically demonstrated in Chapter Nine.

Trance: A state of consciousness characterised by loosening of familiar habitual patterns of doing. In this book I define trance as the flow between familiar organisations of emotions, thoughts, embodied patterns, or relationships—a transitional space of internal and interpersonal organisation. Muscular relaxation, meditation, absorption in a book or film to the extent of ignoring external stimuli, daydreaming, the moments before falling asleep—all these are examples of common trance states. Trance in itself can be both generative (useful, enriching, expanding) and degenerative (limiting, addictive, and potentially abusive)—depending on the relational context (internal and external) within which it is used and the disciplined cultivation of using this tool.

Transference: The way our previous relationships influence the manner in which we attach and relate in the present time. For example, we may relate to our child's teacher with the same dread and apprehension we felt towards our class one authoritarian teacher. All relationships include transferential components; we cannot but relate through the lenses of how we related before. However, the therapeutic relationship is particularly inviting of certain transference patterns, since it is saturated with feelings, expectations, fears, and hopes and due to its inherent asymmetrical nature. Thus, working with transference has been a central axis of the therapeutic act since the dawn of psychoanalysis.

Transitional space/potential space: Different names for the term coined by psychoanalyst Donald Winnicott, which describe the playing area between fantasy and reality, between inside and outside, between intrapsychic and interpersonal. This space is rich with potential for growth and change, and a significant portion of therapy can happen herein. I believe that the *bodymind* is a transitional space.

True self/false self: Terms coined by psychoanalyst Donald Winnicott. True self was the spontaneous and authentic expression of the person which, when given the opportunity, manifested itself in the world. When the person (and child) felt it was unsafe to show herself or himself as they truly were, the true self was covered by the false self, the presented self which was more acceptable and presentable. *Character armour* could be seen as the musculature of the false self, and the therapeutic endeavour included reclaiming the space for the true self in the client's life.

Vegetotherapy: The therapeutic modality developed by Wilhelm Reich, father of modern body psychotherapy. The method is based on working with the autonomic (vegetative) nervous system.

Wider mind: A concept from the work of anthropologist, linguist, and system theoretician Gregory Bateson, describing the creation of *intersubjective* space, where the mind transcends the boundaries of the skin to include myself and the other within it. The concept is expanded on and discussed in Chapter Five.

REFERENCES

Abrams, D. (1996). *The Spell of the Sensuous: Perception and Language in a More Than Human World*. New York: Pantheon.

Aharon, L. (2013). Review of Yoari Sella's lecture: Being real in the world: The schizoid experience and the borderline experience, between mentalisation and embodiment in therapy and training. *Hebrew Psychology*. Retrieved 19 October 2013 from http://www.hebpsy.net/articles.asp?t=0&id=2958.

Ainsworth, M. D. S., Blehar, M. C., Waters, E., & Wall, S. (1978). *Patterns of Attachment: A Psychological Study of the Strange Situation*. Hilllside, NJ: Lawrence Erlbaum.

Anderson, F. S. (2008). At a loss for words and feelings. In: F. S. Anderson (Ed.), *Bodies in Treatment—The Unspoken Dimension* (pp. 1–25). Hove, UK: Analytic Press.

Anzieu, D. (1989). *The Skin Ego*. London: Yale University Press.

Appel-Opper, J. (2010). Intercultural body-oriented psychotherapy: The culture in the body and the body in the culture. *British Journal of Psychotherapy Integration, 7*(2): 13–23.

Arad, G., Askarov, R., Gihon, A., Lieblich, M., & Medina, L. (2013). Panel presentation: Body psychotherapy. (Paper presented at the Multiplicity and Unity in Body Psychotherapy panel discussion at the book launch of *An Anatomy of Therapy—Body Psychotherapy*, Tel Aviv, 25 April.)

Arden, M. (1993). Thoughts on the healing process. *International Forum of Psychoanalysis, 2*: 149–154.

Aron, L. (1991). The patient's experience of the analyst's subjectivity. In: S. A. Mitchell & L. Aron (Eds.), *Relational Psychoanalysis: The Emergence of a Tradition* (pp. 243–268). New York: Analytic Press, 1999.

Aron, L. (1997). Are we to have a meeting of minds?: A reply to the discussions of a meeting of minds. *Psychoanalytic Dialogues, 7*: 885–896.

Aron, L. (1998). Introduction—The body in drive and relational models. In: L. Aron & F. S. Anderson (Eds.), *Relational Perspectives on the Body* (pp. xix–xxviii). Hillsdale, NJ: Analytic Press.

Aron, L. (1999). Clinical choices and the relational matrix. *Psychoanalytic Dialogues, 9*: 1–29.

Aron, L. (2003). Clinical outbursts and theoretical breakthroughs: A unifying theme in the work of Stephen A. Mitchell. *Psychoanalytic Dialogues, 13*: 273–287.

Aron, L. (2013). Monsters, ghosts and the undecidables: Mutual vulnerability. (Paper presented at the conference, Individual and the Group in the Space of Mutual Vulnerability, Tel Aviv.)

Aron, L., & Starr, K. (2013). *A Psychotherapy for the People: Towards a Progressive Psychoanalysis*. Hove, UK: Routledge.

Asheri, S. (2004). Erotic desire in the therapy room. Dare we embody it? Can we afford not to? Paper presented at the 2004 UKCP conference, London. Retrieved 19 October 2013 from http://www.yobeely.f2s.com/articles/eroticdesire.html.

Asheri, S. (2009). To touch or not to touch: A relational body psychotherapy perspective. In: L. Hartley (Ed.), *Contemporary Body Psychotherapy: The Chiron Approach* (pp. 106–120). Hove, UK: Routledge.

Asheri, S., Carroll, R., Rolef Ben-Shahar, A., Soth, M., & Totton, N. (2012). The body in the world, the world in the body. Relational body psychotherapy panel presentation at the 13th International EABP Congress of Body Psychotherapy. Cambridge: Owl Production.

Atwood, G. E., & Stolorow, R. D. (1977). The life and work of Wilhelm Reich: A case study of the subjectivity of personality theory. *Psychoanalytic Review, 64*: 5–20.

Audergon, J. C. (2005). The body in process work. In: N. Totton (Ed.), *New Dimensions in Body Psychotherapy* (pp. 153–167). Maidenhead, UK: Open University Press.

Avigdori, O. (2010). Resonance—the essence of a phenomenon. *Maamarim—The Israeli archive of papers and articles*. Retrieved 19 October 2013 from http://www.mamrim.co.il/index.php?id=art1&idc=966.

Bacal, H. A. (1995). The essence of Kohut's work and the progress of self psychology. *Psychoanalytic Dialogues, 5*: 353–366.

Bachar, E. (2001). *The Fear of Occupying Space: The Self-Psychology and the Treatment of Anorexia and Bulimia*. Jerusalem: Magness.

Baker, E. F. (1967). *Man in the Trap*. New York: Macmillan.

Baker, E. F. (1977). Medical orgonomy. *Journal of Orgonomy, 11*(2): 188–194.

Balbernie, R. (2007). The move to intersubjectivity: A clinical and conceptual shift of perspective. *Journal of Child Psychotherapy, 33*(3): 308–324.

Balint, E., Mitchell, J., & Parsons, M. (1993). *Before I Was I: Psychoanalysis and the Imagination*. London: Free Association.

Balint, M. (1952). *Primary Love and Psycho-Analytic Technique*. London: Tavistock.

Balint, M. (1968). *The Basic Fault. Therapeutic Aspects of Regression*. London: Tavistock.

Balsam, R. M. (2012). *Women's Bodies in Psychoanalysis*. New York: Routledge.

Bandler, R., & Grinder, J. (1979). *Frogs into Princes*. London: Eden Grove.

Bannay, D. (2010). "248 organs"—When the body is entrapped in the mind. (Paper presented at the "And your body is my gaze, my window, my mirror." Body–mind in the psychoanalytic space: the spring conference of the Israeli Association of Psychoanalytic Psychotherapy, Tel Aviv.)

Bányai, É. I. (1998). The interactive nature of hypnosis: Research evidence for a social-psychobiological model. *Contemporary Hypnosis, 15*(1): 52–63.

Bar-Levav, A. (1998). A rationale for physical touching in psychotherapy. In: E. W. L. Smith, P. R. Clance, & S. Imes (Eds.), *Touch in Psychotherapy: Theory, Research, and Practice* (pp. 52–55). New York: Guilford.

Barry, A. M. (2009). Mirror neurons: How we become what we see. *Visual Communication Quarterly, 16*(2): 79–89.

Bateson, G. (1972). *Steps to an Ecology of Mind*. Chicago, IL: University of Chicago Press.

Bateson, G. (1974). Draft: Scattered thoughts for a conference on "broken power". *Coevolutionary Quarterly, 4*: 26–27.

Bateson, G. (1979). *Mind and Nature: A Necessary Unity*. Cresskill, NJ: Hampton Press, 2002.

Baykushev, S. V. (1969). Hyperventilation as an accelerated hypnotic induction technique. *International Journal of Clinical and Experimental Hypnosis, 17*(1): 20–24.

Beauvoir, S. de, & Parshley, H. M. (1949). *The Second Sex*. London: Vintage, 1997.

Beebe, B. (2004). Faces-in-relation: forms of intersubjectivity in adult treatment of early trauma. *Psychoanalytic Dialogues, 14*(1): 1–51.

Beebe , B., & Lachmann, F. (2002). *Infant Research and Adult Treatment: Co-constructing Interactions*. Hillsdale, NJ: Analytic Press.

Benjamin, J. (1990). Recognition and destruction: An outline of intersubjectivity. In: S. A. Mitchell & L. Aron (Eds.), *Relational Psychoanalysis: The Emergence of a Tradition* (pp. 181–210). New York: Analytic Press, 1999.

Benjamin, J. (1995). *Like Subjects, Love Objects*. New Haven, CT: Yale University Press.

Benjamin, J. (2000). Intersubjective distinctions: Subjects and persons, recognitions and breakdowns. Commentary on paper by Gerhardt, Sweetnam, and Borton. *Psychoanalytic Dialogues, 10*: 43–55.

Benjamin, J. (2006). Crash: What we do when we cannot touch. Commentary on paper by Meira Likierman. *Psychoanalytic Dialogues, 16*: 377–385.

Bergmann, S. H. (1974). *The Dialogical Philosophy from Kierkegaard to Buber (Hebrew ed.)*. Jerusalem: Bialik Institute.

Bernheim, H. (1887). *Hypnosis and Suggestion in Psychotherapy*. C. A. Herter (Trans.). New York: University Books, 1965.

Bion, W. R. (1962). *Learning from Experience*. London: Tavistock.

Bion, W. R. (1963). *Elements of Psycho-Analysis*. London: Heinemann.

Bion, W. R. (1989). *Two Papers: The Grid and the Caesura*. London: Karnac.

Blake, W. (1790). The marriage of heaven and hell. In: M. Mason (Ed.), *William Blake: Selected Poetry*. New York: Oxford University Press.

Bloom, K. (2005). Articulating preverbal experience. In: N. Totton (Ed.), *New Dimensions in Body Psychotherapy* (pp. 56–69). Maidenhead, UK: Open University Press.

Boadella, D. (1976). *In the Wake of Reich*. London: Coventure.

Boadella, D. (1985). *Wilhelm Reich—The Evolution of His Work*. London: Arkana.

Boadella, D. (1987). *Lifestreams: An Introduction to Biosynthesis*. London: Routledge & Kegan Paul.

Boadella, D. (1988). *Lifelines and Light Streams (1987 Frank Lake memorial lecture)*. Oxford: Clinical Theology Association.

Boadella, D. (1992). Words, body and transference. In: B. V. Maul (Ed.), *Body Psychotherapy or the Art of Contact* (pp. 9–11). Berlin: European Association for Body Psychotherapy.

Boadella, D. (2011). Psycho-physical synthesis at the foundations of body psychotherapy: The 100-year legacy of Pierre Janet (1859–1947). In: C. Young (Ed.), *The Historical Basis of Body Psychotherapy* (pp. 49–66). Stow, UK: Body Psychotherapy Publications.

Bohm, D. J. (1957). *Causality and Chance in Modern Physics*. London: Routledge & Kegan Paul, 1984.

Bollas, C. (1978). The aesthetic moment and the search for transformation. *The Annual of Psychoanalysis, 6*: 385–394.

Bollas, C. (1987). *The Shadow of the Object*. New York: Columbia University Press.

Bonduelle, M., & Gelfand, T. (1999). Hysteria behind the scenes: Jane Avril at the Salpêtrière. *Journal of the History of the Neurosciences, 7*(1): 35–42.

Borgogno, F. (2004). Why Ferenczi today? The contribution of Sándor Ferenczi to the understanding and healing of psychic suffering. *International Forum of Psychoanalysis, 13*(1): 5–13.

Boroson, M. (1998). Radar to the infinite: Holotropic breathwork and the integral vision. *The Inner Door, 10*(4): 5–6.

Bowlby, J. (1951). *Maternal Care and Mental Health*. Geneva: World Health Organization.

Bowlby, J. (1965). *Child Care and the Growth of Love*. London: Penguin.

Bowlby, J. (1980). *Attachment and Loss, Vol. 3. Loss: Sadness and Desperation*. New York: Basic.

Bowlby, J. (1988). *A Secure Base: Clinical Applications of Attachment Theory*. Abingdon, UK: Routledge.

Boyesen, G. (Ed.). (1980). *Collected Papers on Biodynamic Psychology*. London: Biodynamic Psychology Publications.

Bretherton, I. (1992). The origins of attachment theory: John Bowlby and Mary Ainsworth. *Developmental Psychology, 28*: 759–775.

Bretherton, I. (1995). Attachment theory and developmental psychopathology. In: D. Cicchetti & S. L. Toth (Eds.), *Emotion, Cognition, and Representation. Rochester Symposium on Developmental Psychopathology* (*Vol. 6*) (pp. 231–260). Rochester, NY: University of Rochester Press.

Bromberg, P. M. (1996). Standing in spaces: The multiplicity of self and the psychoanalytic relationship. *Contemporary Psychoanalysis, 32*: 500–535.

Bromberg, P. M. (1998). *Standing in Spaces*. Hillside, NJ: Analytic Press.

Brown, J., & Mowbray, R. (1994). Primal integration. In: D. Jones (Ed.), *Innovative Therapy: A Handbook* (pp. 13–27). Buckingham, UK: Open University Press.

Brown, J., & Mowbray, R. (1996). Primal integration—Deep personal growth work. *London and South East Connection*, December.

Brown, M. (1989). *The Healing Touch: An Introduction to Organismic Psychotherapy*. Mendocino, CA: LifeRhythm.

Buber, M. (1958). *I and Thou*. R. G. Smith (Trans.). New York: Scribner.

Bucci, W. (1994). The multiple code theory and the psychoanalytic process: A framework for research. *The Annual of Psychoanalysis, 22*: 239–259.

Bucci, W. (1998). Beyond symbolizing: A response to Bornstein's review. *Psychoanalytic Psychology, 15*: 576–581.

Bucci, W. (2001). Pathways of emotional communication. *Psychoanalytic Inquiry, 21*: 40–70.

Bucci, W. (2008). The role of bodily experience in emotional organization. In: F. S. Anderson (Ed.), *Bodies in Treatment—The Unspoken Dimension* (pp. 51–76). Hove, UK: Analytic Press.

Bucci, W. (2011). The interplay of subsymbolic and symbolic processes in psychoanalytic treatment: It takes two to tango—but who knows the steps, who's the leader? The choreography of the psychoanalytic interchange. *Psychoanalytic Dialogues, 21*(1): 45–54.

Butler, J. (1988). Performative acts and gender constitution: An essay in phenomenology and feminist theory. *Theatre Journal, 40*(4): 519–531.

Caligor, E., Kernberg, O. F., & Clarkin, J. F. (2007). *Handbook of Dynamic Psychotherapy for Higher Level Personality Pathology*. Arlington, VA: American Psychiatric Publishing.

Capra, F. (1975). *The Tao of Physics*. Boulder, CO: Shambala.

Capra, F. (1982). *The Turning Point*. London: Flamingo.

Capra, F. (2002). *The Hidden Connections*. London: Flamingo.

Carman, T. (1999). The body in Husserl and Merleau-Ponty. *Philosophical Topics, 27*(2): 205–226.

Carroll, L. (1865). *Alice's Adventures in Wonderland*. London: Penguin, 1994.

Carroll, L. (1871). *Through the Looking Glass: And What Alice Found There*. London: Puffin, 1994.

Carroll, R. (2002). Biodynamic massage in psychotherapy: Re-integrating, re-owning and re-associating through the body. In: T. Staunton (Ed.), *Body Psychotherapy* (pp. 78–100). New York: Taylor & Francis.

Carroll, R. (2009). Self-regulation: An evolving concept at the heart of body psychotherapy. In: L. Hartley (Ed.), *Contemporary Body Psychotherapy* (pp. 89–105). Hove, UK: Routledge.

Casement, P. J. (1982). Some pressures on the analyst for physical contact during the re-living of an early trauma. *International Review of Psychoanalysis, 9*: 279–286.

Casement, P. J. (2000). The issue of touch: A retrospective overview. *Psychoanalytic Inquiry, 20*: 160–184.

Castaneda, C. (1968). *The Teachings of Don Juan*. London: Arkana.

Castaneda, C. (1971). *A Separate Reality*. London: Arkana.

Castaneda, C. (1974). *Tales of Power*. New York: Simon & Schuster.

Cavell, M. (2006). *Becoming a Subject: Reflections in Philosophy and Psychoanalysis*. New York: Oxford University Press.

Cerney, S. M. (1995). Treating the heroic treaters. In: C. R. Figley (Ed.), *Compassion Fatigue: Coping with Secondary Traumatic Stress Disorder in Those Who Treat the Traumatized* (pp. 131–149). New York: Brunner/Mazel.

Chaiklin, S., & Wengrower, H. (2009). *The Art and Science of Dance/Movement Therapy: Life is Dance*. New York: Brunner-Routledge.

Chomsky, N. (1957). *Syntactic Structures*. The Hague, Netherlands: Mouton, 1972.

Cixous, H., & Clement, C. (1986). *The Newly Born Woman*. Minneapolis, MN: University of Minnesota Press.

Coello, Y., & Delevoye-Turrell, Y. (2007). Embodiment, spatial categorisation and action. *Consciousness and Cognition, 16*: 667–683.

Conger, J. P. (1988). *Jung & Reich*. Berkeley, CA: North Atlantic, 2005.

Connelly, D. M. (1994). *Traditional Acupuncture: The Law of the Five Elements (2nd ed.)*. Columbia, SC: Traditional Acupuncture Institute.

Conrad, E. (2008). Continuum: An overview. Retrieved 24 May 2013, from http://www.continuummovement.com/docs/continuum-overview.pdf.

Damasio, A. (1994). *Descartes' Error: Emotion, Reason, and the Human Brain*. New York: Penguin.

Daum, H., & Hartman, A. (2010). *Mind the Road (Hebrew ed.)*. Tel Aviv, Israel: Yediot Aharonot, Sifre Hemed.

Davidson, D. (1970). Mental events. In: *Essays on Actions and Events* (pp. 137–149). Oxford: Oxford University Press, 1981.

Davis, W. (2008a). Functional analysis: A depth body psychotherapy. Retrieved 10 June 2013 from http://www.functionalanalysis.de/download.php?view.8.

Davis, W. (2008b). The biological foundations of the schizoid process. Retrieved 10 June 2013 from http://www.functionalanalysis.de/download.php?view.9.

Davis, W. (2012). In support of body psychotherapy. *International Body Psychotherapy Journal, 11*(2): 59–73.

Descartes, R. (1636). Discourse on method. In: M. D. Wilson (Ed.), *The Essential Descartes*. New York: Meridian, 1983.

Diamond, M. J. (1984). It takes two to tango: Some thoughts on the neglected importance of the hypnotist in an interactive hypnotherapeutic relationship. *American Journal of Clinical Hypnosis, 27*(1): 3–13.

Diamond, N. (2006). Between touches. In: G. Galton (Ed.), *Touch Papers* (pp. 79–96). London: Karnac.

Dilts, R. B., & DeLozier, J. (2000). *Encyclopedia of Systemic NLP and New NLP Coding*. Scotts Valley, CA: NLP University Press.

Dilts, R. B., Grinder, J., Bandler, R., Bandler, L. C., & DeLozier, J. (1980). *Neuro-Linguistic-Programming, Volume 1: The Study of the Structure of Subjective Experience*. Cupertino, CA: Meta Publications.

Dimen, M. (1998). Polyglot bodies: Thinking through the relational. In: L. Aron & F. S. Anderson (Eds.), *Relational Perspectives on the Body* (pp. 65–93). Hillsdale, NJ: Analytic Press.

Doidge, N. (2008). *The Brain that Changes Itself: Stories of Personal Triumph from the Frontiers of Brain Science*. London: Penguin.

Dozier, M., & Bates, B. C. (2004). Attachment state of mind and the treatment relationship. In: L. Atkinson & S. Goldberg (Eds.), *Attachment Issues in Psychopathology and Intervention* (pp. 167–180). Mahwah, NJ: Lawrence Erlbaum.

Dupont, J. (1994). Freud's analysis of Ferenczi as revealed by their correspondence. *International Journal of Psychoanalysis, 75*: 301–320.

Ehrenberg, D. B. (1992). *The Intimate Edge*. New York: W. W. Norton.

Eichhorn, N., & Hilton, R. (2012). Relational somatic psychotherapy: An interview by Nancy Eichhorn with Robert Hilton. In C. Young (Ed.), *About Relational Body Psychotherapy* (pp. 1–5). Stow, UK: Body Psychotherapy Publications.

Eiden, B. (1998). The use of touch in psychotherapy. *Self & Society, A Journal of Humanistic Psychology in Britain, 26*: 1–3.

Eiden, B. (2009). The roots and the development of the Chiron approach. In: L. Hartley (Ed.), *Contemporary Body Psychotherapy: The Chiron Approach* (pp. 13–30). Hove, UK: Routledge.

Eiden, B. (2011). The history of body psychotherapy—an overview. In: C. Young (Ed.), *The Historical Basis of Body Psychotherapy* (pp. 39–48). Stow, UK: Body Psychotherapy Publications.

Eliot, T. S. (1940). Four Quartets—East Coker. In: *Collected Poems 1909–1962*. London: Faber and Faber.

Erickson, B. A. (2006). An American healer. In: B. A. Erickson & B. Keeney (Eds.), *Milton H. Erickson, M.D. An American Healer* (pp. 22–84). Sedona, AZ: Ringing Rock Press.

Erickson, M. H., & Rossi, E. L. (1989). *The February Man: Evolving Consciousness and Identity in Hypnotherapy*. New York: Brunner/Mazel.

Eshel, O. (2005). A bond of love, emotional risk, and daring. *Psychoanalytic Dialogues, 15*: 717–725.

Fairbairn, W. R. D. (1952). *Psychoanalytic Studies of the Personality*. London: Routledge.

Fangarette, H. (1963). *The Self in Transformation: Psychoanalysis, Philosophy, and the Life of the Spirit*. New York: Basic.

Farber, S. K. (2008). Dissociation, traumatic attachment, and self-harm: Eating disorders and self-mutilation. *Clinical Social Work Journal, 36*: 63–72.

Feldenkrais, M. (1977). *Awareness Through Movement: Health Exercises for Personal Growth*. London: Penguin.

Fellows, B. J. (1986). The concept of trance. In: P. L. N. Naish (Ed.), *What is Hypnosis? Current Theories and Research* (pp. 37–58). Milton Keynes, UK: Open University Press.

Fenichel, O. (1945). *The Psychoanalytic Theory of Neurosis*. New York: W. W. Norton.

Ferenczi, S. (1925). Contra-indications to the 'active' psycho-analytic technique. In: *The Theory and Technique of Psychoanalysis II*. New York: Basic, 1953.

Ferenczi, S. (1926). *Further Contribution to the Theory and Technique of Psychoanalysis*. London: Karnac, 1994.

Ferenczi, S. (1929). The principle of relaxation and neocatharsis. In: S. Ferenczi & M. Balint (Eds.), *Final Contributions to the Problems and Methods of Psychoanalysis*. London: Maresfield Reprints, 1980.

Ferenczi, S. (1930). The principle of relaxation and neocatharsis. *International Journal of Psychoanalysis, 11*: 428–443.

Ferenczi, S. (1932). *The Clinical Diary of Sándor Ferenczi*. Cambridge, MA: Harvard University Press, 1988.

Ferenczi, S. (1933). Confusion of tongues between the adult and the child. In: M. Balint & J. Rickman (Eds.), *Collected Papers (Vol. 3)* (pp. 156–167). New York: Basic, 1955.

Ferenczi, S., & Rank, O. (1925). *The Development of Psycho-Analysis*. Whitefish, MT: Kessinger Publishing, 2006.

Field, N. (1996). *Breakdown & Breakthrough*. Hove, UK: Routledge.

Figley, C. R. (1995). Compassion fatigue as secondary traumatic stress disorder: An overview. In: C. R. Figley (Ed.), *Compassion Fatigue: Coping with Secondary Traumatic Stress Disorder in Those Who Treat the Traumatized* (pp. 1–20). New York: Brunner/Mazel.

Fine, L. (2003). *Physician of the Soul, Healer of the Cosmos—Isaac Luria and His Kabbalistic Fellowship*. Stanford, CA: Stanford University Press.

Flemons, D. (2001). Therapist as novelist and/or jazz improviser. In: B. Duncan & J. Sparks (Eds.), *Heroic Clients, Heroic Agencies: Partners for Change* (pp. 235–236). Fort Lauderdale, FL: NSU Press.

Fogel, A. (2009). *The Psychophysiology of Self-Awareness*. New York: W. W. Norton.

Forer, B. R. (1969). The taboo against touching in psychotherapy. *Psychotherapy: Theory, Research, and Practice, 6*(4): 229–231.

Franklin, B. (1785). Report by Dr Benjamin Franklin and the other commissioners, charged by the King of France, with the examination of animal magnetism, as now practiced in Paris. Translated from the French with an historical introduction by W. M. Godwin. In: M. M. Tinterow (Ed.), *Foundations of Hypnosis from Mesmer to Freud*. Springfield, IL: Thomas, 1970.

Freud, S. (1890a). *Psychical (or mental) treatment. S. E., 7*: pp. 282–302. London: Hogarth, 1953.

Freud, S. (1891d). *Hypnosis. S. E., 1*: pp. 103–114. London: Hogarth, 1966.

Freud, S. (1900a). *The Interpretation of Dreams. S. E., 4 & 5*: pp. 1–338, 339–621. London: Hogarth, 1953.

Freud, S. (1905d). *Three Essays on the Theory of Sexuality. S. E., 7*: pp. 130–243. London: Hogarth, 1953.

Freud, S. (1912d). *On the universal tendency to debasement in the sphere of love (contributions to the psychology of love II). S. E., 11*: pp. 177–190. London: Hogarth, 1957.

Freud, S. (1912e). *Recommendations to physicians practising psycho-analysis. S. E., 12*: pp. 109–120. London: Hogarth, 1958.

Freud, S. (1913c). *On beginning the treatment (further recommendations on the technique of psycho-analysis I). S. E., 12*: pp. 121–144. London: Hogarth, 1958.

Freud, S. (1914g). *Remembering, repeating and working-through (further recommendations on the technique of psycho-analysis II). S. E., 12*: pp. 145–156. London: Hogarth, 1958.

Freud, S. (1915e). *The unconscious. S. E., 14*: 159–215. London: Hogarth, 1957.

Freud, S. (1917a). *A difficulty in the path of psycho-analysis. S. E., 17*: pp. 135–144. London: Hogarth, 1955.

Freud, S. (1920g). *Beyond the Pleasure Principle. S. E., 18*: 1–64. London: Hogarth, 1955.

Freud, S. (1921c). *Group Psychology and the Analysis of the Ego. S. E., 18*: pp. 65–143. London: Hogarth, 1955.

Freud, S. (1923b). *The Ego and the Id. S. E., 19*: pp. 1–66. London: Hogarth, 1961.

Freud, S. (1925d). *An Autobiographical Study. S. E., 20*: pp. 1–74. London: Hogarth, 1959.

Freud, S. (1926e). *The Question of Lay Analysis. S. E., 20*: pp. 183–250. London: Hogarth, 1959.

Freud, S. (1933a). *New Introductory Lectures on Psycho-Analysis, Lecture XXXI. S. E., 22*: pp. 1–182. London: Hogarth, 1964.

Freud, S., & Breuer, J. (1895). *Studies on Hysteria. S. E., 2*. London: Hogarth, 1955.

Friedman, R. (2013). Concerning the interface of musical and therapetuic aspects of resonance. Lesson 15 in the Introduction to Relational Body Psychotherapy course, the Post Graduate Programme in Relational Body Psychotherapy, the Israeli Centre for Body–Mind Medicine. Ramat Hasharon.

Fromm, E. (1942). *The Fear of Freedom*. London: Routledge & Kegan Paul.

Fromm, E. (1957). *The Art of Loving*. London: Thorsons, 1995.

Gabbard, G. O., & Lester, E. P. (1995). *Boundaries and Boundary Violations in Psychoanalysis*. New York: Basic.

Gallese, V. (2001). The 'shared manifold' hypothesis. From mirror neurons to empathy. *Journal of Consciousness Studies, 8*: 33–50.

Gallese, V., Fadiga, L., Fogassi, L., & Rizzolatti, G. (1996). Action recognition in the premotor cortex. *Brain, 119*: 593–609.

Gallese, V., Ferrari, P. F., & Umiltà, M. A. (2002). The mirror matching system: A shared manifold for intersubjectivity. *Behavioral and Brain Sciences, 25*(1): 35–36.

Gendlin, E. T. (1962). *Experiencing and the Creation of Meaning*. New York: Free Press of Glencoe.

Gendlin, E. T. (1978). *Focusing*. New York: Bantam.

Gendlin, E. T. (1998). *Focusing-Oriented Psychotherapy: A Manual of the Experiential Method*. New York: Guilford.

Gezundhajt, H. (2007). An evolution of the historical origins of hypnotism prior to the twentieth century: Between spirituality and subconscious. *Contemporary Hypnosis, 24*(4): 178–194.

Ghent, E. (1990). Masochism, submission, surrender: Masochism as a perversion of surrender. In: S. A. Mitchell & L. Aron (Eds.), *Relational Psychoanalysis: The Emergence of a Tradition* (pp. 211–242). New York: Analytic Press, 1999.

Gilbert, C. (1999). Breathing: The legacy of Wilhelm Reich. *Journal of Bodywork & Movement Therapies, 3*(2): 97–106.

Gilligan, C. (2004). Knowing and not knowing: Reflections on manhood. *Psychotherapy and Politics International, 2*(2): 99–114.

Gilligan, S. G. (1987). *Therapeutic Trances*. Philadelphia, PA: Brunner/Mazel.

Gilligan, S. G. (1996). The relational self: An expanding of love beyond desire. In: S. G. Gilligan (Ed.), *The Legacy of Milton H. Erickson: Selected Papers of Stephen Gilligan* (pp. 254–281). Phoenix, AZ: Zeig, Tucker & Theisen, 2002.

Gilligan, S. G. (1997). *The Courage to Love: Practice and Principles of Self-Relations Psychotherapy*. New York: W. W. Norton.

Gilligan, S. G. (2012). *Generative Trance: The Experience of Creative Flow*. Bethel, CT: Crown House Publishing.

Gilligan, S. G., & Simon, D. (2004). *Walking in Two Worlds*. Phoenix, AZ: Zeig, Tucker & Theisen.

Goble, F. G. (1970). *The Third Force: The Psychology of Abraham Maslow*. New York: Grossman.

Gödel, K. (1931). *On Formally Undecidable Propositions of "Principia Mathematica" and Related Systems*. London: Oliver and Boyd, 1962.

Goldberg, L. (1949). *What Are the Gazells Doing? (Ma Osot Ha'ayalot, Hebrew edition)*. Bnei Brak, Israel: Sifriat Poalim.

Goldberg, L. (1973). *Poems, Vol. 2 (Shirim, Hebrew edition)*. Bnei Brak, Israel: Sifriat Poalim.

Gomez, L. (1997). *An Introduction to Object Relations*. London: Free Association.

Goodman, M., & Teicher, A. (1988). To touch or not to touch. *Psychotherapy, 25*: 492–500.

Goodrich-Dunn, B. (2004). Somatic psychotherapies: A road map. *Psychotherapy Networker, July/August*: 42–43.

Gould, S. J. (1996). *The Mismeasure of Man (revised and expanded ed.)*. New York: W. W. Norton.

Grand, I. J. (1998). Psyche's body: Towards a somatic psychodynamics. In: D. H. Johnson & I. J. Grand (Eds.), *The Body in Psychotherapy: Inquiries in Somatic Psychology* (pp. 171–193). Berkeley, CA: North Atlantic.

Gravitz, M. A. (2004). The historical role of hypnosis in the theoretical origins of transference. *International Journal of Clinical and Experimental Hypnosis, 52*(2): 113–131.

Greenberg, J. R., & Mitchell, S. A. (1983). *Object Relations in Psychoanalytic Theory*. Cambridge, MA: Harvard University Press.

Greene, E., & Goodrich-Dunn, B. (2013). *The Psychology of the Body (2nd edition)*. Philadelphia, PA: Lippincott Williams & Wilkins.

Groddeck, G. (1931). Psychic conditioning and the psychoanalytic treatment of organic disorders. In: L. Schnacht (Ed.), *The Meaning of Illness: Selected Psychoanalytic Writings by Georg Groddeck*. London: Maresfield Library, 1977.

Grof, S. (1975). *Realms of the Human Unconscious: Observation from LSD Research*. New York: Viking.

Grof, S. (1980). *LSD Psychotherapy*. Pomona, CA: Hunter House.

Grof, S. (1988). *The Adventure of Self-Discovery*. New York: State University of New York Press.

Grof, S., & Bennett, H. Z. (1993). *The Holotropic Mind*. New York: Harper Collins.

Hadad, E., & Rolef Ben-Shahar, A. (2012). The things we're taking home with us: Understanding therapist's self-care in trauma work. *International Journal of Psychotherapy, 16*(1): 50–61.

Hadar, B. (1997a). Therapeutic attitudes toward the body: Exploring relations between psychoanalysis, dance and movement psychotherapy and bioenergetic analysis. Part I (Hebrew ed.). *Sihot, 11*(2): 125–131.

Hadar, B. (1997b). Therapeutic attitudes toward the body: Exploring relations between psychoanalysis, dance and movement psychotherapy and bioenergetic analysis. Part II (Hebrew ed.). *Sihot, 11*(3): 206–213.

Halsen, A. W. (1995). Body psychotherapy in Norway. *Nordic Journal of Psychiatry, 49*(6): 101–105.

Harlow, H. F., & Zimmermann, R. R. (1959). Affectional responses in the infant monkey; orphaned baby monkeys develop a strong and persistent attachment to inanimate surrogate mothers. *Science, 130*(3373): 421–432.

Hartley, L. (2005). Embodying the sense of self: Body–mind centering and authentic movement. In: N. Totton (Ed.), *New Dimensions in Body Psychotherapy* (pp. 128–141). Maidenhead, UK: Open University Press.

Hartley, L. (Ed.) (2009). *Contemporary Body Psychotherapy*. Hove, UK: Routledge.

Heckler, R. S. (1984). *The Anatomy of Change: East/West Approaches to Body/Mind Therapy*. Boulder, CO: Shambhala.

Heller, M. C. (2006). A topography of the mind. *USA Body Psychotherapy Journal, 5*(2): 61–87.

Heller, M. C. (2012). *Body Psychotherapy: History, Concepts, Methods*. London: W. W. Norton.

Hendricks, G. (1995). *Conscious Breathing: Breathwork for Health, Stress Release, and Personal Mastery*. New York: Bantam.

Hendricks, M. N. (2001). Focusing-oriented/experiential psychotherapy. In: D. J. Cain & J. Seeman (Eds.), *Humanistic Psychotherapies: Handbook of Research and Practice* (pp. 221–252). Washington, DC: American Psychological Association.

Heuer, G. (2005). 'In my flesh I shall see god': Jungian body psychotherapy. In: N. Totton (Ed.), *New Dimensions in Body Psychotherapy* (pp. 102–114). Maidenhead, UK: Open University Press.

Hilton, R. (2012a). Bioenergetics as a relational somatic psychotherapy. In: C. Young (Ed.), *About Relational Body Psychotherapy* (pp. 19–34). Stow, UK: Body Psychotherapy Publications.

Hilton, R. (2012b). The ever changing constancy of body psychotherapy. *International Body Psychotherapy Journal, 11*(2): 74–93.

Hinshelwood, R. D. (2002). The di-vidual person: On identity and identifications. In: V. Sinason (Ed.), *Attachment, Trauma and Multiplicity* (pp. 212–230). Hove, UK: Routledge.

Hoffman, I. Z. (1996). The intimate and ironic authority of the psychoanalyst's presence. *Psychoanalytic Quarterly, 65*: 102–136.

Holmes, J. (1996). *Attachment, Intimacy, Autonomy: Using Attachment Theory in Adult Psychotherapy.* Northvale, NJ: Jason Aronson.

Houston, G. (1995). *The Now Red Book of Gestalt.* London: Gaie Houston & Rochester Terrace.

Huxley, A. (1932). *Brave New World.* London: Flamingo, 1994.

Irigaray, L. (1993). *Je, tu, nous: Toward a Culture of Difference.* New York: Routledge.

Jakoby, C. R. (2011). Insecure base: Post traumatic stress disorder as an attachment disorder. (Diploma in Body Psychotherapy thesis, Reidman College, Tel Aviv.)

Johnson, D. H. (Ed.) (1995). *Bone, Breath & Gesture: Practices of Embodiment.* Berkeley, CA: North Atlantic.

Johnson, D. H. (1998). Who walks? In: D. H. Johnson & I. J. Grand (Eds.), *The Body in Psychotherapy: Inquiries in Somatic Psychology* (pp. 1–16). Berkeley, CA: North Atlantic.

Johnson, S. M. (1994). *Character Styles.* New York: W. W. Norton.

Jones, E., Trilling, L., & Marcus, S. (1961). *The Life and Work of Sigmund Freud.* New York: Basic.

Joseph, S. M. (2007). Jung and Kabbalah: Imaginal and noetic aspects. *Journal of Analytical Psychology, 52*: 321–341.

Judith, A. (1996). *Eastern Body Western Mind.* Berkeley, CA: Celestial Arts.

Juhan, D. (1998). *Job's Body: A Handbook for Bodywork (expanded ed.).* New York: Station Hill.

Jung, C. G. (1920). *Collected Papers on Analytical Psychology* (C. E. Long, Trans. 2nd ed.). London: Bailliere, Tindall & Cox.

Jung, C. G. (1934). The archetypes of the collective unconscious. R. F. C. Hull (Trans.). In: S. H. Read, M. Fordham, & G. Adler (Eds.), *The Collected Works of C. G. Jung (Vol. 9, Part 1).* (pp. 3–41). Princeton, NJ: Princeton University Press, 1980.

Jung, C. G. (1949). Preface. In R. W. (Trans) (Ed.), *I Ching—The Book of Changes* (pp. 1–27). London: Penguin.

Jung, C. G. (1988). *Nietzsche's Zarathustra: Notes of the Seminar Given in 1934–1939 by C. G. Jung.* Edited by J. L. Jarrett. Princeton, NJ: Princeton University Press.

Jung, C. G., & Douglas, C. (1931–35). *Visions—Notes on the Seminar Given in 1930–1934.* Princeton, NJ: Princeton University Press, 1997.

Jung, C. G., von Franz, M. L., Henderson, J. L., Jacobi, J., & Jaffé, A. (Eds.) (1964). *Man and His Symbols.* London: Arkana.

Kandel, E. R. (1998). A new intellectual framework for psychiatry. *Psychiatry, Psychoanalysis, and the New Biology of Mind* (pp. 33–58). Arlington, VA: American Psychiatric Publishing, 2005.

Kandel, E. R. (Ed.) (2005). *Psychiatry, Psychoanalysis, and the New Biology of Mind.* Arlington, VA: American Psychiatric Publishing.

Kant, I. (1781). *Critique of Pure Reason.* P. Guyer & A. W. Wood (Trans.). Cambridge: Cambridge University Press, 1998.

Kaplan, A. G. (1975). Sex in psychotherapy: the myth of Sándor Ferenczi. *Contemporary Psychoanalysis, 11*: 175–187.

Kaplan, J. T., & Iacoboni, M. (2006). Getting a grip on other minds: Mirror neurons, intention understanding, and cognitive empathy. *Social Neuroscience, 1*(3): 175–183.

Karcher, S. (2007). Re-enchanting the mind: Oracles, reading, myth, and mantics. *Psychological Perspectives, 50*(2): 198–219.

Karle, H. W. A., & Boys, J. H. (1987). *Hypnotherapy: A Practical Handbook*. London: Free Association.

Kartin-Korman, O. (2011). "I shall know not fear for thou art with me": The therapist's acknowledgment of providence as influencing therapeutic positioning. (Diploma in Body Psychotherapy thesis, Reidman College, Tel Aviv.)

Kashi-Kark, A. (2011). Knowing pain: The effects of body psychotherapy treatment on a person dealing with chronic pain. (Diploma in Body Psychotherapy thesis, Reidman College, Tel Aviv.)

Keeney, B. (1983). *Aesthetics of Change*. New York: Guilford.

Keeney, B. (1994). *Shaking Out the Spirits*. New York: Station Hill.

Keeney, B. (2005). *Bushman Shaman: Awakening the Spirit through Ecstatic Dance*. Rochester, VT: Destiny.

Keeney, B. (2007). *Shaking Medicine: The Healing Power of Ecstatic Movement*. Rochester, VT: Destiny.

Keet, C., Sella, Y., & Ziv-Beiman, S. (2013). One body, different angels. (Paper presented at the book launch of Asaf Rolef Ben-Shahar's "An Anatomy of Therapy", Tel Aviv, 25 April.)

Keith-Spiegel, P., & Koocher, G. P. (1985). *Ethics in Psychology: Professional Standards and Cases*. New York: Random House.

Keleman, S. (1981). *Your Body Speaks its Mind*. Berkeley, CA: Center Press.

Keleman, S. (1985). *Emotional Anatomy*. Berkeley, CA: Center Press.

Keleman, S. (1987). *Embodying Experience—Forming a Personal Life*. Berkeley, CA: Center Press.

Keleman, S. (2012). Forming an embodied life: The difference between being bodied and forming an embodied life. *International Body Psychotherapy Journal, 11*(1): 51–56.

Keleman, S., & Adler, S. (2000). Couples therapy as a formative process. *Journal of Couples Therapy, 10*(2): 49–59.

Kernberg, O. F. (1970). A psychoanalytic classification of character pathology. *Journal of the American Psychoanalytic Association, 18*: 800–822.

Kertay, L., & Reviere, S. L. (1993). The use of touch in psychotherapy: Theoretical and ethical considerations. *Psychotherapy: Theory Research, Practice, Training, 30*(1): 32–40.

Kertay, L., & Reviere, S. L. (1998). Touch in context. In: E. W. L. Smith, P. R. Clance, & S. Imes (Eds.), *Touch in Psychotherapy: Theory, Research, and Practice* (pp. 16–35). New York: Guilford.

Kessel, L. (2013). Couple therapy and relational body psychotherapy: Healing childhood wounds. *Body, Movement and Dance in Psychotherapy, 8*(3): 172–182.

King, A. (2011). Touch as relational affirmation. *Attachment: New Directions in Psychotherapy and Relational Psychoanalysis, 5*: 108–124.

Kipling, R. (2002). In the neolithic age. In: *Rudyard Kipling: The Complete Verse (revised ed.)*. London: Kyle Cathie.

Klein, M. (1946). Notes on some schizoid mechanisms. In: *Envy and Gratitude and Other Works 1946–1963* (pp. 1–24). London: Hogarth, 1975.

Klein, M. (1960). *Our Adult World and Its Roots in Infancy*. London: Tavistock.

Klein, M. (1963). On the sense of loneliness. In: *Envy and Gratitude and Other Works 1946–1963* (pp. 300–313). London: Hogarth, 1975.

Klein, M. (1975). *Envy and Gratitude and Other Works 1946–1963*. London: Hogarth.

Klisic, L. (1992). The orgasm concept. In: B. V. Maul (Ed.), *Body Psychotherapy or the Art of Contact* (pp. 212–214). Berlin: European Association for Body Psychotherapy.

Knoblauch, S. (1997). Beyond the word in psychoanalysis the unspoken dialogue. *Psychoanalytic Dialogues, 7*(4): 491–516.

Knoblauch, S. (1999). The third, minding and affecting: Commentary on paper by Lewis Aron. *Psychoanalytic Dialogues, 9*(1): 41–51.

Knoblauch, S. (2000). *The Musical Edge of Therapeutic Dialogue*. Hillsdale, NJ: Analytic Press.

Knoblauch, S. (2005). Body rhythms and the unconscious: Toward an expanding of clinical attention. *Psychoanalytic Dialogues, 15*(6): 807–827.

Knoblauch, S. (2011). Contextualizing attunement within the polyrhythmic weave: The psychoanalytic samba. *Psychoanalytic Dialogues, 21*(4): 414–427.

Knoblauch, S. (2012). Body rhythms and the unconscious: Expanding clinical attention with the polyrhythmic wave. In: L. Aron & A. Harris (Eds.), *Relational Psychoanalysis Vol. 5: Evolution of Process* (pp. 183–204). Hove, UK: Routledge.

Kohut, H. (1959). Introspection, empathy, and psychoanalysis—An examination of the relationship between mode of observation and theory. *Journal of the American Psychoanalytic Association, 7*L 459–483.

Kohut, H. (1982). Introspection, empathy, and the semi-circle of mental health. *International Journal of Psychoanalysis, 63*: 395–407.

Kohut, H., Goldberg, A., & Stepansky, P. E. (1984). *How Does Analysis Cure?* Chicago, IL: University of Chicago Press.

Kook, A. I. (1990). *Orot Hakodesh (Sacred Lights) (Hebrew ed.)*. Jerusalem: Mosad Harav Kook.

Korzybski, A. (1924). Time-binding: The General Theory. (Paper presented at the International Mathematical Congress, Toronto, Canada.)

Krantz, A. M. (2012). Let the body speak: Commentary on paper by Jon Sletvold. *Psychoanalytic Dialogues, 22*(4): 437–448.

Kristeva, J. (2001). *Strangers to Ourselves*. New York: Columbia University Press.

Kuhn, T. S. (1962). *The Structure of Scientific Revolutions (2nd ed.)*. Chicago, IL: University of Chicago Press.

Kurtz, R. (2007). *Body-Centred Psychotherapy—The Hakomi Method (revised ed.)*. Mendocino, CA: LifeRhythms.

Lake, F. (1979). *Studies in Constricted Confusion: Exploration of a Pre- and Perinatal Paradigm*. Oxford: Clinical Theology Association.

Lash, J. (1989). *The Tai Chi Journey*. Shaftesbury, UK: Element.

Lawrence, D. H. (1928). *Psychoanalysis and the Unconscious*. London: Martin Secker.

Lawry, S. S. (1998). Touch and clients who have been sexually abused. In: E. W. L. Smith, P. R. Clance, & S. Imes (Eds.), *Touch in Psychotherapy: Theory, Research, and Practice* (pp. 201–210). New York: Guilford.

Lerner, Y. (2011). It all starts in the genes. *Atmosphere, 160*.

Levinas, E. (1986). *Of God Who Comes to Mind*. B. Bergo (Trans.). Stanford, CA: Stanford University Press, 1998.

Levine, P. A. (2005). Panic, biology and reason: Giving the body its due. In: N. Totton (Ed.), *New Dimensions in Body Psychotherapy* (pp. 30–39). Maidenhead, UK: Open University Press.

Levine, P. A., & Frederick, A. (1997). *Waking the Tiger*. Berkeley, CA: North Atlantic.

Levy, R. (2012). The body's voice (in Hebrew). *A Different Life (Haim Acherim), 183*.

Levy, R. (2013). Relational body psychotherapy as a transpersonal encounter: Mutual surrender. *Hebrew Psychology*. Retrieved 19 October 2013 from http://www.hebpsy.net/articles.asp?t=0&id=3002

Lewis, T., Amini, F., & Lannon, R. (2000). *A General Theory of Love*. New York: Random House.

Lichtenberg, J. D. (1991). What is a selfobject? *Psychoanalytic Dialogues, 1*: 455–479.

Liotti, G. (2004). Trauma, dissociation, and disorganized attachment: Three strands of a single braid. *Psychotherapy: Theory Research, Practice, Training, 11*(4): 472–486.

Lipkies, L. (2012). The language of crying in body psychotherapy. (Diploma in Body Psychotherapy thesis, Reidman College, Tel Aviv.)

Loewald, H. W. (1977). Primary process, secondary process and language. *Papers on Psychoanalysis* (pp. 178–206). New Haven, CT: Yale University Press, 1980.

Loewald, H. W. (1986). Transference-countertransference. *Journal of the American Psychoanalytic Association, 34*: 275–287.

Lopez, G. (2011). Why verbal psychotherapy is not enough to treat post traumatic stress disorder: A biosystemic approach to stress debriefing. *Body, Movement and Dance in Psychotherapy, 6*(2): 129–143.

Lowen, A. (1958). *The Language of the Body*. New York: Macmillan.

Lowen, A. (1965). *Love and Orgasm*. New York: Signet.

Lowen, A. (1974). The body in personality theory: Wilhelm Reich and Alexander Lowen. In: A. Burton (Ed.), *Operational Theories of Personality*. New York: Brunner/Mazel.

Lowen, A. (1975). *Bioenergetics*. New York: Arkana.

Maar, D. (1942–43). I rested in the arms of my arms. In: M. A. Caws (Ed.), *Surrealist Love Poems* (pp. 82). London: Tate, 2001.

Machado, A. (1983). *Times Alone: Selected Poems of Antonio Machado*. R. Bly (Trans.). Middletown, CT: Wesleyan University Press.

Macnaughton, I. (Ed.) (1998). *Embodying the Mind & Minding the Body*. North Vancouver, Canada: Integral Press.

Mahler, M. S., & McDevitt, J. B. (1982). Thoughts on the emergence of the sense of self, with particular emphasis on the sense of body self. *Journal of the American Psychoanalytic Association, 30*: 827–844.

Malan, D. (1963). *A Study of Brief Psychotherapy*. New York: Plenum.

Malchiodi, C. A. (2007). *Expressive Therapies*. New York: Guilford.

Maoz, G. (2010). Sabina Spielrein: A Greek tragedy or a myth about the development of psychoanalysis. (Paper presented at the Israeli Jungian Society.) Available at: http://israjung.co.il/maozgad/sabina/sabina.doc

Marcher, L., & Fich, S. (2010). *Body Encyclopedia: A Guide to the Psychological Functions of the Muscular System*. Berkeley, CA: North Atlantic.

Maroda, K. J. (1998). *Seduction, Surrender and Transformation*. London: Analytic Press.

Marx, K. (1852). *The Eighteenth Brumaire of Louis Bonaparte*. New York: International Publishers, 1963.

Maslow, A. H. (1943). A theory of human motivation. *Psychological Review, 50*: 370–396.

Masson, J. (1985). *The Complete Letters of Sigmund Freud to Wilhelm Fleiss*. London: Belknap.

McDougall, J. (1989). *Theatres of the Body: A Psychoanalytic Approach to Psychosomatic Illness*. London: Free Association.

McFarlane, A. C., Atchison, M., Rafalowicz, E., & Papay, P. (1994). Physical symptoms in post-traumatic stress disorder. *Journal of Psychosomatic Research, 38*(7): 715–724.

McLaughlin, J. T. (1991). Clinical and theoretical aspects of enactment. *Journal of the American Psychoanalytic Association, 39*: 595–614.

Menninger, K. (1958). *Theory of Psychoanalytic Technique*. New York: Basic.

Merleau-Ponty, M. (1962). *The Primacy of Perception*. Evanston, IL: Northwestern University Press.

Mesmer, F. A. (1766). Dissertation on the discovery of animal magnetism. In: G. Bloch (Ed.), *Mesmerism: A Translation of the Original Scientific and Medical Writing of F. A. Mesmer* (pp. 43–70). Los Altos, CA: Kaufmann, 1986.

Messler-Davies, J. (1994). Love in the afternoon: A relational reconsideration of desire and dread in the countertransference. *Psychoanalytic Dialogues, 4*: 153–170.

Meyer, W. S. (2005). The 'mother' returns to psychoanalysis: Sandor Ferenczi, welcome home. *Smith College Studies in Social Work, 75*(3): 15–31.

Milgram, S. (1974). *Obedience to Authority: An Experimental View*. London: Tavistock.

Miller, A. (1981). *The Drama of the Gifted Child*. New York: Basic.

Mindell, A. (1982). *Dreambody*. Henley-on-Thames, UK: Routledge & Kegan Paul.

Mindell, A. (2004). *The Quantum Mind and Healing*. Charlottesville, VA: Hampton Roads.

Mitchell, J. (1974). *Psychoanalysis and Feminism: With a New Introduction*. London: Penguin, 2000.

Mitchell, S. A. (1988). *Relational Concepts in Psychoanalysis*. Harvard, MA: Harvard University Press.

Mitchell, S. A. (1993). *Hope and Dread in Psychoanalysis*. New York: Basic.

Mitchell, S. A. (1998). From ghosts to ancestors: The psychoanalytic vision of Hans Loewald. *Psychoanalytic Dialogues, 8*: 825–855.

Mitchell, S. A. (2000). *Relationality: From Attachment to Intersubjectivity*. Hillsdale, NJ: Analytic Press.

Mitchell, S. A. (2002). *Can Love Last?* New York: W. W. Norton.

Mitchell, S. A. (2004). My psychoanalytic journey. *Psychoanalytic Inquiry, 24*(4): 531–541.

Mitchell, S. A. (2005). *Influence and Autonomy in Psychoanalysis*. Hillsdale, NJ: Analytic Press.

Mitchell, S. A., & Aron, L. (1999). Preface. In: S. A. Mitchell & L. Aron (Eds.), *Relational Psychoanalysis: The Emergence of a Tradition* (pp. ix–xx). New York: Analytic Press.

Moving Center School (2013). Retrieved 24 May 2013, from www.movingcenterschool.com

Myss, C. M. (1996). *Anatomy of the Spirit: The Seven Stages of Power and Healing*. London: Bantam.

Ochberg, F. M. (1991). Post-traumatic therapy. *Psychotherapy: Theory, Research, Practice, Training, 28*(1): 5–15.

Odent, M. (1994). Preventing violence or developing the capacity to love: Which perspective? Which Investment? Retrieved 19 October 2013 from http://birthpsychology.com/free-article/preventing-violence-or-developing-capacity-love-which-perspective-which-investment

Ogden, P., & Minton, K. (2000). Sensorimotor psychotherapy: One method for processing traumatic memory. *Traumatology, 6*(3): 149–173.

Ogden, P., Minton, K., & Pain, C. (2006). *Trauma and the Body: A Sensorimotor Approach to Psychotherapy*. New York: W. W. Norton.

Ogden, T. H. (1985). On potential space. *International Journal of Psychoanalysis, 66*: 129–141.

Ogden, T. H. (1992). The dialectically constituted/decentred subject of psychoanalysis. I. The Freudian subject. *International Journal of Psychoanalysis, 73*: 517–526.

Ogden, T. H. (1994a). The analytic third—working with intersubjective clinical facts. *International Journal of Psychoanalysis, 75*: 3–20.

Ogden, T. H. (1994b). *Subjects of Analysis*. Northvale, NJ: Jason Aronson.

Ogden, T. H. (1995). Analysing forms of aliveness and deadness of the transference-countertransference. *International Journal of Psychoanalysis, 76*: 695–710.

Ogden, T. H. (1997). Reverie and interpretation. *Psychoanalytic Quarterly, 4*: 567–595.

Oger, D. (2012). *Step into Your Life*. Brussels: Universitas.

Orange, D. M., & Stolorow, R. D. (1998). Self-discolsure from the perspective of intersubjectivity theory. *Psychoanalytic Inquiry, 18*: 530–537.

Orbach, S. (2003a). The John Bowlby memorial lecture: The body in clinical practice. Part I: There is no such thing as a body. *British Journal of Psychotherapy, 20*(1): 3–16.

Orbach, S. (2003b). There is no such thing as a body. In: K. White (Ed.), *Touch, Attachment and the Body* (pp. 17–34). London: Karnac.

Orbach, S. (2004a). The John Bowlby memorial lecture: The body in clinical practice. Part II: When touch comes to therapy. In: K. White (Ed.), *Touch, Attachment and the Body* (pp. 35–47). London: Karnac.

Orbach, S. (2004b). Review essay: Beyond the fear of intimacy. *Psychoanalytic Dialogues, 14*: 397–404.

Orbach, S. (2004c). What can we learn from the therapist's body? *Attachment & Human Development, 6*(2): 141–150.

Orbach, S. (2009). *Bodies*. London: Profile.

Orr, L. (2002). *The Story of Rebirthing Breathwork*. Tangent, OR: Leonard Orr.

Orr, L., & Ray, S. (1977). *Rebirthing in the New Age*. Millbrae, CA: Celestial Arts.

Oschman, J. L. (2000). *Energy Medicine: The Scientific Basis*. Edinburgh: Churchill Livingstone.

Osho (1976). *When the Shoe Fits: Talks on the Stories of Chuang Tzu*. Poona, India: Rajneesh Foundation.

Oster, N. (2011). Body psychotherapy as a diagnostic lens in examining child-development, in comparison with classic theories. (Diploma in Body Psychotherapy thesis, Reidman College, Tel Aviv.)

Osterville, Z. (1995). *Open Solutions (Pitronot Ptuchim) (Hebrew ed.)*. Jerusalem: Shoken.

Painter, J. W. (1984). *Deep Bodywork and Personal Development*. Mill Valley, CA: Bodymind.

Payne, H. (Ed.). (1992). *Dance Movement Therapy*. London: Routledge.

Payne, H. (2006). *Dance Movement Therapy: Theory, Research and Practice (2nd ed.)*. London: Routledge.

Pearlman, L. A., & Mac Ian, P. S. (1995). Vicarious traumatization: An empirical study of the effects of trauma work on trauma therapists. *Professional Psychology: Research and Practice, 26*(6): 558–565.

Pérez-Álvarez, M., & García-Montes, J. M. (2007). The Charcot effect: The invention of mental illnesses. *Journal of Constructivist Psychology, 20*: 309–336.

Perls, F. S. (1948). Theory and technique of personality integration. *American Journal of Psychotherapy, 2*(4): 565–586.

Perls, F. S. (1969). *Gestalt Therapy Verbatim*. Moab, UT: Real People Press.

Perls, F. S., Goodman, P., & Hefferline, R. E. (1951). *Gestalt Therapy: Excitement and Growth in the Human Personality*. London: Souvenir Press, 1972.

Pert, C. B. (1997). *Molecules of Emotion*. London: Pocket.

Pizer, B. (1999). Seduction, surrender and transformation—review. *Journal of the American Psychoanalytic Association, 48*: 969–975.

Pizer, B. (2002). Blowin' in the wind—Considering the impact of "inadvertent touch": Commentary on paper by Graham Bass. *Psychoanalytic Dialogues, 12*: 837–846.

Pizer, B. (2003). When the crunch is a (k)not: A crimp in relational dialogue. *Psychoanalytic Dialogues, 13*: 171–192.

Pizer, B. (2006). Risk and potential in analytic disclosure: Can the analyst make "the wrong thing" right? *Contemporary Psychoanalysis, 42*: 31–40.

Pizer, S. A. (1992). The negotiation of paradox in the analytic process. *Psychoanalytic Dialogues, 2*(2): 215–240.

Pizer, S. A. (2012). The analyst's generous involvement: Recognition and the tension of tenderness. (Paper presented at "Affective Relatedness and Therapeutic Action", the relational training programme, Psychotherapy School at the Faculty of Medicine, Tel Aviv University.)

Platek, S. M., Critton, S. R., Myers, T. E., & Gullup, G. G. J. (2003). Contagious yawning: The role of self-awareness and mental state attribution. *Cognitive Brain Research, 17*: 223–227.

Preece, R. (2000). *The Alchemical Buddha: Introducing the Psychology of Buddhist Tantra*. Chagford, UK: Mudra.

Preston, S. D., & de Waal, F. B. M. (2002). Empathy: Its ultimate and proximate bases. *Behavioral and Brain Sciences, 25*: 1–72.

Priestman, A. (2013). The quietly ferocious struggle: A review of Nick Totton's contribution to and thinking about training in psychotherapy. *Psychotherapy and Politics International, 11*(1): 61–69.

Pulver, S. E. (1963). Delusions following hypnosis. *International Journal of Clinical and Experimental Hypnosis, 11*(1): 11–22.

Rachman, A. W. (2001). Beyond neutrality: The curative function of analyst self-disclosure. In: J. Reppen & J. Schulman (Eds.), *Way Beyond Freud: Post-Modern Conceptions of Psychoanalysis* (pp. 127–142). London: Opengate.

Rachman, A. W., & Ceccoli, V. C. (1996). Analyst self-disclosure in adolescent groups. In: P. Kymissis & D. A. Halperin (Eds.), *Group Therapy with Children and Adolescents* (pp. 155–173). Washington, DC: American Psychiatric Press.

Racker, H. (1968). *Transference and Countertransference*. New York: International Universities Press.

Ramberg, L. (2006). In dialogue with Daniel Stern: A review and discussion of The Present Moment in Psychotherapy and Everyday Life. *International Forum of Psychoanalysis, 15*(1): 19–33.

Rappoport, E. (2012). Creating the umbilical cord: Relational knowing and the somatic third. *Psychoanalytic Dialogues, 22*(3): 375–388.

Raubolt, R. R. (1985). Humanistic analysis: Integrating action and insight in psychotherapy. *Journal of Contemporary Psychotherapy, 15*: 46–57.

Rauch, S. L. (2005). A descriptive study on the differences between body psychotherapists and traditional counselors. (Doctor of Philosophy thesis, University of North Carolina, Charlotte.) Retrieved 19 October 2013 from http://www.hakomiinstitute.com/Resources/research/Rauch-disseration.doc

Ray, F. K. (2001). Ethics in therapy: Moving from the mind to the heart. *Journal of Systemic Therapies, 20*(4): 25–36.

Reich, W. (1930). *The Sexual Revolution*. (T. P. Wolfe, Trans.). New York: Octagon, 1971.

Reich, W. (1933a). *Character Analysis*. New York: Noonday, 1972.

Reich, W. (1933b). *The Mass Psychology of Fascism*. New York: Orgone Institute Press, 1946.

Reich, W. (1942). *The Function of the Orgasm*. V. R. Carfagno (Trans.). London: Souvenir Press, 1973.

Reich, W. (1948). *The Discovery of the Orgone (Vol. 2): The Cancer Biopathy*. Kildonan, Isle of Arran, UK: Banton, 1998.

Reich, W. (1960). *Selected Writings*. New York: Farrar, Straus & Giroux, 1979.

Reich, W. (1967). *Reich Speaks of Freud*. London: Penguin.

Reis, R. (2011). Deciphering the complete autistic encapsulation as a plasmatic defence mechanism. (Diploma in Body Psychotherapy thesis, Reidman College, Tel Aviv.)

Renik, O. (1993). Analytic interaction: Conceptualizing technique in light of the analyst's irreducible subjectivity. *Psychoanalytic Quarterly, 62*(4): 553–571.

Rilke, R. M. (1996). *Rilke's Book of Hours: Love Poems to God*. A. Barrows & J. Macy (Trans.). New York: Riverhead.

Rinpoche, T. W. (1998). *The Tibetan Yogas of Dream and Sleep*. Ithaca, NY: Snow Lion Publications.

Rizzolatti, G., Fadiga, L., Fogassi, L., & Gallese, V. (1996). Premotor cortex and the recognition of motor actions. *Cognitive Brain Research, 3*: 131–141.

Roffman, A. E. (2003). Embodiment and coordination. *Journal of Systemic Therapies, 22*(4): 57–71.

Rogers, C. R. (1951). *Client-Centered Therapy*. Boston, MA: Houghton Mifflin.

Roisman, G. I., Padrón, E., Sroufe, L. A., & Egeland, B. (2002). Earned-secure attachment status in retrospect and prospect. *Child Development, 73*(4): 1204–1219.

Rolef Ben-Shahar, A. (2001a). Holistic approach to psychotherapy. *Rapport, 53* (Autumn): 46–49.

Rolef Ben-Shahar, A. (2001b). A myth of transition. *AnchorPoint, 15*(9): 3–13.

Rolef Ben-Shahar, A. (2002a). Hypnosis and bodywork part I: Trancework. *AnchorPoint, 16*(7): 18–22.

Rolef Ben-Shahar, A. (2002b). Hypnosis and bodywork part II: Trancework in the body. *AnchorPoint, 16*(8): 30–35.

Rolef Ben-Shahar, A. (2003). Dare I touch? *Rapport, 59* (Spring): 17–19.

Rolef Ben-Shahar, A. (2008a). Embodied trances, relational hypnosis. *British Journal of Psychotherapy Integration, 5*(1): 17–29.

Rolef Ben-Shahar, A. (2008b). Resonance: The gift of connection. *Self & Society, A Journal of Humanistic Psychology in Britain, 36*(1): 45–48.

Rolef Ben-Shahar, A. (2008c). The woodpecker. *Attachment: New Directions in Psychotherapy and Relational Psychoanalysis, 2*(2): 216–224.

Rolef Ben-Shahar, A. (2009). Trees in shades of grey: Trauma, attachment and dissociation in the personal, clinical and socio-political settings. *Attachment: New Directions in Psychotherapy and Relational Psychoanalysis, 3*(2): 121–143.

Rolef Ben-Shahar, A. (2010a). Blanche Wittman's breasts. *Psychotherapy and Politics International, 8*(3): 213–226.

Rolef Ben-Shahar, A. (2010b). From ballroom dance to five rhythms. *USA Body Psychotherapy Journal, 9*(1): 41–50.

Rolef Ben-Shahar, A. (2010c). Surrender to flow: A unifying theory of trance, relationality and embodiment. (PhD dissertation, American Pacific University, Kailua-Kona, Hawaii.)

Rolef Ben-Shahar, A. (2010d). Sustaining an erection. *Psychotherapy and Politics International, 8*(2): 96–112.

Rolef Ben-Shahar, A. (2011a). Salsa lessons and the emergent self. *USA Body Psychotherapy Journal, 10*(2): 22–31.

Rolef Ben-Shahar, A. (2011b). Something old, something new, something borrowed, something blue: Individual selves and dyadic selves in relational body psychotherapy. *USA Body Psychotherapy Journal, 10*(1): 58–67.

Rolef Ben-Shahar, A. (2012a). About touching psychotherapists. *Somatic Psychotherapy Today*, Winter: 27–29.

Rolef Ben-Shahar, A. (2012b). Do cry for me Argentina: the challenges trauma work poses for holistic psychotherapy. *Body, Movement and Dance in Psychotherapy, 7*(1): 7–12.

Rolef Ben-Shahar, A. (2012c). The relational turn and body psychotherapy II: Something old, something new, something borrowed, something blue: Individual selves and dyadic selves in relational body psychotherapy. In: C. Young (Ed.), *About Relational Body Psychotherapy* (pp. 129–154). Stow, UK: Body Psychotherapy Publications.

Rolef Ben-Shahar, A. (2012d). The relational turn and body psychotherapy IV. Gliding on the strings that connect us - Resonance in relational body psychotherapy. *International Body Psychotherapy Journal, 11*(1): 12–24.

Rolef Ben-Shahar, A. (2012e). A therapeutic anatomy: A historical and theoretical review of body psychotherapy. *Attachment: New Directions in Psychotherapy and Relational Psychoanalysis, 6*(1): 73–93.

Rolef Ben-Shahar, A. (2013a). *An Anatomy of Therapy: Body Psychotherapy (Hebrew ed.)*. Haifa, Israel: Pardes.

Rolef Ben-Shahar, A. (2013b). A cup, grasping my fingers. *Somatic Psychotherapy Today,* Spring: 40–42.

Rolef Ben-Shahar, A. (2013c). Fairy wings and the psychotherapeutic act: Who's regulating whom. *Somatic Psychotherapy Today, 3*: 50–53.

Rolef Ben-Shahar, A. (2013d). The target audience of pain: systemic, embodied, and relational aspects of working with pain. (Paper presented at the "Pain—in light of medical psychology" conference, Rambam Medical Centre, Haifa, Israel.)

Rolef Ben-Shahar, A. (2013e). Three hot potatoes, or Nick Totton's courage in inconveniencing the field of psychotherapy. *Psychotherapy and Politics International, 11*(1): 5–17.

Rolef Ben-Shahar, A., & MacDonald, G. (2011). Meeting through grace: Relational body psychotherapy. *Attachment: New Directions in Psychotherapy and Relational Psychoanalysis, 5*: 45–69.

Rolef Ben-Shahar, A., & Rolef Ben-Shahar, T. T. (2005). The music box. *AnchorPoint, 18*(10): 11–17.

Rolef Ben-Shahar, A., & Wood, K. (2009). Let there be light: Creating differentiation and safety with a highly dissociative client. *USA Body Psychotherapy Journal, 8*(1): 32–43.

Rolf, I. P. (1977). *Rolfing: The Integration of Human Structures*. London: Harper & Row.

Rosen, M., & Brenner, S. (2003). *Rosen Method Bodywork: Accessing the Unconscious through Touch*. Berkeley, CA: North Atlantic.

Rosenberg, J. L., Rand, M. L., & Asay, D. (1985). *Body, Self, & Soul: Sustaining Integration*. Atlanta, GA: Humanics.

Ross, G. (2003). *Beyond the Trauma Vortex: The Media's Role in Healing Fear, Terror, and Violence*. Berkeley: CA: North Atlantic.

Rossi, E. L. (1973). Psychological shocks and creative moments in psychotherapy. In: E. L. Rossi (Ed.), *The Collected Papers of Milton H. Erickson on Hypnosis* (*Vol. IV—Innovative Hypnotherapy*) (pp. 447–464). New York: Irvington, 1989.

Rossi, E. L., & Cheek, D. B. (1988). *Mind-Body Therapy*. New York: W. W. Norton.

Rothschild, B. (2000). *The Body Remembers: The Psychophysiology of Trauma and Trauma Treatment*. New York: W. W. Norton.

Rothschild, B. (2004). Applying the brakes—In trauma treatment, creating safety is essential. *Psychotherapy Network*, Jan-Feb.

Rothschild, B., & Rand, M. L. (2006). *Help for the Helper: The Psychophysiology of Compassion Fatigue and Vicarious Trauma*. New York: W. W. Norton.

Rubenfeld, I. (2000). The Rubenfeld Synergy Method: The six 'ahas'. *The Gestalt Review, 4*(4): 319–329.

Rubenfeld, I. (2001). *The Listening Hand: How to Combine Bodywork and Psychotherapy to Heal Emotional Pain*. London: Pitakus.

Ruiz, D. M. (1997). *The Four Agreements: A Practical Guide to Personal Freedom*. San Rafael, CA: Amber-Allen.

Rumi (1995). *Rumi—Selected Poems*. C. Banks (Trans.). London: Penguin.

Saint-Exupéry, A. de (1943). *Le Petit Prince*. Paris: Editions Gallimard, 1973.

Satir, V. (1988). *The New Peoplemaking*. Palo Alto, CA: Science and Behavior.

Schafer, R. (1992). *Retelling a Life: Narration and Dialogue in Psychoanalysis*. New York: Basic.

Schneck, J. M. (1966). A study of alterations in body sensations during hypnoanalysis. *International Journal of Clinical and Experimental Hypnosis, 14*(3): 216–231.

Schopenhauer, A. (1818). *The World as Will and Representation (Vol. I)*. New York: Dover, 1958.

Schore, A. (1994). *Affect Regulation and the Origin of the Self*. Hove, UK: Lawrence Erlbaum.

Schore, A. (2002). Advances in neuropsychoanalysis, attachment theory, and trauma research: Implications for self psychology. *Psychoanalytic Inquiry, 22*(3): 433–484.

Schore, A. (2003). *Affect Regulation and Repair of the Self*. Hove, UK: Lawrence Erlbaum.

Schwieger, C. H. -J. (1998). *Charakter als Überlebensstrategie. Persönlichkeitsentwicklung in der Bioenergetik*. Munich, Germany: Kösel—Verlag.

Searles, H. F. (1959). Oedipal love in the countertransference. *International Journal of Psychoanalysis, 40*: 180–190.

Searles, H. F. (1979). *Countertransference and Related Subjects*. New York: International Universities Press.

Seaward, B. L. (2005). *Quiet Mind, Fearless Heart: The Taoist Path through Stress and Spirituality*. Hoboken, NJ: John Wiley & Sons.

Seligman, M. E. P. (1975). *Helplessness: On Depression, Development, and Death*. San Francisco, CA: W. H. Freeman.

Sella, Y. (2003). The body as a source of creation and provision of meaning. (Paper presented at "The body in psychotherapy": A shared conference for the Psychology Department and the South-East Asia Studies Department, Tel Aviv University, Tel Aviv.)

Sella, Y. (2005a). Body-oriented psychotherapy: A renewed challenge (in Hebrew). *Psychoactualia: The Israeli Psychological Association (IPA) quarterly*, November.

Sella, Y. (2005b). Recovering and eliciting precursors of meaning: A psychodynamic perspective of the body in psychotherapy. In: N. Totton (Ed.), *New Dimensions in Body Psychotherapy* (pp. 87–101). Maidenhead, UK: Open University Press.

Sella, Y. (2011). Verbum caro hic factum est: A philosophical-linguistic look at Didier Anzieu's "The Skin Ego" (Hebrew ed.). *Merhavim: The journal of the Israeli Association for Psychoanlaytic Psychotherapy, 1*. Retrieved 19 October 2013 from http://www.psygroups.com/iapp/wp-content/uploads/2011/04/yorai-sela-f.pdf

Shahar-Levy, Y. (2004). *A Body-Movement-Mind Paradigm: for Psychophysical Analysis of Emotive Movement and Movement Therapy (2nd ed.)*. Jerusalem: Printiv.

Shahar-Levy, Y. (2005). A basic typology of the emotive language (in Hebrew). *Sihot, 19*(3): 237–246.

Shalit, R. (2011). Efficiency of psychotherapy involving altered states of consciousness. (Diploma in Body Psychotherapy thesis, Reidman College, Tel Aviv.)

Shapiro, F. (1989). Efficacy of the eye movement desensitization and reprocessing procedure in the treatment of traumatic memories. *Journal of Traumatic Stress, 2*: 199–223.

Shapiro, F. (2001). *Eye Movement Desensitization and Reprocessing (2nd ed.)*. New York: Guilford Press.

Shapiro, F., & Maxfield, L. (2002). Eye movement desensitization and reprocessing (EMDR): Information processing in the treatment of trauma. *Journal of Clinical Psychology, 58*(8): 933–946.

Shapiro, S. A. (1996). The embodied analyst in the Victorian consulting room. *Gender and Psychoanalysis, 1*: 297–322.

Sharaf, M. (1984). *Fury on Earth—Biography of Wilhelm Reich*. London: Arrow.

Sheldrake, R. (1987). Part I—Mind, memory, and archetype: Morphic resonance and the collective unconscious. *Psychological Perspectives, 18*(1): 9–25.

Shiraz, G. (2013). Simplicity and complexity in body psychotherapy. (Paper presented at the Israeli Association of Body Psychotherapy founding conference, Tel Aviv.)

Shlain, L. (1998). *The Alphabet versus the Goddess*. New York: Viking/Penguin.

Sills, F. (2009). *Being and Becoming*. Berkeley, CA: North Atlantic.

Sinason, V. (Ed.). (2002). *Attachment, Trauma and Multiplicity*. Hove, UK: Routledge.

Sinason, V. (2006). No touch please—we're British psychodynamic practitioners. In: G. Galton (Ed.), *Touch Papers* (pp. 49–60). London: Karnac.

Slavin, J. H. (2013). Moments of truth and perverse scenarios in psychoanalysis: Revisiting Davies' "Love in the Afternoon". *Psychoanalytic Dialogues, 23*(2): 139–149.

Sletvold, J. (2012). Training analysts to work with unconscious embodied expressions: Theoretical underpinnings and practical guidelines. *Psychoanalytic Dialogues, 22*(4): 410–429.

Smith, E. W. L. (1985). *The Body in Psychotherapy*. Jefferson, NC: McFarland.

Soth, M. (2005). Embodied countertransference. In: N. Totton (Ed.), *New Dimensions in Body Psychotherapy* (pp. 40–55). Maidenhead, UK: Open University Press.

Soth, M. (2009). From humanistic holism via the 'integrative project' towards integral-relational body psychotherapy. In: L. Hartley (Ed.), *Contemporary Body Psychotherapy: The Chiron Approach* (pp. 64–88). Hove, UK: Routledge.

Spotnitz, H. (1972). Touch countertransference in group psychotherapy. *International Journal of Group Psychotherapy, 22*: 455–463.

Stern, D. B. (1983). Unformulated experience: from familiar chaos to creative disorder. In: S. A. Mitchell & L. Aron (Eds.), *Relational Psychoanalysis: The Emergence of a Tradition* (pp. 77–107). New York: Analytic Press, 1999.

Stern, D. B. (Ed.). (2010). *Partners in Thought: Working with Unformulated Experience, Dissociation, and Enactment*. Hove, UK: Routledge.

Stern, D. N. (1985). *The Interpersonal World of the Infant*. New York: Basic.

Stern, D. N. (1991). *Diary of a Baby*. London: Fontana.

Stern, D. N. (2002). *The First Relationship: Infant and Mother*. Cambridge, MA: Harvard University Press.

Stern, D. N. (2004). *The Present Moment in Psychotherapy and Everyday Life*. New York: W. W. Norton.

Stolorow, R. D., & Atwood, G. E. (1992). *Contexts of Being: The Intersubjective Foundations of Psychological Life*. Hillsdale, NJ: Analytic Press.

Sullivan, H. S. (1940). *Conceptions of Modern Psychiatry*. New York: W. W. Norton.

Sullivan, H. S. (1953). *The Interpersonal Theory of Psychiatry*. New York: W. W. Norton, 1997.

Sullivan, H. S. (1954). *The Psychiatric Interview*. H. S. Perry & M. L. Gawel (Eds.). New York: W. W. Norton.

Sumedho, A. (1992). *Cittaviveka: Teachings from the Silent Mind*. Hemel Hempstead, UK: Amaravati Publications.

Summers, F. (2002). Object-relations psychotherapy. In: M. Hersen & W. Sledge (Eds.), *Encyclopedia of Psychotherapy* (*Vol. 2*) (pp. 235–244). Oxford: Academic Press.

Suttie, I. D. (1935). *The Origins of Love and Hate*. London: Kegan Paul.

Svensen, A. R., & Bergland, A. (2007). Learning through bodily experience: A possibility to enhance healthcare students' ability to empathize? *Advances in Physiotherapy, 9*(1): 40–47.

Tennyson, A. Lord (1849). In memoriam. In: W. J. Rolfe (Ed.), *The Works of Alfred, Lord Tennyson, Vol. IV*. Boston, MA: Dana Estates, 1892.

Torraco, P. (1998). Jean's legacy: On the use of physical touch in long-term psychotherapy. In: E. W. L. Smith, P. R. Clance, & S. Imes (Eds.), *Touch in Psychotherapy: Theory, Research, and Practice* (pp. 220–237). New York: Guilford.

Tosone, C. (1997). Sándor Ferenczi: Forerunner of modern short-term psychotherapy. *Journal of Analytic Social Work, 4*(3): 23–41.

Totton, N. (1998). *The Water in the Glass: Body and Mind in Psychoanalysis*. London: Rebus.

Totton, N. (2000). *Psychotherapy and Politics*. London: SAGE.

Totton, N. (2003). *Body Psychotherapy: An Introduction*. Maidenhead, UK: Open University Press.

Totton, N. (2005). Embodied relational therapy. In: N. Totton (Ed.), *New Dimensions in Body Psychotherapy* (pp. 168–181). Maidenhead, UK: Open University Press.

Totton, N. (2006). A body psychotherapist's approach to touch. In: G. Galton (Ed.), *Touch Papers* (pp. 145–162). London: Karnac.

Totton, N. (2010). *The Problem with the Humanistic Therapies*. London: Karnac.

Totton, N., & Edmondson, E. (1988). *Reichian Growth Work: Melting the Blocks to Life and Love*. Bridport, UK: Prism Press.

Totton, N., & Edmondson, E. (2009). *Reichian Growth Work: Melting the Blocks to Life and Love (2nd ed.)*. Ross-on-Wye, UK: PCCS.

Totton, N., & Jacobs, M. (2001). *Character and Personality Types*. Buckingham, UK: Open University Press.

Totton, N., & Priestman, A. (2012). Embodiment & relationship: Two halves of one whole. In: C. Young (Ed.), *About Relational Body Psychotherapy* (pp. 35–53). Stow, UK: Body Psychotherapy Publications.

Trevarthen, C. (1974). Conversations with a 2-month-old. *New Scientist, 2*: 230–235.

Trevarthen, C. (1993). The self born in intersubjectivity: The psychology of an infant communicating. In: U. Neisser (Ed.), *The Perceived Self: Ecological and Interpersonal Sources of Self-Knowledge*. New York: Cambridge University Press.

Trevarthen, C. (2004). Intimate contact from birth. In: K. White (Ed.), *Touch: Attachment and the Body* (pp. 1–15). London: Karnac.

Trevarthen, C., & Aitken, K. J. (2001). Infant intersubjectivity: research, theory, and clinical applications. *Journal of Child Psychology and Psychiatry, 42*(1): 3–48.

Tronick, E. Z. (2004). Why is connection with other so critical? The formation of dyadic states of consciousness and the expansion of individual's states of consciousness: Coherence governed selection and the co-creation of meaning out of messy meaning making. In: J. Nadel & D. Muir (Eds.), *Emotional Development—Recent Research Advances* (pp. 293–316). Oxford: Oxford University Press.

Tronick, E. Z., Bruschweiler-Stern, N., Harrison, A. M., Lyons-Ruth, K., Morgan, A. C., Nahum, J. P., Sander, L., & Stern, D. N. (1998). Dyadically expanded states of consciousness and the process of therapeutic change. *Infant Mental Health Journal, 19*(3): 277–353.

Turp, M. (1999). Touch, enjoyment and health: In infancy. *European Journal of Psychotherapy & Counselling, 2*(1): 23–39.

Turp, M. (2000). Touch, enjoyment and health: In adult life. *European Journal of Psychotherapy & Counselling, 3*(1): 61–76.

United States Association for Body Psychotherapy (2007). Ethics guidelines. Retrieved 4 August 2013, from http://www.usabp.org/associations/1808/files/USABPethics.pdf

Van der Kolk, B. A. (1996). The body keeps the score: Approaches to the psychobiology of posttraumatic stress disorder. In: B. A. Van der Kolk, A. C. McFarlane, & L. Weisæth (Eds.), *Traumatic*

Stress: The Effects of Overwhelming Experience on Mind, Body, and Society (pp. 214–241). New York: Guilford.

Van Dusen, W. (1958). Wu Wei, no-mind, and the fertile void. In: J. O. Stevens (Ed.), *Gestalt Is: A Collection of Articles about Gestalt Therapy and Living* (pp. 87–93). Moab, UT: Real People Press, 1975.

Wallach, Y. (1992). *The Subconscious Opens like a Fan*. Tel Aviv, Israel: Hakibbutz Hameuchad.

Warnecke, T. (2008). The well tempered therapist: Psychotherapy integration and the personality of the therapist. *British Journal of Psychotherapy Integration, 5*(2): 16–20.

Warnecke, T. (2009). The borderline relationship. In: L. Hartley (Ed.), *Contemporary Body Psychotherapy: The Chiron Approach* (pp. 194–211). Hove, UK: Routledge.

Weil, S. (1947). *Gravity and Grace*. London: Routledge.

West, W. (1994). Clients' experience of bodywork psychotherapy. *Counseling Psychology Quarterly, 7*(3): 287–303.

Whitaker, C. A. (2000). Hypnosis and family depth therapy. *The Family Journal: Counselling and Therapy for Couples and Families, 8*(1): 7–13.

Wilkinson, H. (2000). An inspired resurrection of Freudian drive theory: But does Nick Totton's Reichian 'bodymind' concept supersede Cartesian dualism? *International Journal of Psychotherapy, 5*(2): 153–166.

Williams, M. (1922). *The Velveteen Rabbit or How Toys Become Real*. London: Egmont, 2004.

Winnicott, D. W. (1949). Mind and its relation to the psyche-soma. In: D. W. Winnicott (Ed.), *Through Paediatrics to Psychoanalysis: Collected Papers* (pp. 243–254). London: Karnac, 1958.

Winnicott, D. W. (1952). Anxiety associated with insecurity. In: D. W. Winnicott (Ed.), *Through Paediatrics to Psychoanalysis: Collected Papers* (pp. 97–100). London: Karnac, 1958.

Winnicott, D. W. (1954). Metapsychological and clinical aspects of regression within the psychoanalytical set-up. In: D. W. Winnicott (Ed.), *Through Paediatrics to Psychoanalysis: Collected Papers* (pp. 258–294). New York: Basic, 1975.

Winnicott, D. W. (1958a). The capacity to be alone. In: D. W. Winnicott (Ed.), *The Maturational Processes and the Facilitating Environment: Studies in the Theory of Emotional Development* (pp. 29–36). London: Karnac, 1990.

Winnicott, D. W. (1958b). A letter to Victor Smirnoff. In: R. F. Rodman (Ed.), *The Spontaneous Gesture: Selected Letters of D. W. Winnicott* (pp. 120–124). London: Harvard University Press.

Winnicott, D. W. (1960a). Ego distortion in terms of true and false self. In: D. W. Winnicott (Ed.), *The Maturational Processes and the Facilitating Environment* (pp. 140–152). London: Karnac, 1990.

Winnicott, D. W. (1960b). The theory of the parent-infant relationship. In: D. W. Winnicott (Ed.), *The Maturational Processes and the Facilitating Environment* (pp. 37–55). London: Karnac, 1990.

Winnicott, D. W. (1962). Ego integration in child development. In: D. W. Winnicott (Ed.), *The Maturational Processes and the Facilitating Environment* (pp. 56–63). London: Karnac, 1990.

Winnicott, D. W. (1963). Communicating and not communicating leading to a study of certain opposites. In: D. W. Winnicott (Ed.), *The Maturational Processes and the Facilitating Environment* (pp. 179–192). London: Karnac, 1990.

Winnicott, D. W. (1971a). *Playing and Reality*. New York, Basic.

Winnicott, D. W. (1971b). Playing: Creative activity and the search for the self. In: D. W. Winnicott (Ed.), *Playing and Reality* (pp. 53–64). New York: Basic.

Winnicott, D. W. (1987). *Babies and Their Mothers*. London: Free Association.

Winnicott, D. W. (1988). *Human Nature*. New York: Schochen.

Withers, R. (2008). Descartes' dreams. *Journal of Analytical Psychology, 53*: 691–709.

Wittgenstein, L. (1921). *Tractatus logico philosophicus*. Jerusalem: The Magnes Press.

Wittgenstein, L. (1953). *Philosophical Investigations (2nd ed.)*. G. E. M. Anscombe (Trans.). Oxford: Blackwell, 1958.

Wolf, N. S., Gales, M. E., Shane, E., & Shane, M. (2001). The developmental trajectory from amodal perception to empathy and communication: The role of mirror neurons in this process. *Psychoanalytic Inquiry, 21*(1): 94–112.

Woolger, R. J. (1988). *Other Lives, Other Selves*. New York: Bantam.

Wrye, H. K. (1998). The embodiment of desire: Relinking the bodymind within the analytic dyad. In: L. Aron & F. S. Anderson (Eds.), *Relational Perspectives on the Body* (pp. 97–116). Hillsdale, NJ: Analytic Press.

Yardley, L. K. (1990). *The Heart of Huna*. Honolulu, HI: Advanced Neuro Dynamics.

Yarom, N. (2001). *The Body Speaks (Hebrew ed.)*. Or Yehuda, Israel: Dvir.

Yarom, N. (2013). *Body Dialects: Illuminating Mental Phenomena as Expressed in the Body (Hebrew ed.)*. Haifa, Israel: Pardes.

Young, C. (2011a). The history and development of body psychotherapy: An American legacy of Reich. In: C. Young (Ed.), *The Historical Basis of Body Psychotherapy* (pp. 83–100). Stow, UK: Body Psychotherapy Publications.

Young, C. (2011b). The science of body psychotherapy today: Part 1: A background history. In: C. Young (Ed.), *About the Science of Body Psychotherapy* (pp. 25–50). Stow, UK: Body Psychotherapy Publications.

Young, C. (Ed.). (2011c). *About the Science of Body Psychotherapy*. Stow, UK: Body Psychotherapy Publications.

Young, C. (Ed.). (2011d). *The Historical Basis of Body Psychotherapy*. Stow, UK: Body Psychotherapy Publications.

Young, C. (Ed.). (2012). *About Relational Body Psychotherapy*. Stow, UK: Body Psychotherapy Publications.

Young, I. M. (2005). *On Female Body Experience: "Throwing Like a Girl" and Other Essays*. New York: Oxford University Press.

Zack, S. (2013). *Lost in Translation: SIlence as an Unknown Language*. (MA thesis, Lesley University, Israel.)

Zahm, S. G., & Gold, E. K. (2002). Gestalt therapy. In: M. Hersen & W. Sledge (Eds.), *Encyclopedia of Psychotherapy* (pp. 863–872). Oxford: Academic Press.

Ziehl, S. (2000). *Character Structure—Integrating Reichian and post-Reichian Perspectives*. (Paper presented at the Deep Bodywork Training Material conference, London.)

Ziehl, S. (2005). Bodywork as poetry. *Open Centre, 29*(1). Retrieved 19 October 2013 from http://www.entelia.com/bodyworkaspoetry.shtml

Ziv-Beiman, S. (2013). Therapist self-disclosure as an integrative intervention. *Journal of Psychotherapy Integration, 23*(1): 59–74.

INDEX

For Product Safety Concerns and Information please contact our EU
representative GPSR@taylorandfrancis.com
Taylor & Francis Verlag GmbH, Kaufingerstraße 24, 80331 München, Germany

www.ingramcontent.com/pod-product-compliance
Lightning Source LLC
LaVergne TN
LVHW080805011026
849160LV00015B/1531
* 9 7 8 1 7 8 2 2 0 0 9 4 9 *